D1245280

Prescription for the Boards
USMLE Step 2

Third Edition

DREXEL UNIVERSITY
HEALTH SCIENCES LIBRARIES
HAHNEMANN LIBRARY

DREXEL UNIVERSITY
HEALTH SCIENCES LIBRARIES
HAHNEMANN LIBRARY

Prescription for the Boards
USMLE Step 2

Third Edition

Kate C. Feibusch, M.D., M.P.H.

Physician, Family Practice
Concern America
Las Cruces, Petén, Guatemala
University of California, San Francisco, School of Medicine
Class of 1996

Radhika Sekhri Breaden, M.D., M.P.H.

Physician, Internal Medicine
Kaiser Permanente
Portland, Oregon
University of California, San Francisco, School of Medicine
Class of 1996

Cheryl Bader, M.D., M.P.H.

Physician, Obstetrics and Gynecology
Kaiser Medical Center
Santa Clara, California
University of California, San Diego, School of Medicine
Class of 1996

Stephen N. Gomperts, M.D., Ph.D.

Resident, Neurology
Massachusetts General Hospital
Brigham and Women's Hospital
Boston, Massachusetts
University of California, San Francisco, School of Medicine
Class of 2001

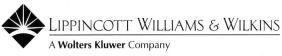

LIPPINCOTT WILLIAMS & WILKINS
A **Wolters Kluwer** Company
Philadelphia · Baltimore · New York · London
Buenos Aires · Hong Kong · Sydney · Tokyo

Executive Editor: Neil Marquardt
Managing Editor: Daniel Pepper
Marketing Manager: Scott Lavine
Senior Production Editor: Karen M. Ruppert
Compositor: Peirce Graphic Services
Printer: Quebecor

Copyright © 2002 Lippincott Williams & Wilkins

351 West Camden Street
Baltimore, MD 21201
530 Walnut St.
Philadelphia, PA 19106

All rights reserved. This book is protected by copyright. No part of this book may be reproduced in any form or by any means, including photocopying, or utilized by any information storage and retrieval system without written permission from the copyright owner.

The publisher is not responsible (as a matter of product liability, negligence, or otherwise) for any injury resulting from any material contained herein. This publication contains information relating to general principles of medical care that should not be construed as specific instructions for individual patients. Manufacturers' product information and package inserts should be reviewed for current information, including contraindications, dosages, and precautions.

Printed in the United States of America
First Edition, 1996
Second Edition, 1998

Library of Congress Cataloging-in-Publication Data

Prescription for the boards : USMLE step 2 / Kate C. Feibusch . . . [et al.].—3rd ed.
    p. cm.
   Includes index.
   ISBN 0-7817-3400-2
    1. Medicine—Examinations, questions, etc. I. Feibusch, Kate C.

   R834.5 .P67 2002
   616'.0076—dc21

                         2002066071

The publishers have made every effort to trace the copyright holders for borrowed material. If they have inadvertently overlooked any, they will be pleased to make the necessary arrangements at the first opportunity.
To purchase additional copies of this book, call our customer service department at **(800) 638-3030** or fax orders to **(301) 824-7390**. International customers should call **(301) 714-2324**.

Visit Lippincott Williams & Wilkins on the Internet: http://www.LWW.com. Lippincott Williams & Wilkins customer service representatives are available from 8:30 am to 6:00 pm, EST.

02 03 04 05 06
1 2 3 4 5 6 7 8 9 10

We dedicate this book to the army of committed individuals
without whom it would not have been possible:
Our teachers

Contents

Preface

Have you looked at the 12-page outline the United States Medical Licensing Examination (USMLE) provides as a study guide? It is overwhelming, to say the least. We all had mixed feelings about studying for the Step 2 exam. On the one hand, it is a great opportunity to review medicine before residency. On the other hand, who has the time?

Prescription for the Boards USMLE Step 2, third edition, turns that overwhelming outline into a useful study tool by providing "just enough" information about each topic. As one student put it, the Step 2 is "like seeing 800 patients in a day." Therefore, our descriptions are patient-oriented, and we have tried to limit the information to the amount expected at this point in your medical career—and that's plenty! Finally, because some things just have to be memorized in the day or so before the exam, we have written "cram pages" full of memorizable facts. They are designed to be photocopied, personalized, and used for—what else—cramming!

Prescription for the Boards USMLE Step 2 we see as a work in progress, and we look forward to receiving your input to shape future editions. If we use your comments in promotion materials, we'll send you a coupon for $10 toward any Lippincott Williams & Wilkins medical book. Happy studying, and good luck on the boards!

K.C.F.
R.S.B.
C.D.B.
S.N.G.

Acknowledgments

This book would not have been possible without the encouragement and support of many people. We convey our deep gratitude to Patty Mintz for launching us on this journey and to Evan Schnittman for believing in us all along. Thanks also to Daniel Pepper and Karen Ruppert at Lippincott Williams & Wilkins for their encouragement (and flexibility!) and to Jane Bangley McQueen and the staff at Silverchair Science + Communications for sharing our passion to make everything look just right. Special thanks go to our family and friends for their unwavering support over these many months: Julie Kiser, Mira Moore, and Marianne Feibusch; Matthew Breaden and Neelam Sekhri; Marc, Mira, and Miles Bader; and Joan Autio, Ed and Barbara Gomperts, and Susan Rozanova. Thanks also to Gloria Hwang, Scott Williams, Elizabeth Hoge, and Steven Hetts for their invaluable input on the new Step 2 format and content.

Finally, we extend our thanks to each other for the months of hard work. *Now* what will we do with all our free time?

> It is not often that someone comes along who is a true friend and a good writer.
>
> —E. B. White, *Charlotte's Web*

Remember Goat Rock!

Introduction:
The Inside Scoop

Rx: Test-taking tips
Sig: Take advice prn for optimal success

Another standardized test? Ugh, again?

Take heart, this one might not be so bad, and it really does give you an opportunity to review important material before internship.

Using This Book

How you use this book depends on your goals for the Step 2 exam. Many of the students we've talked to say that simply passing the boards is most important to them. If you are one of these students, this book can provide a quick overview of the topics you should be familiar with before taking the Step 2 exam. On the other hand, students entering highly competitive residencies, international medical graduates, and students who want a broad review before beginning residency will find that this book has comprehensive summaries of important topics and can serve as the basis for a more complete review.

We hope this book will be useful in passing on the accumulated tips and strategies that medical students from across the country have shared with us. On that note, we ask that you send us your feedback about anything and everything regarding the Step 2 so that we can share the information with future Step-2 takers. Your input may help shape future editions of this book! To contact us, please send email to *book comments@lww.com* or write to:

Scott Lavine, Marketing
Manager, Lippincott Williams & Wilkins
351 West Camden Street
Baltimore, MD 21201-2436

How We've Organized This Book

The United States Medical Licensing Examination (USMLE) publishes a rather overwhelming 12-page "content outline" that lists the topics covered on the exam. Our book is based on this outline. For each disease listed, we include a brief description, the characteristic signs and symptoms, pertinent studies and methods of diagnosis, and brief treatment information. Information on prevention or screening is included when applicable. We've tried to incorporate information that will help you answer the many case-based questions on the exam. The outline also includes a number of "symptoms, signs, and ill-defined conditions" that don't fit well into the signs/symptoms–diagnosis–treatment model. We've defined these words and included brief differential diagnoses. Finally, we've included information about normal physiology in many chapters because many students have indicated that the test questions have occasionally asked the student to decide whether a particular case presentation was "normal" or not, especially in obstetrics/gynecology and pediatrics.

At the end of the book, we've included some "cram pages"—pages that you can rip out and use to test yourself in the days (and hours) before the exam. We encourage you to add your own "cram facts" to this list. Write us if you'd like to share some especially helpful ones!

Description of the USMLE Step 2

The USMLE Step 2 is the second part of a three-step process to gain medical licensing in the United States. The Step 2 is typically taken in the fourth year of medical school. The subjects tested on the USMLE Step 2 include medicine, surgery, obstetrics and gynecology, pediatrics, psychiatry, preventive medicine, and public health.

In 1999, the Step 2 was transitioned from a paper-based format to a computer-based format (known as CBT). With the start of the computerized Step 2 exam, it became possible to offer the test throughout the year, instead of only twice a year. Also, the Step 2 has gone from a 2-day examination to a 9-hour examination. Students who have taken the computer-based test feel that it is better than the paper-based test because it is more flexible to schedule and now lasts only 1 day, although that 1 day is quite a long one! Students who have taken the computer-based Step 1 exam also state that the Step 2 differs from the Step 1 in that the 1 day of testing is much longer than each day of Step 1 testing, so it is important to pace yourself.

The National Board of Medical Examiners (NBME) is also changing the way it distributes the Step 2 application materials. Beginning in 2001, applicants will receive information for all three USMLE Step examinations on a compact disc (CD), which includes the USMLE Bulletin of Information, Content Description, and Sample Test Materials as well as the forms and guidelines for registration. These materials will be available at medical schools and sent to individuals upon request. Portions of the registration materials and updated information are available at http://www.usmle.org and http://www.nbme.org. You can also contact the NBME to request an information packet at the following address:

> National Board of Medical Examiners (NBME)
> Department of Licensing Examination Services
> Office of Registration
> 3750 Market Street
> Philadelphia, PA 19104-3190
> Telephone: (215) 590-9700
> Fax: (215) 590-9457
> E-mail: webmail@mail.nbme.org

Setting the Date for the Test

Once your application materials are received and processed, you are provided with a period of a few months in which you must schedule to take the test. Most students state that it is fairly easy to schedule the test if you call to set the date fairly soon after you receive your registration materials; if you wait to schedule until the middle or end of your testing period, you may have little or no choice of the testing date. Also, some students state that there is no guarantee that there will be any openings at all, depending on the season!

The date can also be changed if necessary—many students appreciate this flexibility as it has allowed greater choice in application completion and residency interview scheduling.

Approximately 3 to 6 weeks after the examination, your score report will arrive in the mail. The score report contains both your overall score on the Step 2 and a profile of your performance in each subject area (Figure 1).

Test Description

The Step 2 test has about 400 multiple choice test items. It is divided into eight 60-minute blocks. The eight blocks are administered in a one 9-hour testing session, including 45 minutes of break time and a 15-minute optional tutorial.

During the time allotted in each block, you may answer the questions in any order, review your responses, and change answers. When you have completed a block, or when the time allotted has expired, you cannot go back to change answers. After you complete a testing block, an Item Review Screen will be on the monitor. You may review and change answers as desired if you have remaining time left in your testing block.

The test session ends when you have completed or run out of time for all the blocks. After you have started taking the examination, you cannot cancel or reschedule that examination, unless a technical problem requires it. If you experience a computer problem during the test, be sure to notify the test center immediately!

Test Format

The computer-based Step 2 uses the same basic question types as the paper-based test (primarily multiple choice one-best-answer questions), although the computer-based format has required a change in the layout of some of the test questions.

There are a few different types of question formats used in the USMLE Step 2. It is important to be familiar with them because they may require different approaches.

Single One Best Answer

Multiple choice, or "one best answer," is the standard question type. Generally, a brief case description is followed by several answer options. The majority of the questions on the Step 2 are in this multiple-choice format (Figure 2).

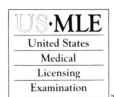

US·MLE
United States
Medical
Licensing
Examination ™

UNITED STATES MEDICAL LICENSING EXAMINATION™

USMLE Step 2 is administered to students and graduates of U.S. and Canadian medical schools by the
NATIONAL BOARD OF MEDICAL EXAMINERS® (NBME®)
3750 Market Street, Philadelphia, Pennsylvania 19104-3190.
Telephone: (215) 590-9700

STEP 2 SCORE REPORT

Pass, I. William

123 Melrose Place
Beverly Hills, CA 90210

USMLE ID: 1-234-567-8

Test Date: August 2000

The USMLE is a single examination program for all applicants for medical licensure in the United States; it replaces the Federation Licensing Examination (FLEX) and the certifying examinations of the National Board of Medical Examiners (NBME Parts I, II, and III). The program consists of three Steps designed to assess an examinee's understanding of and ability to apply concepts and principles that are important in health and disease and that constitute the basis of safe and effective patient care. **Step 2** is designed to assess whether an examinee possesses the medical knowledge and understanding of clinical science considered essential for the provision of patient care under supervision, including emphasis on health promotion and disease prevention. Results of the examination are reported to medical licensing authorities in the United States and its territories for use in granting an initial license to practice medicine. The two numeric scores shown below are equivalent; each state or territory may use either score in making licensing decisions. These scores represent your results for the administration of Step 2 on the test date shown above.

PASS	This result is based on the minimum passing score set by USMLE for Step 2. Individual licensing authorities may accept the USMLE-recommended pass/fail result or may establish a different passing score for their own jurisdictions.

200	This score is determined by your overall performance on the examination. The score scale is based on the performance of students in medical schools accredited by the Liaison Committee on Medical Education (LCME) who took the NBME comprehensive Part II examination for the first time in September 1991 and were in their final year of medical school at the time they were tested. The scale was defined to have a mean of 200 and a standard deviation of 20 for this group. Most examinees receive a score between 140 and 260. A score of 167 is set by USMLE to pass Step 2. The standard error of measurement (SEM)+ for this scale is five points.

82	This score is also determined by your overall performance on the examination. A score of 82 on this scale is equivalent to a score of 200 on the scale described above. A score of 75 on this scale, which is equivalent to a score of 167 on the scale described above, is set by USMLE to pass Step 2. The SEM+ for this scale is one point.

+Your score is influenced by both your general understanding of clinical science and the specific set of items selected for this Step 2 examination. The SEM provides an estimate of the range within which your scores might be expected to vary by chance if you were tested repeatedly using similar tests.

279LD429

Fig. 1-1. Sample Score Report

INTRODUCTION

INFORMATION PROVIDED FOR EXAMINEE USE ONLY

The Performance Profiles below are provided solely for the benefit of the examinee.
The USMLE will not provide or verify the Performance Profiles for any other person, organization, or agency.

USMLE STEP 2 PERFORMANCE PROFILES

PHYSICIAN TASK PROFILE	Lower Performance	Borderline Performance	Higher Performance
Health & Health Maintenance			XXXXXXXXXXX
Understanding Mechanisms of Disease		XXXXXXXXX	
Diagnosis			XXXXXXX
Principles of Management		XXXXXXXXXXX	

ICD-9 DISEASE PROCESS PROFILE

	Lower Performance	Borderline Performance	Higher Performance
Normal Growth & Development; Principles of Care			XXXXXX*
Infectious & Parasitic Diseases			XXXXXXXXXX
Neoplasms		XXXXXXXXXXXXX	
Immunologic Disorders			XXXXXXXXXXXXXXX
Diseases of Blood & Blood Forming Organs		XXXXXXXXXXXXX	
Mental Disorders			XXXXXXXXXXXXXX
Diseases of the Nervous System & Special Senses		XXXXXXXXXXX	
Cardiovascular Disorders		XXXXXXXXXXX	
Diseases of the Respiratory System		XXXXXXXXXXXXX	
Nutritional & Digestive Disorders			XXXXXXXXXXXXX
Gynecologic Disorders			XXXXXXXXX*
Renal, Urinary & Male Reproductive Systems		XXXXXXXXXXXXXXXX	
Disorders of Pregnancy, Childbirth & Puerperium		XXXXXXXXXXXXXXXX	
Musculoskeletal, Skin & Connective Tissue Diseases			XXXXXXXXXXXXX
Endocrine & Metabolic Disorders		XXXXXXXXXXXXXX	
Injury & Poisoning		XXXXXXXXXXXXXXXX	

DISCIPLINE PROFILE

	Lower Performance	Borderline Performance	Higher Performance
Medicine			XXXXXXX
Obstetrics & Gynecology			XXXXXXXXXXX
Pediatrics		XXXXXXXXXXX	
Preventive Medicine & Public Health			XXXXXXXXX
Psychiatry			XXXXXXXXXXX
Surgery		XXXXXXX	

The above Performance Profiles are provided to aid in self-assessment. The shaded area defines a borderline level of performance for each content area; borderline performance is comparable to a HIGH FAIL/LOW PASS on the total test.

Performance bands indicate areas of relative strength and weakness. Some bands are wider than others. The width of a performance band reflects the precision of measurement; narrower bands indicate greater precision. The band width for a given content area is the same for all examinees. An asterisk indicates that your performance band extends beyond the displayed portion of the scale.

Additional information concerning the topics covered in each content area can be found in the *USMLE Step 2 General Instructions, Content Description, and Sample Items.*

293JC155

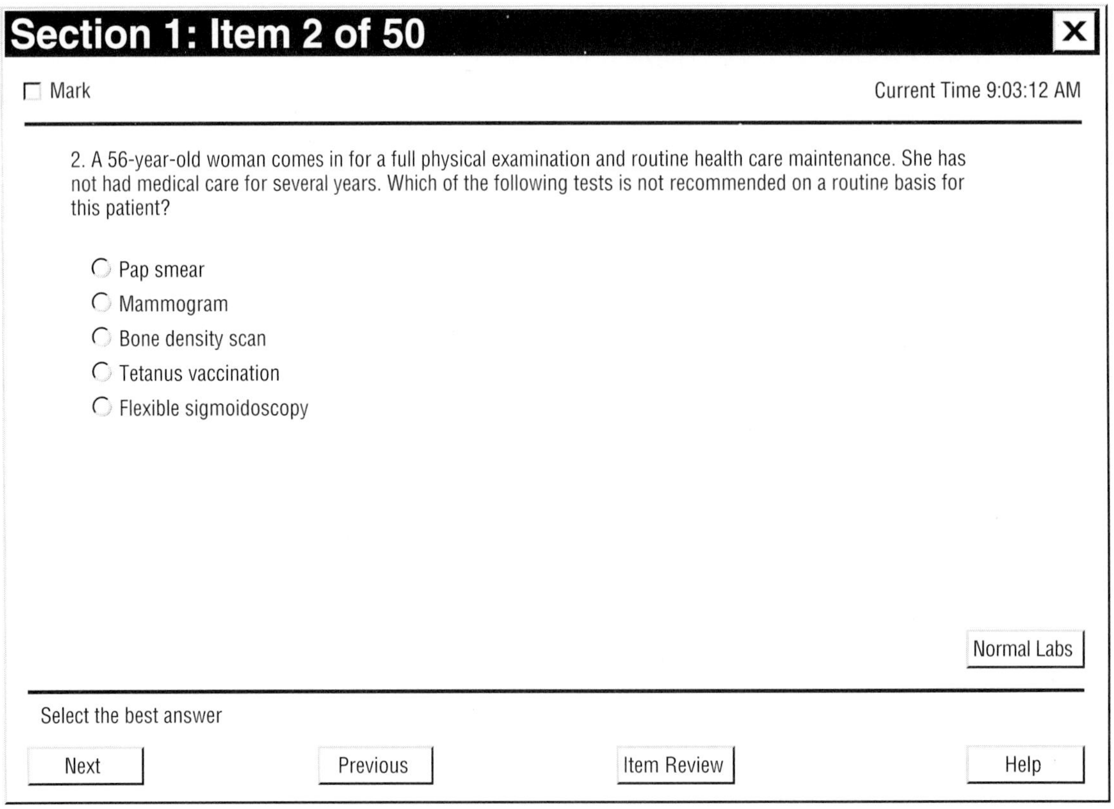

Section 1: Item 2 of 50 ☒

☐ Mark   Current Time 9:03:12 AM

---

2. A 56-year-old woman comes in for a full physical examination and routine health care maintenance. She has not had medical care for several years. Which of the following tests is not recommended on a routine basis for this patient?

○ Pap smear

○ Mammogram

○ Bone density scan

○ Tetanus vaccination

○ Flexible sigmoidoscopy

| Normal Labs |

Select the best answer

| Next | | Previous | | Item Review | | Help |

Fig. 1-2. Single one best answer.

Photos and Diagrams

Multiple choice questions are occasionally accompanied by photos or diagrams. The computerized USMLE examinations now have many more of these types of questions as compared to the paper-based version.

In the paper-based Step 2 examination, these questions could often be answered without reviewing the accompanying diagram or photo. However, in the computer-based test, the entire question is sometimes based on understanding the figure represented. Commonly seen figures include **histology slides, blood smears, chest x-rays, abdominal CT scans, ECGs, and physiology graphs** (e.g., blood flow). Estimates indicate that about 5%–10% of test questions contain photos or diagrams (Figure 3).

Single Best Answer Matching Sets

These types of questions actually consist of a series of questions that use the same list of possible answers. There are between 4 and 26 response options. As you answer the questions in this type of format, the options may be used once, more than once, or not at all. You should respond to each question independently. Approximately 5%–10% of questions were in single best answer matching set format (Figure 4).

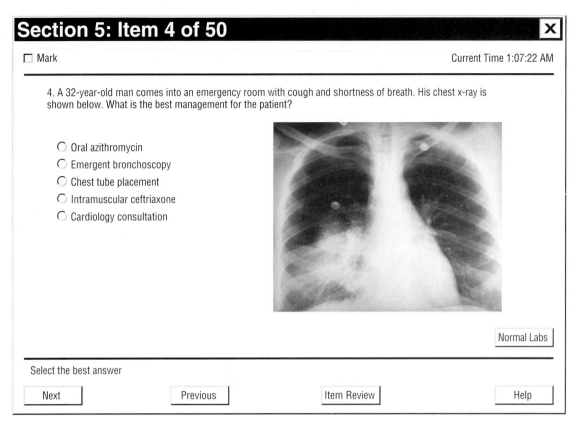

Fig. 1-3. Question with photo.

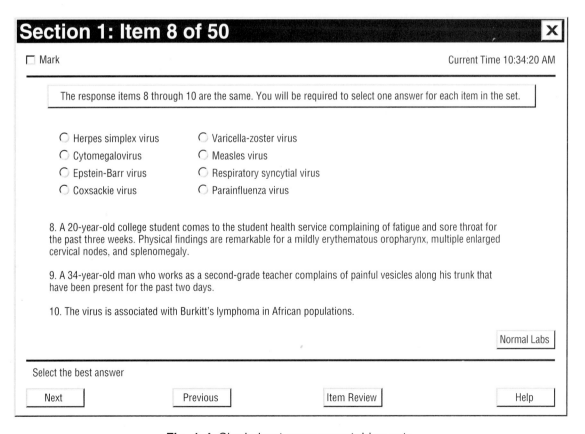

Fig. 1-4. Single best answer matching sets.

INTRODUCTION

Multiple Answer Matching Sets

For this type of question, you are required to choose multiple answers for each case. You may use the answers once, more than once, or not at all. For this type of question, try to generate the answers before looking at the list of answers, then review the answer list.

Unlike in the paper format of the Step 2, you may receive partial credit if some of your answers are correct. However, if you choose more than the indicated number of answers, the question will automatically be marked completely wrong.

This type of question is often used for **vitamins, drugs, diagnostic tests, and preventive health measures.** Approximately 2%–5% of questions are in this format (Figure 5).

Break Time

The computer-based Step 2 is taken in "blocks" of approximately 60 minutes each. Your entire testing session is scheduled for a fixed amount of time, which includes 45 minutes of break time. The 45 minutes of break time can be divided up; for example, you can take a short break at your seat after you complete a block or you can take a longer break for a meal outside the test center after you have completed a few blocks. If you don't use the optional 15-minute tutorial time or you finish a particular test block early, you can use the extra time for breaks—you cannot use the extra time to complete other blocks of the test.

Section 3: Item 18 of 50 ☒

☐ Mark   Current Time 11:24:50 AM

The response items 18 through 19 are the same. Each item will state the number of options to select. Choose exactly this number.

- ○ Iron   ○ Zinc   ○ Folate
- ○ Vitamin A   ○ Vitamin D
- ○ Thiamine   ○ Magnesium
- ○ Fluoride   ○ Vitamin B12

18. A 54-year-old homeless man is brought to the emergency room after a fall. His nutritional history is unclear. Lab studies reveal macrocytic anemia with low ferritin levels (SELECT 4 SUPPLEMENTS)

19. A mother brings her 6-month-old male infant in for a well-baby checkup. She has been breast-feeding him since birth. His weight is in the 45th percentile for his age. (SELECT 2 SUPPLEMENTS)

Normal Labs

Select the best answer

| Next | Previous | Item Review | Help |

Fig. 1-5. Multiple answer matching sets.

Your minimum 45 minutes of break time is being used for all between-block pauses, including the time you take to enter your identification number for the next block, for a quick stretch, or for a bathroom break.

After you complete each test block, the computer will ask you whether you want to take a break or continue. You need to monitor your total break time to make sure that it does not exceed your available break time. If you take too much break time, the time left to complete the remaining test blocks will be reduced.

Most students stated that they used less than the allotted break time. However, past test-takers warn that the break time is usually not sufficient to purchase lunch outside of the test center unless the shop is extremely close! Plan to bring your own lunch and snacks.

The Typical Step 2 Test Day

In 2000, the Step 2 test was administered at Sylvan Test Centers, which vary from city to city. The test centers are used for several other classes and programs other than the Step 2 exam, so most test-takers tell us that the centers can be variable in noise level. Almost all test-takers suggested that you drive to your test center on a "dry run" prior to your test date so you can check out the parking, the surrounding businesses, and the test center itself.

After you arrive at the test center on the morning of the test, you will need to show your scheduling permit and an acceptable form of government-issued identification. You will be assigned a locker for your belongings and offered a set of earplugs as well as an erasable writing board.

Students typically state that they arrive at the test center at around 7 am and leave around 5 pm. Several students stated that the check-in process took longer than they expected. Otherwise, most other aspects of the test-taking process proceeded smoothly. You may find several other test-takers scheduled to take the test concurrently.

Studying for the Exam

Different students have different goals, so the amount of time students spend studying for the exam varies. An informal study of two top West Coast schools showed that the average time spent studying for the Step 2 was approximately 28 hours at one school and 62 hours at the other. The range of reported study time at both schools was quite wide—from taking it cold with no preparation (what confidence!) to approximately 180 hours of study time.

Obviously, the "right" amount of time to study depends on your experience, strengths, confidence, and goals. After you have registered for the Step 2, try to anticipate how much time you are willing to commit to studying. Students spend approximately half of their time in "leisurely study" of a few hours per week in the months before the exam. An "intense" period of study begins during the week or two before the exam. Think about how much time you want to spend in each of these study periods.

Our Advice

After talking to many medical students, we have put together some suggestions and tips for the Step 2 exam. Here are our recommendations.

- **Practice with the computer-based USMLE sample items.** The USMLE provides a computerized sample of questions that are similar to those on the Step 2 and may even be taken from previous administrations of the test. The questions are included in the USMLE Step 2 registration or can be downloaded from their website at www.usmle.org.

  Most students agree that using these questions is the single most important way to prepare for the actual exam. Some students take the sample exam before they begin studying to reveal areas of weakness, whereas others prefer to use it toward the end to simulate the exam and establish pacing. Either way, you'll get a feel for the content, style, and speed of the test.

  As of September 2000, the test software that is used to deliver the USMLE Step 2 is provided by Prometric, Inc. However, the NBME is developing new software, known as FRED, which should be released in 2001. We strongly suggest that you make sure that you practice with the correct sample test materials, although older USMLE test materials may be helpful for review of question content material. Check the web page at http://www.usmle.org if you have any questions as to which version of the computerized software is being used.

- **Don't forget to study ob/gyn, pediatrics, and surgery.** Many students make the mistaken assumption that internal medicine will be the predominant topic on the exam, with only a little ob/gyn, pediatrics, and other subjects mixed in. There is a large amount of material from these fields on the exam, so make sure that you don't give them short shrift and get caught unprepared on exam day.

  Specific topics that students report are emphasized include **dermatology, trauma, antibiotics** and other **specific drugs,** and **microbiology.**

- **Find review books that suit your style and goals.** Browse through the review books and pick the ones that seem the best for you. But keep in mind how much time you are willing to spend studying—you don't want to waste your time and money with too many books. Review books are there to help you, not to stress you out!

- **Use old notes and syllabi.** If you have some notes from clinical and preclinical rotations, dig them out and use them! If you do this, remember to review the study outline from the USMLE registration packet to find any topics that were overlooked or overemphasized in your particular syllabus.

- **Refer to more complete texts when you need detailed information.** Because all students have different experiences, interests, and weaknesses, there will be times when the overview you read in a review book is not enough for you to master a topic. Keep some of the "big" texts, such as Harrisons's or Cecil's nearby. Also, consider using some of your Step 1 books when reviewing bugs and drugs, as well as some of your clinical pocket handbooks (such as *The Washington Manual* or your "scut monkey" handbooks) to review details on treatment.

- **Spend a little time studying the classic pictures of skin conditions, radiology findings, and histology.** We have tried to include some of the classic "pictures" that you may see on the test, but this is, of course, notoriously difficult to predict! For good sources of pictures, we recommend dermatology atlases, radiology texts, and histology slide books.

Use of the USMLE Scores for Resident Selection

Although the NBME has stated that the Step 2 exam is not designed for use in resident selection and may not be accurate in predicting future performance, many residency programs ignore this advice. Some programs use Step 2 scores as part of their screening and selection process.

Because letters of recommendation and clerkship evaluations vary so much from school to school, some programs use Step 2 scores as a nationally standardized way to evaluate the performance of each applicant. Certain specialties even require that the Step 2 exam be taken in the fall so that they will receive the scores in time to use them as a part of your application. Residency requirements vary, so it is important to identify the requirements of programs that interest you before it is too late to register for the exam.

Percentile Information

As of May 1999, percentile information is no longer provided with the USMLE score reports. The reason for this is that the percentiles can only be calculated based on each individual examinee group—that is, different groups will have different mean scores and variability, so the percentiles will vary and cannot be compared directly to each other. (By the way, this is also a statistical concept that is a testable fact in epidemiology on the boards! Go to Chapter 16 and make sure you understand this if you are not sure!)

More Information on Applying for Residency

Other books with more information about residency applications include *Getting into a Residency: A Guide for Medical Students* (Galen Press) and *First Aid for the Match* (Appleton & Lange). Both describe the application process in great detail and contain lots of tips for success.

References

Iserson K. *Getting into residency.* Tucson, AZ: Galen Press, 1993.

National Board of Medical Examiners. Report on 1995 examinations. *The National Board Examiner,* Winter 1995.

National Board of Medical Examiners. *1995 Step 2 general instructions and content outline.* Philadelphia: NBME, 1995.

O'Donnell MJ, Obenshain SS, Erdmann JB. Background essential to the proper use of results of Step 1 and Step 2 of the USMLE. *Acad Med* 1993;68:734–739.

1
Gastroenterology

Nutritional Disorders

Obesity

Obesity and other diet-related diseases are the second most common cause of premature death in the United States. One third of American adults are overweight or obese. Prevalence increases with age and is higher among African-American women and people of low socioeconomic status.

Obesity results from a caloric intake that is chronically greater than expenditure. Many factors may contribute to the development of obesity, including genetics, social influences, metabolic and endocrine factors, psychiatric components, developmental factors, and physical activity.

SIGNS & SYMPTOMS

Obese individuals have increased morbidity and mortality from cardiovascular disease (including coronary artery disease, peripheral vascular disease, and congestive heart failure), hypertension, type 2 diabetes, and sleep apnea. They are also more prone to osteoarthritis, gallbladder disease, urinary stress incontinence, infertility, and venous stasis disease. Overweight teenagers may develop slipped capital femoral epiphysis (see Chapter 8). Obesity has a protective effect against osteoporosis.

DIAGNOSIS

Individuals with a body mass index [BMI: weight in kg/(heights in meters)^2] greater than 25 are considered overweight and those with a BMI over 30 are obese unless they have a high muscle mass.

TREATMENT

Weight loss of even 5%–10% can reduce symptoms and improve comorbid diseases in obese individuals. Weight reduction requires decreasing caloric intake and increasing energy expenditure. Behavior modification and lifestyle changes are key components of therapy. Medications can augment (but not replace) a diet and exercise plan. Surgery, which may be indicated for severe obesity, involves decreasing the patient's stomach capacity with a vertical banded gastroplasty or performing a gastric bypass procedure.

Anorexia Nervosa

Anorexia nervosa is a condition of extreme weight loss resulting from a severe disturbance in body image and a fear of obesity. The typical patient is a teenage girl, often of higher socioeconomic status, who is intelligent and a perfectionist. This disorder may be mild, but it has a 6% mortality rate among hospitalized patients. **Bulimia** is a related disorder of binge eating, which may be followed by induced vomiting and laxative use.

SIGNS & SYMPTOMS

The anorexic patient becomes increasingly cachectic and may have amenorrhea, bradycardia, low blood pressure, hypothermia, edema, and lanugo hair growth (fine hair covering the entire body, usually seen only in a fetus or premature infant). Patients remain physically active despite their wasted state. Depression and manipulative behavior are common. Cardiac, fluid, and electrolyte abnormalities can be severe, and ventricular arrhythmias can lead to sudden death. Dental decay may be present in bulimic patients because of the effects of gastric acid in the vomitus.

Loss of more than 15% of body weight in a thin patient who denies illness and has a fear of obesity.

Immediate short-term interventions (hospitalization and acute psychiatric care) are often critical to ensure the patient's safety; however, tube or IV feeds are rarely needed. Long-term psychiatric care and family counseling are often successful in treating this disorder.

Vitamin Deficiencies

In developed countries where a variety of foods is available, vitamin deficiencies generally result from chronic alcohol use, medication misuse, food faddism, or long-term parenteral nutrition. All are treated with vitamin replacement and maintenance.

Fat-soluble Vitamins

- **Vitamin A** (retinol) is found in egg yolk, dairy products, liver, and fish. It is also formed by the body from beta-carotene, which is found in yellow, orange, and leafy green vegetables. Vitamin A is a component of photoreceptor pigments in the retina and helps maintain normal epithelium. Deficiency results in **night blindness, conjunctival dryness,** and **corneal keratinization,** which may result in perforation. Other signs include dry skin and keratinization of lung, gastrointestinal, and urinary epithelium.

  Excess beta-carotene stains the skin orange. Vitamin A toxicity causes mouth sores, anorexia, vomiting, and increased intracranial pressure with papilledema and headaches.

- **Vitamin D** (calciferol) is made in the skin upon exposure to sunlight. It is also found in supplemented dairy products and fish. Vitamin D enhances calcium and phosphate absorption from the gut. Vitamin D deficiency leads to **rickets** in children and **osteomalacia** in adults. X-rays show several characteristic deformities, including long-bone bowing in children and demineralization in adults.

  Vitamin D toxicity causes hypercalcemia and calcifications in the kidney, eyes, and joints.

- **Vitamin E** maintains cell membranes by protecting lipids from oxidation. Vitamin E is found in vegetable oils, nuts, legumes, and whole grains. Deficiency results from vitamin-insufficient infant formulas, protein-energy malnutrition, and some malabsorption syndromes with steatorrhea. Deficiency causes **red blood cell hemolysis,** which may lead to anemia in infants, and **neurologic changes,** such as gait changes, areflexia, and decreased vibration, and position sense.

  Toxicity is rare.

- **Vitamin K** is supplied by leafy green vegetables and is also produced by normal intestinal bacteria. It is a cofactor in the synthesis of clotting factors II, VII, IX, and X, so its deficiency results in **spontaneous bleeding** or prolonged oozing. Prothrombin time (PT) is increased more than partial thromboplastin time (PTT), although both may be affected. Injections of vitamin K may be given if rapid correction of the deficiency is needed.

  Toxicity can cause hemolysis but is rare.

Water-soluble Vitamins

- **Thiamine** (vitamin B_1) contributes to carbohydrate metabolism as a coenzyme. It is found in grains, but it is removed in the production of highly polished rice. Certain conditions, including pregnancy and hyperthyroidism, increase the need for vitamin B_1 and can cause secondary deficiency. Deficiency is manifested as **beriberi,** classified as either "dry beriberi," with bilateral, symmetric peripheral neuropathy, or "wet beriberi," a cardiovascular disease of high-output heart failure. CNS involvement causes **Wernicke-Korsakoff syndrome,** a condition particularly common in alcoholics in which nystagmus, ataxia, confusion, and confabulation may progress to coma and death.

- **Riboflavin** (B_2) is a component of the coenzymes flavin adenine dinucleotide (FAD) and flavin mononucleotide (FMN). Deficiency of riboflavin occurs with insufficient milk or animal protein consumption. **Cheilosis** (swollen, cracked, bright red lips) and **angular stomatitis** (fissuring at the angles of the mouth), seborrheic dermatitis, corneal vascularization, and anemia are seen.

- **Niacin** is a coenzyme in carbohydrate metabolism that is found in protein and dairy products as well as in many cereals and vegetables. Deficiency occurs when maize (milled corn) is a diet staple, or in the setting of diarrhea, cirrhosis, alcoholism, or isoniazid (INH) use. Deficiency leads to **pellagra,** which is characterized by "the four Ds": diarrhea, dermatitis, dementia, and death. The dermatitis presents as dark, scaly lesions on sun-exposed skin.

  High-dose niacin can be used to lower low-density lipoproteins (LDL—"bad" cholesterol) and raise high-density lipoproteins (HDL—"good" cholesterol). Flushing is a common side effect, which can be partially prevented with aspirin.

- **Pyridoxine** (B_6) is used in the metabolism of amino acids and the synthesis of heme. It is found in many foods, so deficiency is rare but may occur because of alcoholism or interactions with medications, especially INH. As with other B vitamin deficiencies, seborrheic dermatosis, cheilosis, and glossitis, severe deficiency causes peripheral neuropathy, lymphopenia, and anemia. Infants may have seizures.

  Vitamin B_6 toxicity causes sensory neuropathy.

- **Cobalamin** (B_{12}) is important for DNA synthesis and myelin formation. It is found in meat, eggs, and milk. Once ingested, vitamin B_{12} binds to intrinsic factor from the parietal cells, and the complex is absorbed. **Pernicious anemia,** in which the destruction of parietal cells results in insufficient amounts of intrinsic factor, leads to vitamin B_{12} deficiency. Vitamin B_{12} body stores are depleted slowly over many months to years. **Megaloblastic anemia, neurologic disturbances,** and **ataxia** are the keys to diagnosis, which is confirmed by the Schilling test. Intramuscular injections of vitamin B_{12} may be necessary.

- **Folate** is found in leafy green vegetables and citrus fruits and is used in DNA synthesis. Deficiency generally results from inadequate nutrition, seen often in the elderly, alcoholics, and the poor. Folate body stores are depleted quickly over only a few months. **Megaloblastic anemia without neurologic changes** suggests this diagnosis.

- **Vitamin C** (ascorbic acid) is needed for the formation of collagen and the maintenance of connective tissue, bone, and teeth, wound healing, and iron absorption. Its deficiency, **scurvy,** is often due to dietary insufficiency and appears up to 1 year after the deficient state starts. Splinter hemorrhages, swollen and friable gums, myalgias, and hemarthroses occur, followed by tooth loss, secondary infections, gangrene, and spontaneous hemorrhages. Anemia is also common.

Disorders of the Mouth and Esophagus

Dental Caries

Tooth decay results when microorganisms gradually disintegrate the tooth surface, eventually affecting the pulp as well. Dietary carbohydrates, particularly sucrose, provide the substrate for bacterial production of lactic acid, which erodes the tooth enamel. Only advanced lesions produce symptoms, usually pain from eating hot, cold, or sugary foods. Dental fillings are recommended for treatment of caries.

While the teeth are developing, usually from birth to age 13 years, ingestion of fluoride lends some protection against the formation of caries. In many regions of the United States, water is fluoridated. Children outside of these areas should take fluoride supplements and use fluoride compounds applied directly to the teeth, such as mouth rinses and toothpaste.

Salivary Gland Disorders

Enlarged, painful salivary glands may result from ductal stones, termed sialolithiasis, which are usually found in the submandibular glands. Pain with eating is common. Use of sialagogues (e.g., lemon drops), warm compresses, and massage are often successful in removing the stone, but excision may be needed.

Painless swelling of the parotid glands occurs with mumps, sarcoidosis, cirrhosis, neoplasms, or infection. In a dehydrated person, oral bacteria are not sufficiently washed away and may ascend into the ducts, causing infection and swelling. Hydration and antibiotics are the usual treatment.

Dysphagia

Difficulty swallowing can be divided into problems with oropharyngeal transport and problems with esophageal transport. Oropharyngeal problems are usually caused by neurologic or muscular disorders (e.g., stroke, multiple sclerosis, myasthenia gravis). Esophageal dysphagia can be due to obstructive or motor lesions. Obstructive disorders, such as tumors, strictures, and rings, first affect the patient's swallowing of solids; whereas motor disorders, such as achalasia (see next section), spasms, and scleroderma, affect solids and liquids equally.

SIGNS & SYMPTOMS

Nasal regurgitation or cough secondary to tracheal aspiration occurs if the lesion is pre-esophageal. Patients with esophageal lesions report that "food gets stuck." Supraclavicular lymphadenopathy may indicate cancer.

DIAGNOSIS

Chronology, including whether onset involved solids, liquids, or both, is the key in diagnosing the location and type of dysphagia. Barium swallow studies, upper endoscopy, esophageal manometry, and esophageal pH monitoring may be useful. Dysphagia is a different diagnosis from **globus hystericus,** a "lump in the throat," which is usually psychogenic.

Patients with stroke and other neuromuscular disorders may benefit from therapy. Obstruction may be correctable with surgery.

Achalasia

Achalasia, a neuromuscular disorder of the esophagus, involves impairment of peristalsis and lower esophageal sphincter relaxation. Etiology of the disorder is unknown. Gradual onset most commonly begins between 20 and 40 years of age. A small minority of patients presenting with achalasia have a malignancy of the gastroesophageal junction.

Gradual onset dysphagia of both solids and liquids is the major symptom. Regurgitation is common. At night, this causes cough and aspiration.

Barium swallow studies show a dilated esophagus, with a classic beak-like lower portion. Peristalsis is absent. Endoscopy with biopsy is used to rule out stricture and carcinoma.

Pneumatic dilation or botulinum toxin injection often relieves the obstruction, and both can be repeated if necessary. Otherwise, laparoscopic myotomy (the surgical division of the involved muscle) is useful, although this may result in gastroesophageal reflux. Simultaneous fundoplication is often performed (see next section).

Esophageal Reflux

Also known as **gastroesophageal reflux disease** (GERD), esophageal inflammation results when low pressures at the lower esophageal sphincter allow reflux of gastric contents into the esophagus. In addition to inflammation and ulceration, patients may develop strictures, **Barrett's esophagus** (columnar metaplasia sometimes leading to adenocarcinoma), bleeding, and aspiration. This condition is common in overweight patients and may be seen in infants, who present with vomiting, failure to thrive, anemia, or pulmonary symptoms.

Heartburn is described as burning pain behind the sternum that rises from the stomach toward the mouth. It generally occurs when the patient lies down after eating and is relieved by sitting up, drinking fluids, and taking antacids. Reflux may cause atypical symptoms, such as sore throat, cough, asthma, and non-cardiac chest pain.

The history often suggests reflux. Endoscopy, motility studies, or a pH probe can all be used to confirm the diagnosis.

Patients should elevate the head of their beds, lose weight, and change their diets to decrease intake of fat, alcohol, chocolate, caffeine, and late-night snacks, all of which can exacerbate symptoms. If these steps are unsuccessful, medical treatment includes antacids, H_2-receptor antagonists, or a short-term trial of metoclopramide (Reglan) or a proton pump blocker (omeprazole, lansoprazole). A surgical procedure, such as Nissen fundoplication, which wraps stomach tissue around the lower esophageal sphincter to tighten it, may help in severe disease.

Esophageal Cancer

Esophageal cancer is usually a squamous cell carcinoma, but adenocarcinoma, related to Barrett's esophagus and chronic GERD, now accounts for almost half of cases. Heavy alcohol and tobacco use are risk factors for squamous cell carcinoma. Most patients have metastases to the lymph nodes at the time of presentation, and local extension with invasion of nearby structures is also common.

The initial symptom is dysphagia, leading to weight loss. Patients first experience difficulty swallowing solids, which gradually progresses to difficulty swallowing liquids as well. Weakness, anemia, pain, regurgitation, and aspiration are also noted. Coughing or hoarseness may be present if the laryngeal nerves are involved.

Typically, barium swallow shows a lumen narrowed by an irregular mass. Constricting bands are seen with annular lesions. Esophagoscopy with biopsy is necessary for tissue diagnosis. CT scan may show extension and metastases.

Some combination of surgery, radiation, and chemotherapy. Prognosis is poor.

Hiatal Hernia

Hiatal hernia is a common disorder that involves protrusion of part of the stomach above the diaphragm. A sliding hiatal hernia involves upward displacement of both the gastroesophageal junction and the stomach through the diaphragm, while a paraesophageal hiatal hernia results when part of the stomach is pushed through the diaphragm next to a normally located esophagus and gastroesophageal junction.

If the lower esophageal sphincter is displaced upward, it is exposed to lower pressures in the thoracic cavity and may not be able to remain closed. Gastroesophageal reflux results. Many cases, however, are asymptomatic.

X-rays and barium studies show a portion of the stomach above the diaphragm.

GASTROENTEROLOGY

The only therapy needed for sliding hiatal hernias is control of reflux, if present. A paraesophageal hernia can incarcerate and strangulate. This complication can be prevented by surgical reduction. Surgery is also indicated for recurrent or intractable symptoms and often involves a Nissen fundoplication.

Disorders of the Stomach and Intestine

Gastritis

Gastritis, an inflammation of the gastric mucosa, can be classified as *erosive* or *nonerosive.* Erosive gastritis is usually due to NSAID use, alcohol, severe illness, or trauma. This so-called stress gastritis involves rapidly developing, superficial lesions.

Nonerosive gastritis, caused by *Helicobacter pylori,* is present in 30%–50% of the population and may cause gland atrophy or metaplasia. Complete atrophy of the fundal mucosa with loss of parietal cells results in pernicious anemia.

Mild dyspepsia is the presenting symptom. With stress gastritis in hospitalized patients, blood in the nasogastric aspirate or hematemesis ("coffee grounds" emesis) is often the first sign. Because the lesions are superficial, significant bleeding does not usually occur. Nonerosive gastritis is usually asymptomatic.

Endoscopy should be done promptly to rule out bleeding from more serious lesions such as ulcers or esophageal varices. In erosive gastritis, petechiae and erosions may be seen. In nonerosive gastritis, the stomach appears normal but biopsy shows inflammation with neutrophils and lymphocytes.

Avoidance of NSAIDs and alcohol may be sufficient treatment for erosive gastritis. Antacids and H$_2$-blockers are also commonly used. Prophylactic H$_2$-blockers prevent stress gastritis in intensive care unit patients.

Peptic Ulcer Disease

Ulcerative corrosion of the epithelium occurs more frequently in the duodenum than in the stomach. Although gastric acid is the injurious agent, *H. pylori* plays an important role in weakening the epithelium and making it susceptible to damage. NSAID use and smoking are other risk factors. Few ulcer patients have higher-than-normal acid secretion.

Burning or gnawing epigastric pain may be alleviated by food or antacids, depending on the location of the ulcer (Table 1-1). Nausea and epigastric tenderness are common. Fecal occult blood is present in one-third of patients. Ulcers may be complicated by bleeding, perforation, or obstruction.

The ulcer may be seen on an upper GI series, but endoscopy with biopsy identifies active *H. pylori* infection or malignancy, which is a particular concern in cases of gastric ulcer without history of NSAID use. Tests of active *H. pylori* infection rely on the fact that *H. pylori* produces urease. Biopsy tissue is

GASTROENTEROLOGY

Table 1-1. Gastric ulcers versus duodenal ulcers

	Gastric ulcer	*Duodenal ulcer*
Frequency	25% of PUD	75% of PUD
Age	Older	Younger
Major risk factor	NSAIDs	*Helicobacter pylori*
Pain	Varies, often not relieved by eating	Improves with food, worse 2 to 4 hr later

NSAIDs, nonsteroidal anti-inflammatory drugs; PUD, peptic ulcer disease.

assessed for urease using pH-sensitive media. The noninvasive ^{14}C and ^{13}C urea breath tests are used to document *H. pylori* eradication after therapy. Serum antibodies are sometimes useful but cannot distinguish between active and resolved infection. Serum gastrin levels can be measured to exclude hypersecretory states such as **Zollinger-Ellison syndrome** (gastrinoma).

TREATMENT

Antibiotic combinations to treat *H. pylori* infection include tetracycline, metronidazole, amoxicillin, and clarithromycin. Bismuth subsalicylate (Pepto-Bismol) or proton pump blockers are added in most regimens. Retreatment may be necessary to eradicate infection. After successful treatment of infection, recurrence of the ulcer is rare. Nonhealing ulcers should raise suspicions of carcinoma. Chronic H_2-blocker therapy and surgical treatment are now rarely necessary. In patients in whom NSAIDs cannot be stopped, coadministration of H_2-blockers, proton pump inhibitors, or the prostaglandin analog misoprostol help reduce ulcer recurrence. Use of COX-2 selective NSAIDs also helps.

Gastric Carcinoma

Stomach cancer is almost always adenocarcinoma, although squamous cell tumors may invade from the esophagus. Gastric carcinoma can take four forms:

- **Ulcerating carcinoma** is a penetrating, ulcerlike tumor with shallow edges, in contrast to the raised edges seen in peptic ulcer disease.
- **Polypoid carcinoma** involves a bulky, intraluminal tumor that metastasizes late.
- **Superficial spreading carcinoma,** also called *early gastric carcinoma,* is confined to the mucosa and submucosa and has the best prognosis.
- **Linitis plastica** spreads throughout all layers of the stomach, decreasing its elasticity. Prognosis is poor.

H. pylori infection is a risk factor for stomach cancer, and the incidence parallels *H. pylori* prevalence. Older men, African-Americans, Hispanics, and Asian-Americans are most at risk. There is a high incidence of gastric cancer in Japan.

SIGNS & SYMPTOMS

The most common symptoms are abdominal heaviness, early satiety, anorexia, weight loss, and, rarely, melena (black, tarry stools). Vomiting may occur, particularly if pyloric obstruction develops; the vomitus may have a "coffee-ground" appearance because of bleeding. Many gastric carcinoma patients have a positive guaiac test, but less than 20% have a palpable epigastric mass. **Virchow's node,** an enlarged left supraclavicular node, indicates metastasis. A small percentage of gastric carcinomas metastasize to the ovary, causing ovarian masses known as **Krukenberg's tumors.**

Carcinoembryonic antigen (CEA) levels are often elevated, especially when the tumor has spread. Hematocrit is low in many patients because of occult blood loss.

An upper GI series will show most tumors. Gastroscopy and biopsy are particularly necessary with ulcerating lesions to differentiate them from benign ulcers.

Surgical resection is the sole treatment option. Survival rates for early cancer are about 90%, but overall 5-year survival in the United States is only 12%.

Hernias

Hernias occur when intra-abdominal tissue protrudes through a defect in the abdominal wall. Common hernias are found at the umbilicus, along the linea alba, along the femoral sheath, and in the inguinal region. **Indirect inguinal hernias** are congenital defects that result when the processus vaginalis fails to close after the testicle has descended into the scrotum. **Direct inguinal hernias** are caused by a weakness of the abdominal musculature in Hesselbach's triangle. These hernias develop in adults. A **reducible** hernia is one in which the abdominal contents can be manipulated back into the abdominal cavity. An **irreducible** or **incarcerated** hernia may result in bowel obstruction or tissue strangulation.

Patients may be asymptomatic or may report an aching discomfort in the region. A mass may bulge when intra-abdominal pressure increases (i.e., cough, Valsalva).

Clinical inspection. Distinguishing between direct and indirect inguinal hernias requires digital invagination of the skin along the spermatic cord and palpation of the internal inguinal ring. An indirect hernia protrudes at this point, whereas a direct hernia will be felt medial to this ring.

Surgical repair is necessary to prevent bowel incarceration, obstruction, and infarction.

Diverticulosis

Diverticulosis is an acquired condition of multiple diverticula in which the colonic mucosa and submucosa herniate through the muscular layer. Diverticulosis is especially common in developed nations because of a low-fiber diet, resulting in increased intraluminal pressures.

Diverticulosis is generally asymptomatic. Symptoms arise from a lower GI bleed or from diverticulitis (see next section).

Diverticula are seen on barium enema or colonoscopy (Figure 1-1).

A high-fiber diet may reduce the risk of complications. Avoidance of foods that can become impacted in the diverticulum, such as small seeds and peanuts, is advised.

Diverticulitis

Diverticulitis, a complication of diverticulosis, occurs when a diverticulum becomes infected or perforates, causing an abscess or peritonitis. Diverticulitis may be further complicated by formation of fistulas to the bladder, vagina, or skin or by the development of adhesions that cause small bowel obstruction.

Acute lower abdominal pain, usually on the left side, is accompanied by fever, chills, and constipation or loose stools. Occult blood in the stool is common and frank bleeding may occur. A lower abdominal mass may be present on examination.

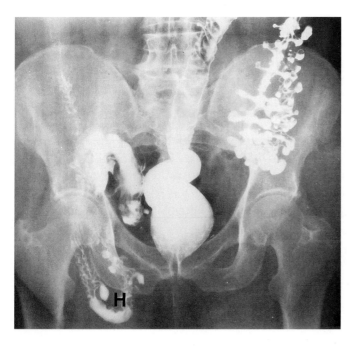

Figure 1-1. Colonic diverticulosis. The diverticulosis is worse on the left side of the colon. Note the inguinal hernia (*H*) on the right. (Reprinted with permission from Daffner R: *Clinical Radiology: The Essentials,* 2nd ed. Baltimore, Williams & Wilkins, 1999, p 309.)

A plain abdominal film showing free air under the diaphragm can confirm perforation. CT scan with water-soluble contrast can be used to locate an abscess during the acute attack. Barium enema x-ray or colonoscopy can be used after the acute attack has completely resolved.

Mild cases may be managed on an outpatient basis with a clear liquid diet and oral antibiotics to cover both gram-negative bacteria and anaerobes. Hospitalization, with nasogastric tube placement, IV antibiotics, and surgical resection, may be needed for severe disease.

Malabsorption

The mucosa of the small bowel has many enzymes required for proper absorption of nutrients. If the enzymes are absent or the mucosa is inflamed, malabsorption occurs. Symptoms of malabsorption are due to increased fecal fat, bacterial fermentation of unabsorbed food, and vitamin and nutrient deficiencies.

- **Lactose intolerance** results from a deficiency of the enzyme lactase, which splits lactose into glucose and galactose. Unsplit lactose in the bowel lumen causes an osmotic diarrhea, and bacterial fermentation of lactose produces excessive gas. Lactase deficiency is thus characterized by bloating and explosive diarrhea after milk intake. Lactase is normally located in the jejunal brush border, so lactase deficiency may result from diseases that alter the jejunal mucosa, such as Crohn's disease, other types of malabsorption diseases, and giardiasis. Viral gastroenteritis can cause temporary lactase deficiency. Lactase deficiency occurs normally in 75% of adults in most ethnic groups but in less than 20% of those of northwestern European descent. Onset is between 10 and 20 years of age, and a lactose-free diet is needed for prevention of symptoms.
- **Celiac sprue** is a hereditary sensitivity to the gliadin component of gluten, a protein found in wheat, barley, and rye. Interaction of gliadin with antibodies initiates an immune reaction that causes jejunal mucosal damage. Failure to thrive, abnormal stools, and bloating are common symptoms in infants, whereas a syndrome of malabsorption and vitamin deficiency is the presentation in adults. Diagnosis is made by finding antiendomysial or antigliadin antibodies in the serum or by biopsy showing a loss of normal villi in the jejunal mucosa. Patients improve on a gluten-free diet but have an increased risk of developing other autoimmune diseases and intestinal lymphoma.
- **Tropical sprue,** a malabsorption syndrome of unknown etiology, is characterized by nutritional deficiencies and small-bowel mucosal abnormalities. It is an acquired disorder found primarily in the Caribbean, South India, and Southeast Asia. Folic acid replacement and tetracycline are often curative.
- **Whipple's disease** is a rare disorder of middle-aged men, caused by infection with the bacillus *Tropheryma whippelli.* Many organs are involved. Symptoms include joint pain, weight loss and other symptoms of malabsorption, fever, cough, lymphadenopathy, congestive heart failure or new murmurs due to myocardial involvement, and neurologic symptoms such as seizures or dementia. Jejunal biopsy is diagnostic, with foamy macrophages containing masses of gram-positive, rod-shaped bacilli that stain with the periodic acid–Schiff (PAS) reagent. Untreated, Whipple's disease is fatal; however, several antibiotics are curative.

General symptoms of malabsorption include weight loss, abdominal distention, flatulence, diarrhea, and steatorrhea (fatty stools). Protein malabsorption can cause hypoproteinemic edema. Symptoms from nutrient deficiencies are common and include glossitis, stomatitis, dermatitis, anemia, and easy bruising (from vitamin K deficiency).

Microcytic anemia reflects iron deficiency, while megaloblastic anemia usually points to folic acid deficiency. Low serum ferritin generally indicates celiac disease or a postgastrectomy state because iron absorption occurs in the duodenum and upper jejunum. A Sudan stain is often positive if fecal fat is present and usually makes a quantitative 72-hour fecal fat study unnecessary.

The triad of weight loss, diarrhea, and anemia strongly suggests malabsorption. Direct measurement of fecal fat is a reliable test, as increased fecal fat always indicates malabsorption. The d-xylose absorption test measures xylose excreted in the urine after an oral load. Abnormal absorption points to mucosal abnormalities. Biopsy is often diagnostic.

Treat the underlying disorder, as discussed in the preceding sections.

Irritable Bowel Syndrome

Irritable bowel syndrome is a common disorder involving chronic GI symptoms, often associated with psychiatric symptoms. Onset is typically in young adulthood.

Patients report chronic, crampy abdominal pain, bloating, flatulence, and diarrhea or constipation. Abdominal pain is usually relieved by defecation.

Irritable bowel syndrome is a diagnosis of exclusion. Malabsorption, thyroid dysfunction, and parasitic infections should be ruled out. Presumptive diagnosis may be made in the context of chronic symptoms without weight change or findings on physical examination.

Dietary bulk supplements, anticholinergics to decrease spasms, antidiarrheals, and tricyclic antidepressants may be helpful.

Crohn's Disease

Also called *regional enteritis* or *granulomatous colitis,* Crohn's disease is a chronic and progressive inflammation of the GI tract. Its course is variable and is marked by remissions and exacerbations. Crohn's disease can cause changes anywhere along the GI tract, with lesions most frequently occurring in the distal ileum. Some patients have "skip" lesions, discontinuous lesions with normal bowel in between. A majority of patients have granulomas in the bowel wall or mesenteric lymph nodes. Other characteristics of Crohn's disease are fissures, strictures, ulcers, and transmural involvement, as well as complications including intestinal obstruction, abscess formation, fistulas, colon cancer, and systemic manifestations. As with ulcerative colitis, extracolonic complications include peripheral arthritis, ankylosing spondylitis, uveitis, and primary sclerosing cholangitis.

SIGNS & SYMPTOMS

Manifestations include diarrhea, recurrent abdominal pain, right lower quadrant abdominal mass (due to an inflamed ileum), low-grade fever, malnutrition, weight loss, anemia, and anorectal fissures, fistulas, and abscesses. Oral ulcers are also common.

DIAGNOSIS

On barium study or endoscopy, the small bowel shows edema, ulceration, fistulas, strictures, and "cobblestone" patterns (Figure 1-2). Serologic testing for antineutrophil cytoplasmic antibodies with perinuclear staining (pANCA) and anti-yeast S cerevisiae antibodies (ASCA) may help distinguish between Crohn's and ulcerative colitis in subtle cases (Table 1-2).

TREATMENT

Initially, treatment involves rest, antidiarrheal agents, and dietary changes with supplemental parenteral nutrition if disease is severe. Steroids, sulfasalazine, immunosuppressives, and antibiotics are all used with some success. Surgery is necessary for complications, such as obstruction and fistulas, but surgery for Crohn's disease is palliative and not curative.

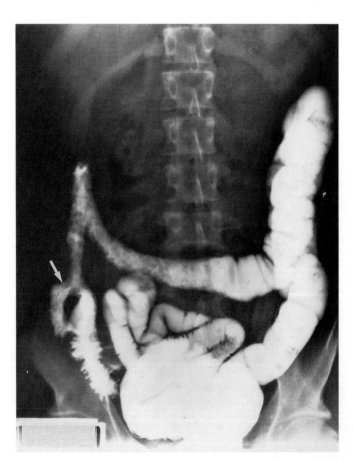

Fig. 1-2. Ilial involvement and fistula formation (*arrow*) in a patient with Crohn's disease. (Reprinted with permission from Daffner R: *Clinical Radiology: The Essentials,* 2nd ed. Baltimore, Williams & Wilkins, 1999, p 318.)

Table 1-2. Ulcerative colitis and Crohn's disease

	Ulcerative colitis	*Crohn's disease*
Location	Continuous disease starting at the rectum and possibly including the colon and distal ileum	Distal ileum is most common site, but entire gastrointestinal tract may be involved, with multiple "skip" areas
Depth of pathology	Mucosa and submucosa	Entire bowel wall, with granulomas
Abdominal mass	Absent	Frequently present in right lower quadrant
Bloody stools	Frequently present	Usually absent
Endoscopic findings	Friable mucosa in rectal area	Aphthous ulcers and "cobblestone" pattern
Radiographic	"Lead pipe" colon without haustrations	"Cobblestone" pattern with small-bowel ulcerations, strictures, and fissures
Serologic testing		
pANCA	60%–70% positive	5%–10% positive
ASCA	10%–15% positive	60%–70% positive
Treatment	Sulfasalazine, steroids, immunosuppressives	Sulfasalazine, steroids, immunosuppressives
	Colectomy is curative	Surgery can treat complications but is not curative
Complications	Perforation	Small bowel abscesses, obstruction, and fistulas
	Hemorrhage	Perianal disease
	Toxic megacolon	Malabsorption
	Colon cancer	Toxic megacolon
		Colon cancer

Ulcerative Colitis

Ulcerative colitis, a chronic, idiopathic inflammation of the colon and rectum, has a variable course of remissions and exacerbations. Ulcerative colitis generally involves the rectum, and in half of cases it is confined solely to this region (**ulcerative proctitis**). Inflammation spreads proximally to the distal ileum in a minority of patients. The affected colon is contiguous, without skip lesions. Ulcers and abscesses form in the mucosa and submucosa and may develop into characteristic pseudopolyps, which occur when inflammatory growths from the intestinal mucosa have a polyplike appearance. Hemorrhage is a frequent complication, and the colon may become dilated and perforate. Patients have an increased risk of colon cancer, and other extracolonic complications are common. These include peripheral arthritis, uveitis, ankylosing spondylitis, and primary sclerosing cholangitis.

SIGNS & SYMPTOMS

Frequent symptoms include rectal bleeding, tenesmus, crampy abdominal pain, and blood or mucus with diarrhea. Patients may experience fever, nausea and vomiting, weight loss, or dehydration.

DIAGNOSIS

Sigmoidoscopy shows dull, granular, friable mucosa, but biopsy of affected areas may be needed to rule out infectious and ischemic colitis. Barium enemas should not be performed in acutely ill patients, but in its chronic state, ulcerative colitis has a typical mucosal irregularity and a "lead pipe" appearance as the colon narrows, shortens, and loses its haustrations (Figure 1-3).

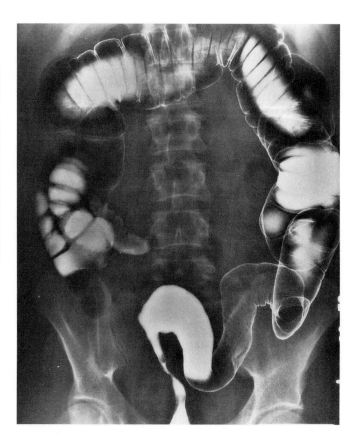

Fig. 1-3. Air contrast barium enema in a patient with ulcerative colitis. Note the narrowing of the rectum and sigmoid. (Reprinted with permission from Daffner R: *Clinical Radiology: The Essentials,* 2nd ed. Baltimore, Williams & Wilkins, 1999, p 300.)

Sulfasalazine, steroids, or immunosuppressives are used to treat mild exacerbations and maintain periods of remission. More severe episodes require hospital admission with a nasogastric tube, parenteral nutrition, IV steroids, and antibiotics. Vigilant surveillance is needed for colon cancer, with annual colonoscopy and biopsies beginning 8–10 years after diagnosis. Folic acid supplements decrease cancer risk. Colectomy may be needed for severe or intractable disease and is curative.

Toxic Megacolon

Dilation, usually of the transverse colon, must exceed 6 cm in diameter for the diagnosis of toxic megacolon to apply. In adults, this condition is often preceded by inflammatory bowel disease (e.g., ulcerative colitis and Crohn's), whereas in children, Hirschsprung's disease (absence of colonic nerve plexus) is the more common etiology. Toxic megacolon can result in septicemia, generalized peritonitis, or perforation and carries a high mortality rate.

Patients are severely ill, with high fever, abdominal pain, distention, and hypotension.

Abdominal x-rays show intraluminal gas along a continuous segment of very dilated bowel.

Patients must be NPO (nothing by mouth) with IV fluid replacement and electrolyte maintenance as needed. Antibiotics and steroids are administered in inflammatory bowel disease. Passage of a rectal tube may alleviate megacolon but can cause a perforation. Surgery may be necessary.

Ischemic Colitis

Ischemic colitis is caused by insufficient blood supply to the colon, leading to inflammation and eventually necrosis. Etiology may be atherosclerotic or embolic. Patients are most often elderly or are younger patients with chronic diseases such as diabetes, lupus, and sickle cell anemia. Reversible ischemic colitis heals with medical management, but irreversible cases require surgical treatment. Mortality is high.

Patients experience an abrupt onset of abdominal pain after eating and may have bloody diarrhea. Classically, the patient's pain is out of proportion to the examination findings.

Endoscopy shows a bloody, edematous, friable mucosa and may reveal ulcers or a gray membrane, in which case stool should be checked for *Clostridium difficile*. Barium x-ray demonstrates a "thumb print" or pseudotumor pattern.

IV fluids and antibiotics are frequently sufficient, although resection of the ischemic portion of the colon is necessary in the case of irreversible damage.

Colonic Polyps

Colonic polyps are small tissue masses projecting into the colonic lumen. Polyps may be sessile or pedunculated, and may be mucosal, submucosal, or muscular in origin. They have a variety of etiologic and histologic types. Neoplastic polyps are adenomas. Non-neoplastic polyps may be inflammatory, hyperplastic, or hamartomatous (juvenile or Peutz-Jeghers).

Adenomatous polyps are found in 50% of 70 year olds. These premalignant adenomas are probably the origin of most large-bowel adenocarcinomas. Cancer is found in only 1% of adenomas less than 1 cm in diameter, but it is found in 45% of adenomas more than 2 cm in diameter, making size an important predictor of histology. Villous adenomas are more frequently malignant than tubular adenomas. Sessile polyps are more often malignant than pedunculated polyps.

Familial adenomatous polyposis is a rare, autosomal-dominant condition involving multiple polyps that eventually develop into colorectal cancer if left untreated.

Polyps are generally asymptomatic. Larger lesions can cause intermittent bleeding and changes in bowel habits, such as increased frequency, constipation, or tenesmus.

GASTROENTEROLOGY

Distal polyps may be felt on digital rectal examination. Barium enema can show colonic lesions suggestive of polyps. Diagnosis is confirmed with colonoscopy.

Biopsy is necessary to rule out cancer. Carcinoma in situ only requires polypectomy. Segmental resection of the colon may be needed if pathology shows invasive adenocarcinoma.

Colon Cancer

The colon is the second most common site of visceral cancer in Western countries. The incidence of colon cancer increases dramatically above age 40 years. The vast majority of these cancers are adenocarcinoma. Risk factors include a personal history of previous colon cancer or adenomatous polyps, a family history of colon cancer, ulcerative colitis, and the autosomal-dominant familial adenomatous polyposis. Increased incidence is seen in higher socioeconomic classes and is probably related to high-fat, high-calorie, low-fiber, and low-calcium diets.

Colon cancer spreads most frequently to regional lymph nodes. Cancer may also spread by direct extension, as seen with the common circumferential growth pattern of left colon lesions, and it can invade nearby structures. Hematogenous spread commonly leads to metastases in the liver or lungs. "Seeding," or transperitoneal metastasis, may cause local implants or generalized abdominal carcinomatosis. The tumor, node, metastasis (TNM) system and Dukes classification are both used for staging.

Adenocarcinoma remains asymptomatic for approximately 5 years. Right-sided colon lesions typically cause weakness secondary to anemia and right-sided discomfort or fullness. Left-sided colon cancer more often causes changes in bowel habits from occlusion of the lumen, with alternating constipation and increased frequency, blood-streaked stool, and stool with decreased diameter ("pencil stools").

In 70% of patients, CEA is elevated in the serum, but this finding is not specific to colon cancer. CEA therefore is not considered an appropriate screening tool, but it can be useful to detect recurrences. CBC often reveals anemia.

Barium enema examination and colonoscopy with biopsy are the principal means of diagnosis. Colon cancer classically appears as an annular, "apple core" filling defect on contrast examination (Figure 1-4).

Surgical resection of the lesion is the first step. Regional lymph node dissection is important to stage disease and help decide about adjuvant radiation or chemotherapy. Even in advanced cases, resection is also often helpful for palliation to prevent obstruction and bleeding. Overall survival is 35%.

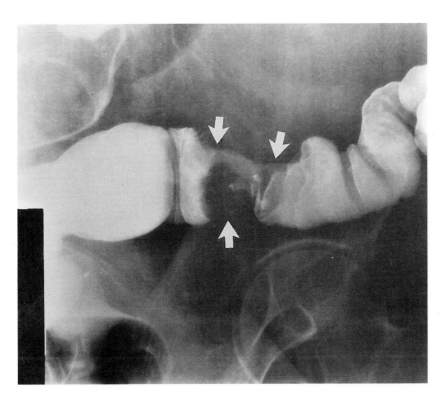

Fig. 1-4. "Apple-core" filling defect in colon cancer. (Reprinted with permission from Daffner R: *Clinical Radiology: The Essentials,* 2nd ed. Baltimore, Williams & Wilkins, 1999, p 304.)

The American Cancer Society recommends annual digital rectal examinations for individuals 40 years of age or older. Annual stool occult blood tests and flexible sigmoidoscopy every 5 years are recommended after age 50. Alternatives to this combination include colonoscopy every 10 years or double contrast barium enema every 5–10 years.

Rectal Cancer

Similar to colon cancer, rectal cancer is usually adenocarcinoma.

The most frequent presenting symptom is persistent hematochezia (blood-streaked stools), which must be evaluated for cancer even in the presence of hemorrhoids. Tenesmus, altered bowel habit, and sensation of incomplete evacuation are also common symptoms.

Distal lesions can be palpated on digital examination. Sigmoidoscopy may be needed to biopsy the lesion.

Surgical resection is performed, often with adjuvant radiation therapy.

Hemorrhoids

Hemorrhoids can be internal (arising from a cushion of veins above the dentate line) or external (arising from veins below the dentate line). They engorge when venous pressure increases, such as with constipation and straining, prolonged sitting, pregnancy, and obesity.

Symptoms include discomfort and small amounts of bright red bleeding.

External hemorrhoids are visible around the anus and internal hemorrhoids can be visualized using an anoscope. Sigmoidoscopy is frequently indicated to rule out causes of bleeding in the rectum or sigmoid colon, despite the presence of hemorrhoids. Colonoscopy or barium enema is indicated if microcytic anemia is present.

Increasing dietary fiber and avoiding prolonged sitting and straining is the first-line treatment. Sclerotherapy, rubber band ligation, and excision are also options.

Anal Fissures

Anal fissures are painful, linear tears in the epithelium of the anal verge, usually in the posterior midline. They generally result from trauma during defecation. Atypical fissures should raise the suspicion of Crohn's disease. Symptoms include intense pain with defecation, which may lead to constipation, and spots of bright red bleeding. Treatment requires softening stools to allow healing. A skin tag (sentinel pile) may develop at the healed site. Patient with recurrent fissures may benefit from a partial sphincterotomy, however fecal incontinence is a risk of this procedure.

Anorectal Abscesses

Abscesses arise from infection of the anal crypts at the dentate line, infection of a prolapsed internal hemorrhoid, and infection of a hair follicle or local abrasion. People with Crohn's disease are particularly prone to abscess and fistula formation.

Symptoms include throbbing rectal pain and, if the abscess is large, systemic signs of infection. Superficial abscesses are indurated, red, and may be fluctuant. Deeper abscesses are tender on digital rectal exam.

Clinical examination.

Treatment requires antibiotics to cover both aerobic and anaerobic gram-negative rods and complete incision and drainage, which may need to be done in the operating room, depending on the extent of the abscess.

Fistulas

Abscesses may be complicated by the formation of a fistula or tract, usually between the anal crypt and the site from which the abscess drains. The patient reports a chronic discharge and has a history of previous abscesses. On exam, the opening may be visible as a red papule with pus coming from it. A cord-like tract can often be palpated and may be able to be probed. Treatment is with fistulotomy, in which the tract is completely opened and allowed to heal from within.

Gastrointestinal Infectious Disorders

Viral Gastroenteritis

Nausea, vomiting, diarrhea, and abdominal cramps in viral gastroenteritis may be due to one of several potential viral agents. The Norwalk virus is a common cause of gastroenteritis outbreaks, particularly in group settings. Rotaviruses cause severe diarrhea in small children and cause significant mortality in the third world. Enteroviruses, particularly Coxsackie virus A1 and echovirus, and adenoviruses are other sources of disease. Viral cultures are rarely clinically indicated. Fecal leukocytes are absent. These syndromes typically resolve without treatment, although hospitalization and rehydration may be needed for severely affected children.

Staphylococcal Gastroenteritis

Staphylococcal gastroenteritis results from eating food containing the toxin produced by *Staphylococcus aureus.* Foods left at room temperature, particularly milk, cream products, and some meat and fish, provide a fertile breeding ground for this organism.

Within 8 hours after eating, patients experience the abrupt onset of vomiting, often with cramping, and diarrhea (Table 1-3). Complete recovery occurs within 24 to 48 hours of onset.

A history of similar illness in others who ate the same food is common. Fecal leukocytes are usually absent. Laboratory studies to distinguish between this and viral gastroenteritis do not change management and are usually not done.

GASTROENTEROLOGY

Table 1-3. Bacterial gastroenteritis

	Incubation	Toxin-mediated	Vomiting	Diarrhea	Stool RBCs/WBCs	Fever	Antibiotics
Staphylococcal gastroenteritis	1–8 hrs	Yes	+++	+	–	–	No
Cholera	12 hrs–7 days	Yes	–	+++	–	–	Decreases duration of symptoms
Shigella	12–72 hrs	No	+	+++	+/+	+	Decreases duration of symptoms
Salmonella gastroenteritis	8–48 hrs	No	+	+–+++	+/+	+	Prolongs excretion of organism; indicated in severe disease
Hemorrhagic colitis	1–7 days	Yes	–	+++	+/–	–	No
Pseudomembranous colitis	0–6 weeks	Yes	–	+++	+/Sometimes	Sometimes	Discontinue other antibiotics if possible; treat if severe

TREATMENT

Fluid and electrolyte maintenance.

Cholera

The enterotoxin from *Vibrio cholerae* causes electrolytes and water to be secreted into the bowel lumen. The organism is spread by fecal contamination of water, seafood, and other products. Endemic cases are found along the Gulf Coast of the United States, as well as in Asia, Africa, and the Middle East. Epidemics, usually caused by fecal contamination of water supplies, can occur in any season and affect children and adults equally.

SIGNS & SYMPTOMS

Huge quantities of "rice-water" stools are passed without pain. Diarrhea is not bloody because the bowel mucosa remains intact. Fever is rare. Severe dehydration leads to thirst, oliguria or anuria, cramps, weakness, and loss of skin tone. Circulatory collapse may cause cyanosis, stupor, renal tubular necrosis, and death.

Metabolic acidosis may be severe because of loss of bicarbonate in the stool.

Stool culture. Fecal WBCs are absent.

Maintaining fluid and electrolyte balance is imperative. Ciprofloxacin or doxycycline reduces duration of symptoms.

Vibrio parahaemolyticus

Vibrio parahaemolyticus is typically acquired by ingestion of undercooked oysters. Watery diarrhea, crampy abdominal pain, and fever occur within 24 hours of eating contaminated shellfish. Symptoms are self-limited and antibiotics are not necessary.

Shigellosis

Shigella species bacteria cause dysentery (bloody diarrhea) after ingestion of even a very small inoculum. Fecal-oral spread and contaminated foods are responsible, and flies act as mechanical vectors. Epidemics occur with overcrowding and insufficient sanitation, and reinfection is possible.

Young children have an acute onset of symptoms, including fever, nausea, vomiting, diarrhea, abdominal pain, and distention. Within 3 days, diarrhea becomes severe and bloody, often with pus or mucus. Dehydration can cause death; otherwise, the acute disease resolves within several days. Adults tend to have a milder illness.

Stool culture. Proctoscopy shows an ulcerated, erythematous mucosal surface. Fecal WBCs are present.

Fluid replacement is critical. Ciprofloxacin or TMP/SMX can shorten the course in severe disease. Antidiarrheals, such as diphenoxylate hydrochloride with atropine sulfate (Lomotil), may prolong the course and should not be given.

GASTROENTEROLOGY

Salmonella Gastroenteritis

Gastroenteritis is the most common of the syndromes caused by *Salmonella*. Infection results from eating foods produced from infected animals, such as meat, milk, poultry, and eggs; from drinking contaminated water; and from fecal-oral transmission.

Symptoms may develop within 2 days of eating infected food. Nausea and cramps are followed by watery or bloody diarrhea, fever, and sometimes vomiting.

Stool culture. Fecal WBCs are present.

Supportive care. Antibiotics are indicated only in severe disease because antibiotics prolong excretion of organisms. Asymptomatic carriers need not be treated unless they are food handlers or health care workers. Prolonged courses (4 weeks) of antibiotics sometimes clear the organism, but follow-up cultures are necessary for verification.

Hemorrhagic Colitis

Hemorrhagic colitis is an infection of enterohemorrhagic *Escherichia coli* O157:H7, which produces a toxin that damages GI mucosa and vascular endothelial cells. Absorption of this toxin leads to damage in vessels of other organs, particularly the kidneys. The organism has a bovine reservoir, so sporadic cases and outbreaks are due to consumption of unpasteurized milk and undercooked beef. Fecal-oral transmission is also possible. (Travelers' diarrhea is most frequently caused by non-hemorrhagic strains of *E. coli*.)

Acute, severe abdominal cramps and watery diarrhea progress rapidly to bloody diarrhea. Fever tends to be low, except when complications arise. An uncomplicated course lasts approximately 1 week, but a small number of cases are complicated by **hemolytic-uremic syndrome** (HUS) or **thrombotic thrombocytopenic purpura** (TTP).

Stool culture. Fecal WBCs are usually absent.

Supportive care, especially with fluid replacement. Antibiotics do not help to reduce symptoms or duration. Complications require aggressive management.

Pseudomembranous Colitis

When antibiotic therapy changes the balance of normal intestinal bacteria, overgrowth of a pathogen can result in pseudomembranous colitis, a form of diarrhea associated with exudative "pseudomembranes" in the colon. The bacterium that most often causes this condition is *Clostridium difficile*. Although therapy with any antibiotic may cause this problem, clindamycin, ampicillin, and the cephalosporins are most frequently involved.

Onset of symptoms usually occurs during a course of antibiotic therapy but may be delayed by as much as 6 weeks. The illness is often mild, but severe bloody diarrhea with abdominal cramping, fever, and dehydration may occur.

Finding *C. difficile* toxin in the stool is diagnostic. Stool culture or sigmoidoscopy with visualization of pseudomembranes may also be used.

Discontinuing antibiotics, if possible, may be sufficient treatment. Metronidazole or oral vancomycin is used in more severe cases.

Amebiasis

Entamoeba histolytica typically infects the colon and may produce abscesses in the liver. Cysts stay viable in soil and water for weeks, and infection occurs when cysts are ingested. Transmission is more common where sanitation is poor and may be via person-to-person contact, fecal contamination of water supplies, or mechanical vectors such as flies.

Symptoms range from mild diarrhea with cramps to severe dysentery, in which trophozoites invade the bowel wall and can cause hemorrhage or perforation and peritonitis. If carried by the blood to the liver, an amebic abscess may develop.

Three sequential ova and parasite (O&P) stool samples are only 80% sensitive and must be analyzed immediately before trophozoites are destroyed. The serologic indirect hemagglutination test may aid in diagnosis.

Metronidazole and paromomycin.

GASTROENTEROLOGY

Giardiasis

Giardiasis occurs when the cyst form of the protozoa *Giardia lamblia* is ingested and the trophozoite emerges in the small bowel and infects the epithelium. Sources of infection include fecal contamination of water (often in mountain streams), day care centers and other close household contacts, and anal-oral sex. Incubation is 1–3 weeks.

SIGNS & SYMPTOMS

Presentation varies widely and many patients are asymptomatic. Diarrhea begins suddenly or gradually and may be mild or severe. Stools are bulky, greasy, and malodorous and may occur daily or every few days, often after breakfast. Patients may have abdominal cramping and lots of gas.

DIAGNOSIS

Cysts, trophozoites, or the Giardia antigen are identified in a stool sample sent for O&P examination. For greater sensitivity, obtain three samples at two-day intervals.

TREATMENT

Metronidazole. Carriers should also be treated.

Pancreatic Disorders

Acute Pancreatitis

Nonbacterial inflammation of the pancreas occurs when extravasated pancreatic enzymes digest the pancreas and surrounding tissues. Acute pancreatitis is most commonly caused by gallstone disease (40%) or alcoholism (40%), but it may also be due to hypercalcemia, hyperlipidemia, drugs, or unidentifiable causes. Complications include pancreatic abscess, pseudocyst formation, necrosis, hemorrhage, and splenic vein thrombosis. Systemic complications also arise and include circulatory shock, disseminated intravascular coagulation (DIC), acute renal failure, respiratory failure, and sepsis.

SIGNS & SYMPTOMS

Acute epigastric pain radiating to the back is the classic symptom and may be accompanied by nausea and vomiting. Grey Turner's sign (bluish discoloration in the flank) or Cullen's sign (periumbilical discoloration) occurs in only 1% to 2% of patients. Severe cases may display fever, left pleural effusion, tachycardia, and hypotension or shock.

LABS

Serum amylase and lipase are increased. Note that these are not prognostic. Ranson's criteria (see box) are used to predict prognosis. X-ray findings frequently include a "sentinel loop" (dilated loop of bowel near pancreas) or the "colon cutoff sign" (gas distending the right colon that abruptly stops near the pancreas).

Elevated amylase and lipase in the appropriate clinical setting establishes the diagnosis. CT scan shows pancreatic enlargement and can identify necrosis and pseudocyst formation.

Treatment includes nasogastric suction, fluid replacement, and narcotic analgesics. The patient must be NPO to reduce pancreatic stimulation.

Chronic Pancreatitis

Long-term pancreatic inflammation is usually due to chronic alcoholism. Complications of chronic pancreatitis include common bile duct or gastric outlet obstruction, ascites, and pseudocysts.

The most common symptom is chronic or recurrent epigastric pain. The patient may also have signs of pancreatic insufficiency, with malabsorption (weight loss and steatorrhea) and diabetes mellitus.

Ranson's Criteria

The presence of three or more are associated with increased mortality.

On admission

1. Age >55 years old
2. Serum glucose >200 mg/dL
3. Serum lactic dehydrogenase >350 IU/L
4. Serum aspartate transaminase (AST) >250 units
5. WBC count >16,000/mL

Within 48 hours

1. Hematocrit drops >10%
2. Blood urea nitrogen (BUN) rises >5 mg/dL
3. Serum calcium <8 mg/dL
4. PaO_2 <60 mm Hg
5. Base deficit >4 mEq/L
6. Fluid sequestration estimated at >6 L

GASTROENTEROLOGY

Serum amylase and lipase are elevated during acute attacks, but amylase may be normal if the pancreas is fibrotic. Pancreatic calcification can be seen on x-ray. Endoscopic retrograde cholangiopancreatography (ERCP) can establish the diagnosis.

Alcohol intake should be stopped. Narcotics may be given for analgesia, although addiction is a common problem. Pancreatic insufficiency is treated with enzyme supplements. Surgery to dilate the pancreatic duct may be palliative.

Pancreatic Pseudocyst

The term pseudocyst describes a walled-off fluid collection with a high enzyme concentration that arises from the pancreas. It is called a pseudocyst because its walls consist of inflamed membranous material, not epithelial tissue as in a true cyst. As a complication of pancreatitis, pseudocysts are generally sterile, although infection can lead to abscess formation. Other complications include rupture and hemorrhage.

Symptoms can appear up to 6 weeks after an episode of acute pancreatitis and include epigastric mass, pain, and mild fever.

Leukocytosis and persistent increased serum amylase are seen.

The cyst can be visualized on ultrasound or CT scan.

Of pancreatic pseudocysts, 40% resolve spontaneously, so conservative management in the first 4 to 6 weeks is appropriate unless the cyst is expanding rapidly or causing pain. If needed, surgical management involves drainage or excision.

Cancer of the Exocrine Pancreas

Adenocarcinomas of the pancreas are usually ductal in origin and are most often located in the head of the pancreas (80%). Middle-aged men are the typical patients. Symptoms are generally not evident until the tumor has spread locally or metastasized, and 5-year survival is less than 2%.

Most patients experience weight loss and abdominal pain that may radiate to the back. Obstructive jaundice occurs if the tumor is in the head of the pancreas and impinges on the bile duct. A palpable, nontender gallbladder in a jaundiced patient is a classic sign (Courvoisier's sign). If the tumor is in the body or tail, splenic vein obstruction may result, causing splenomegaly or gastric and esophageal varices.

Hyperglycemia is evident in 10%–20% of patients. Bilirubin and alkaline phosphatase are elevated if bile obstruction occurs.

CT, MRI, or ERCP locates the tumor, and biopsy confirms the diagnosis.

Resection is indicated for localized disease, but patients usually present with advanced disease and treatment is generally palliative. Exocrine pancreas insufficiency and diabetes mellitus are treated medically. No chemotherapy has been shown to be effective.

Cancer of the Endocrine Pancreas

Pancreatic islet-cell tumors may be nonfunctioning (leading primarily to symptoms of biliary and duodenal obstruction) or functioning (with increased secretion of one of the pancreatic hormones). Some are found in syndromes of **multiple endocrine neoplasia** (see Chapter 4). The functioning tumors are the following:

- **Insulinoma,** a rare tumor, causes insulin hypersecretion, and symptoms result from hypoglycemia. CNS changes begin with headaches, confusion, motor weakness, visual problems, and personality changes, and can progress to seizures and coma. **Whipple's triad** confirms that hypoglycemia is the source of the symptoms. It requires that symptoms occur while fasting, that hypoglycemia is present, and that carbohydrate intake relieves the symptoms. Diagnosis is supported when fasting insulin levels remain high, and, if necessary, a C-peptide assay confirms that the insulin is endogenous. (C-peptide is manufactured with the insulin molecule and is then cleaved. If it is present, the insulin is endogenous; if absent, the insulin is exogenous.) Only 10% of insulinomas are malignant, so surgical cure rates are high.
- In **Zollinger-Ellison syndrome,** gastrin-producing tumors cause excess acid secretion and peptic ulceration. Multiple, small tumors are frequently present, and half of these tumors are malignant. Aggressive peptic ulcers, often in atypical sites, may bleed, perforate, or cause obstruction. Serum gastrin is the most reliable diagnostic measure. Proton pump inhibitors (omeprazole, lansoprazole) relieve symptoms, but surgical resection may be needed for cure.
- **VIPoma** is a non-beta islet-cell tumor that produces vasoactive intestinal peptide (VIP),

GASTROENTEROLOGY

which affects blood flow to the GI tract. Also called *WDHA,* VIPoma usually involves **watery diarrhea, hypokalemia,** and **achlorhydria.** Diarrhea may be present for years before diagnosis and may be accompanied by dehydration. Weakness, nausea, vomiting, and abdominal cramps are also common. Unexplained secretory diarrhea suggests VIPoma, but diagnostic tests are unreliable. Exploratory laparotomy is the best means of diagnosis, although resection may not be curative.

- **Glucagonoma,** a tumor of the alpha islet cells, is rare and slow growing. Eighty percent of patients are women, and 80% of tumors are malignant. Weight loss, anemia, and diabetes are present. **Necrolytic migratory erythema** is a characteristic exfoliating lesion of the extremities. Elevated glucagon levels and angiography suggest the diagnosis, and resection is indicated. Prognosis is poor.

Biliary and Liver Disorders

Cholelithiasis

Cholelithiasis, stones in the gallbladder, is a common disorder and is usually asymptomatic. Incidence increases with age. Other risk factors include female gender, multiparity, and obesity. These can be remembered as "the four Fs": female, fertile, forty, and fat. Native Americans have a particularly high rate of cholelithiasis. Most patients (75%) have cholesterol stones. Other stones contain primarily calcium or bile pigments from hemoglobin breakdown.

SIGNS & SYMPTOMS

Biliary colic results from transient blockage of the cystic duct. This episodic pain in the right upper quadrant may be accompanied by nausea and vomiting. It is frequently precipitated by fatty meals. Only 2% of patients with asymptomatic gallstones develop symptoms each year.

DIAGNOSIS

Ultrasound. X-ray is not helpful because only a small percentage of gallstones are radiopaque.

TREATMENT

Laparoscopic cholecystectomy is performed on symptomatic patients and as prophylaxis for patients with large stones (>3cm) or a calcified gallbladder. Calcification of the gallbladder is associated with carcinoma.

Cholecystitis

Cholecystitis is an inflammation of the gallbladder usually associated with gallstones; however, **acalculous cholecystitis** may occur in patients on total parenteral nutrition or in critically ill patients with no oral intake. Symptoms may be acute or chronic, causing scarring of the gallbladder. Some frequent complications include choledocholithiasis (stones in the common bile duct), cholangitis (inflammation of the bile duct), pancreatitis (due to obstruction of the common bile duct), ileus, empyema, and perforation. Chronic, mild cholecystitis can lead to acute, severe cholecystitis or gallbladder adenocarcinoma.

Biliary colic starts suddenly and often occurs after a large, fatty meal. Patients with acute cholecystitis have severe right upper-quadrant pain, pain referred to the right scapula, and low fever. Vomiting is common. One-third of patients have a palpable gallbladder. Pain is steady and abates slowly. Patients tend to curl up and shift position frequently. A positive Murphy's sign of inspiratory arrest during palpation over the gallbladder reflects likely cholecystitis. Milder symptoms of chronic cholecystitis may occur in episodes or almost continuously.

Leukocytosis and mildly increased serum bilirubin and alkaline phosphatase often occur with acute cases. Increased amylase indicates a stone in the common bile duct and associated pancreatitis.

Ultrasound can show the presence of gallstones but is not as accurate as an HIDA (hepatic iminodiacetic acid) scan. This procedure uses radioisotopes, which are taken up by the liver and excreted in the bile. If the gallbladder is not visualized, cystic duct obstruction is present.

Initial treatment is with hydration, antibiotics, and pain control. Laparoscopic cholecystectomy is the treatment of choice, although open cholecystectomy, percutaneous cholecystostomy, lithotripsy, and stone dissolution are also options.

Cholangitis

Bacterial infection of the bile ducts is symptomatic only when accompanied by biliary obstruction. Frequent causes are choledocholithiasis, biliary strictures, and neoplasm. Bacteria are generally of enteric origin.

Charcot's triad is classic: biliary colic, jaundice, and fever. There is often a previous history of biliary colic as well.

Leukocytosis, increased serum bilirubin, and increased alkaline phosphatase are present. Bacteremia is common.

Ultrasound is usually diagnostic but may be supplemented with ERCP or CT scan.

IV antibiotics are administered. Surgical correction of the obstruction is usually necessary.

Biliary Tract Neoplasm

Cancer of the gallbladder is typically diagnosed unexpectedly in up to 2% of patients undergoing surgery for cholelithiasis or other biliary tract disease. It spreads by direct extension into the liver or peritoneum.

Jaundice, anorexia, weight loss, fever, and abdominal pain that radiates to the back are typical symptoms. The gallbladder may be palpable.

Elevated conjugated bilirubin is most striking. Alkaline phosphatase and serum cholesterol are also elevated.

Diagnosis is made by using endoscopic retrograde cholangiography with biopsy or during surgery.

Unless the tumor is well localized and can be completely excised (<10% of the time), prognosis is poor.

Hepatic Abscess

Most frequently due to enteric bacteria or amebae, hepatic abscesses usually form after spread of infection from biliary or abdominal infections. An underlying malignancy is present in 40% of patients. Complications include formation of multiple abscesses, rupture, septicemia, and liver failure.

Onset may be insidious, but symptoms eventually include spiking fevers, chills, right upper-quadrant pain, and tender hepatomegaly. Jaundice is often seen with multiple abscesses.

Ultrasound, CT scan, or MRI shows abscesses. Serum indirect hemagglutination tests for *Entamoeba histolytica* help identify the causative organism.

GASTROENTEROLOGY

Percutaneous suction catheters are used to drain the abscess if the patient does not respond quickly to antibiotics. Surgical treatment is only rarely indicated.

Subphrenic Abscess

Subphrenic abscesses, abscesses under the diaphragm and above the transverse colon, result from direct contamination after abdominal surgery, peritonitis, or extension from an adjacent site. Fifty percent occur on the right, 25% on the left, and 25% in multiple sites.

Approximately 1 to 2 months after abdominal surgery, patients develop fever and other nonspecific symptoms. Abdominal pain and tenderness may be present, often with paralytic ileus. Cough, dyspnea, and chest or shoulder pain result from diaphragmatic irritation, and decreased breath sounds, rales, rhonchi, and dullness to percussion of the chest may be present.

Leukocytosis and anemia are common.

Chest x-ray shows ipsilateral pleural effusions and an elevated hemidiaphragm. Abdominal films may show gas in the abscess, displaced organs, or a soft-tissue mass. Ultrasound or CT scan generally confirms the diagnosis.

Surgical or percutaneous drainage and antibiotics.

Jaundice

Yellowing of the skin and sclera is due to elevated serum bilirubin. Jaundice may be categorized as prehepatic, hepatic, or posthepatic in origin. The most common cause of **prehepatic jaundice** is hemolysis, because hemoglobin breakdown causes increased bilirubin production. Two other prehepatic disorders are Gilbert's disease and the Crigler-Najjar syndrome. **Hepatic jaundice** may be hepatocellular (acute hepatitis, chronic cirrhosis) or cholestatic (primary biliary cirrhosis, toxic drug jaundice, cholestatic jaundice of pregnancy). Biliary obstruction is the most common cause of **posthepatic jaundice** because of a tumor, gallstones, or biliary stricture.

Yellow skin, scleral icterus, and pruritus are the most common symptoms. Patients may have hepatomegaly and signs of cirrhosis. Patients with choledocholithiasis (stones blocking the bile duct) may also have biliary colic, fever, and chills. Hepatitis may cause tenderness over the liver. With posthepatic obstruction, patients may note light stools and cola-colored urine because of urinary excretion of bile metabolites.

Increased bilirubin is in the unconjugated form with prehepatic disease. A mixture of conjugated and unconjugated bilirubin is typical of hepatocellular disease. Conjugated bilirubin is increased in intrahepatic cholestasis and posthepatic disease. Some loss in the urine (bilirubinuria) occurs because conjugated bilirubin is water soluble. With posthepatic obstruction, serum AST and lactic dehydrogenase (LDH) will also be elevated. Alkaline phosphatase may be elevated in cases of intrahepatic cholestasis, cholangitis, or extrahepatic obstruction.

LABS

Ultrasound is commonly used to diagnose liver and biliary disorders.

DIAGNOSIS

Treat the underlying disorder. The most common disorders are discussed separately in the following sections.

TREATMENT

Viral Hepatitis

Any inflammatory process in the liver is referred to as hepatitis, including viral, alcoholic, or drug-induced hepatitis. The five major hepatatrophic viruses are discussed here. Acute infection may precede chronic hepatitis, which is diagnosed when the disease lasts more than 6 months. Chronic hepatitis can lead to liver failure, cirrhosis, and cancer. These five viruses are currently the most well established:

- **Hepatitis A virus** (HAV) is spread by fecal-oral contact and contaminated food, with shellfish a common culprit. Epidemics may be water- or food-borne, and sporadic cases are common as well. Fecal shedding begins before the onset of symptoms. Infection is acute, often subclinical, and confers lifelong immunity (Figure 1-5A).
- **Hepatitis B virus** (HBV) causes hepatitis B, sometimes with a concurrent infection of the hepatitis D virus. The Dane particle, which is the infective agent of HBV, is transmitted through contact with infected body fluids. Injection drug use, sexual contact, and vertical transmission in pregnancy are the most common modes of spread. (Transfusions are a less frequent source of infection now that donor blood is routinely screened.) Hepatitis B is endemic in parts of Asia. HBV can cause subclinical infection, acute or chronic hepatitis, or cirrhosis, and it is associated with hepatocellular carcinoma.

The HBV surface antigen (HBsAg) appears first during the incubation and then usually disappears. After a window period known as the "core" window, anti-HBs antibody appears, increasing during the patient's recovery and lasting a lifetime (Figure 1-5B). When anti-HBs does not develop, HBsAg persists and the patient becomes a carrier (Figure 1-5C). Anti-HBc, the antibody against HBV core antigen, can be detected in serum, usually as symptoms begin. (HBV core antigen is found only in liver cells.)

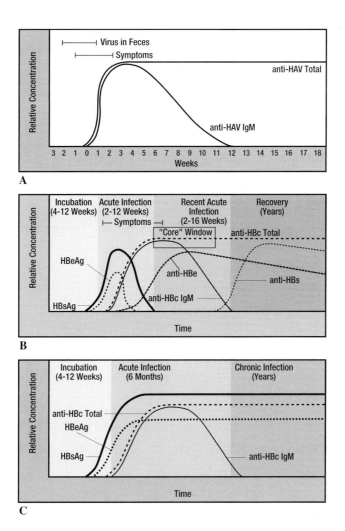

Fig. 1-5. Hepatitis serologic profiles. **A:** Hepatitis A serologies. **B:** Typical hepatitis B serologies. **C:** Hepatitis B chronic carrier serologies. (Redrawn from Wallach J: *Interpretation of Diagnostic Tests,* 6th ed. Boston: Little, Brown, 1996, p 194.)

Anti-HBc immunoglobulin M (IgM) develops first, followed by immunoglobulin G (IgG), which is present throughout the patient's life. The e antigen (HBeAg) reflects viral replication and greater infectivity; high levels of anti-HBe indicate a good prognosis (Table 1-4).

- **Hepatitis C virus** (HCV) is the most common source of posttransfusion hepatitis, but IV drug use is also a common mechanism of infection. HCV may have been responsible for many diagnoses of "idiopathic" hepatitis in the past. Most patients become chronic carriers. They may have subclinical disease or may develop chronic hepatitis, cirrhosis, or hepatocellular carcinoma. Screening donated blood for HCV has dramatically reduced the incidence of posttransfusion hepatitis.

- **Hepatitis D virus** (delta agent) can replicate only when HBV is present, so it occurs only as a coinfection of HBV. Manifestations of this agent are either more severe hepatitis or an exacerbation of chronic disease.

GASTROENTEROLOGY

Table 1-4. Hepatitis B serologies

	HBsAg incubation or active disease	Anti-HBc (IgM) Active disease	Anti-HBs Immunity	HBeAg Infectivity	Anti-HBe Good prognosis, low infectivity
Late incubation or early symptoms	+	–	–	+	–
Acute infection	+	+ (IgM)	–	+	–
Acute infection with good prognosis	+	+ (IgM)	–	–	+
Past infection or vaccinated	–	–	+	–	–
Chronic infection	+	+ (IgM)	–	+	–

- **Hepatitis E virus** is a major cause of waterborne hepatitis in underdeveloped countries. It is spread by fecal-oral contact and is associated with high mortality among pregnant women.

SIGNS & SYMPTOMS

Severity of hepatitis ranges from subclinical to fulminant liver failure. A prodrome of malaise, fever, nausea, and vomiting is followed by darkening of the urine (bilirubinuria) and jaundice. Jaundice may persist while other symptoms fade. Full recovery of acute infection generally requires approximately 4 weeks.

LABS

Alanine aminotransferase (ALT) and AST are elevated, bilirubin is high, and alkaline phosphatase may be mildly increased. WBC count is usually normal to low.

DIAGNOSIS

In HAV, IgM antibody is present during the illness, and the presence of IgG indicates prior infection. For HBV, HBsAg is present before onset of symptoms, and anti-HBs antibody indicates a resolved infection. During the symptomatic phase, anti-HBc IgM is the only antibody present in the serum. Presence of anti-HCV antibody or HCV RNA is diagnostic of HCV infection.

TREATMENT

Acute hepatitis usually resolves with only supportive care. Chronic infection develops in 5% to 10% of HBV cases and 80% of HCV cases, and this may lead to cirrhosis or hepatocellular carcinoma. Chronic infection can be treated with alfa interferon (with ribavirin for HCV) but treatment is poorly tolerated and successful less than 50% of the time.

PREVENTION

Immunoglobulin should be given to close contacts of patients with hepatitis A. Hepatitis A vaccine is recommended for travelers to developing countries, patients with liver disease, and caregivers. Hepatitis B immunoglobulin (HBIG) is given following needlestick exposure to HBV-infected blood if the exposed person is unvaccinated or had an inadequate anti-HBs response to vaccine. Vaccination against HBV is very effective and is recommended for all children and high-risk adults (e.g., health care providers, homosexual males, and IV drug users). It is given as a series of three injections over 6 months.

GASTROENTEROLOGY

Alcohol-related Hepatic Disease

Alcoholic liver damage occurs in three progressive stages. Hepatic steatosis, or fatty liver, is the first stage. Fat deposits in the liver cause hepatomegaly and mild enzyme changes, but this pathology is reversible with cessation of alcohol intake. The second stage of disease is alcoholic hepatitis. Biopsies show characteristic changes in tissue, including inflammation and necrosis. The third stage is cirrhosis, discussed in further detail in the following section. Risk of liver damage increases with duration and quantity of alcohol consumption as well as with HBV and HCV coinfection.

SIGNS & SYMPTOMS

Alcohol-related changes may be clinically silent or may cause an enlarged, tender liver, anorexia, nausea and vomiting, ascites, splenomegaly, fever, and encephalopathy.

LABS

Elevated ALT, AST, gamma-glutamyl transpeptidase (GGT), alkaline phosphatase, and bilirubin are commonly seen. In contrast to viral hepatitis, AST levels are generally higher than ALT levels. PT is prolonged because of a reduction in hepatic production of clotting factors, especially factors II, VII, IX, and X, which have the shortest half-lives.

DIAGNOSIS

Diagnosis is usually made from clinical signs and laboratory tests. If necessary, a biopsy can confirm diagnosis.

TREATMENT

Cessation of alcohol intake and supportive care are the keys to treatment.

Alcohol Use

Typically, alcohol consumption is associated with liver disease and cirrhosis, but its effects are more far reaching.

GI problems associated with alcohol include gastritis, peptic ulcer disease, hepatitis, cirrhosis, and pancreatitis. Cancers associated with alcohol use include oropharyngeal, stomach, hepatocellular, and colon cancer. Cardiovascular diseases include cardiomyopathy and arrhythmias. Nutritional deficiencies and anemia are also seen more often in chronic alcohol users. Aspiration pneumonia is common in alcoholics.

Depression and suicide are often alcohol-related, as are many neurologic disorders, such as delirium, dementia, Wernicke's disease, Korsakoff's disease, and other neuropathies.

Alcohol has been established as the primary cause of injury-related death, including motor vehicle accidents and drowning. Complications resulting from alcohol use during pregnancy include premature labor, low birth weight, and fetal alcohol syndrome (discussed in more detail in Chapter 8).

Cirrhosis

In cirrhosis, insults to liver tissue cause necrosis and fibrosis. The development of regenerative nodules follows, replacing healthy liver cells. Alcohol is the most common cause of cirrhosis in the United States, and 15% of alcoholics develop the condition. Other causes of cirrhosis include hepatitis C and B infection, chronic obstruction of the common bile duct, autoimmune disease, chronic heart disease, and metabolic disorders. After diagnosis, 30% of patients die within 1 year. Cirrhosis is the third leading cause of death in 45 to 65 year olds in the United States.

SIGNS & SYMPTOMS

Patients may be asymptomatic for years or may experience nonspecific symptoms of weakness, weight loss, and malaise. Reduced bile salt excretion can cause fat malabsorption and deficiencies of the fat-soluble vitamins (vitamins A, D, E, K). A dramatic upper GI hemorrhage from esophageal varices may be the presenting symptom. Common physical examination findings of chronic liver disease include hepatomegaly, splenomegaly, jaundice, wasting, ascites, vascular spiders on the upper half of the body, caput medusae (superficial venous collaterals visible on the abdominal wall), palmar erythema, Dupuytren's palmar contractures, peripheral neuropathy, testicular atrophy, and gynecomastia. Cirrhosis is frequently complicated by portal hypertension, ascites, bleeding varices, hepatic encephalopathy, and hepatoma.

LABS

Decreased serum albumin (due to decreased synthetic activity by the liver), anemia, thrombocytopenia, and increased PT (due to decreased vitamin K absorption and decreased liver synthesis of clotting factors).

DIAGNOSIS

Diagnosis can be made from clinical presentation and confirmed by biopsy.

TREATMENT

Cirrhosis is incurable and irreversible, but the disease generally does not progress if the offending agent is removed. Liver transplantation may improve the long-term prognosis.

Portal Hypertension

Elevated pressure in the portal vein is generally due to cirrhosis, other liver disease, or extrahepatic portal vein occlusion. Ascites, secondary hypersplenism, and variceal bleeds occur because of increased pressure in the portal venous system. Hepatic encephalopathy occurs because the liver cannot adequately filter toxins from the blood. Diagnosis and treatment of portal hypertension depend on the presenting symptoms, and these complications are discussed in detail in the following sections.

Esophageal Varices

Esophageal varices are tortuous, collateral veins, usually esophageal or gastric, that expand to circumvent congested hepatic blood flow. They may rupture, causing upper GI bleeding. The 50% death rate from bleeding varices reflects severe hemorrhage in the presence of existing severe liver disease.

Varices are asymptomatic until rupture leads to hemorrhage with hematemesis or melena (black, tarry stool).

The diagnosis is suggested by an upper GI bleed in the context of cirrhosis or portal hypertension, and it is confirmed by esophagoscopy.

For bleeding varices, controlling bleeding and replacing fluid and blood loss are crucial. The most common measures to control bleeding include octreotide, balloon tamponade, endoscopic sclerotherapy, transjugular intrahepatic portosystemic shunt (TIPS), and invasive surgical treatment, such as emergency portosystemic shunt placement. Several of these procedures may also be performed as prophylactic or therapeutic treatment in nonbleeding patients. Beta-blockers have also been shown to decrease portal pressure and incidence of rebleeding. Despite intervention, prognosis is poor.

Hepatic Encephalopathy

Hepatic encephalopathy is a reversible metabolic condition seen in patients with chronic liver disease and those with portocaval shunts. Decreased detoxification by the liver, because of liver failure or because blood is shunted around the liver, leads to exposure of the brain to toxins absorbed from the gut. Possible agents responsible for this effect are ammonia, amino acid neurotransmitters, and other neurotoxins. Altered mental status is exacerbated by increased protein absorption, whether dietary or from an upper GI bleed, by azotemia from dehydration, and by some medications.

Altered consciousness, ranging from lethargy to coma, and abnormal neuromuscular activity, such as asterixis (a wrist-flapping tremor).

Clinical presentation and elevated serum ammonium.

Eliminate or control the precipitating factor. Reduce dietary protein and administer lactulose, neomycin, or metronidazole to decrease intestinal absorption of ammonia.

Ascites

Ascites, fluid collection in the peritoneal cavity, is most frequently a complication of hepatic disease. It results from a combination of sodium and water retention by the kidneys, low plasma osmotic pressure due to hypoalbuminemia, and elevated hydrostatic pressure in hepatic sinusoids or portal veins.

Abdominal fluid collection can be demonstrated by the presence of a fluid wave or shifting dullness on abdominal exam.

Paracentesis is used to sample the ascitic fluid. The serum-ascites albumin gradient is a useful tool in identifying ascites associated with portal hypertension. In portal hypertensive ascites, serum albumin concentration exceeds ascites fluid albumin concentration by at least 1.1 g/dL. An increased concentration of albumin in the ascitic fluid suggests infection or malignancy (e.g., ovarian cancer), as does an LDH level exceeding 60% of the serum level. An increased ascitic fluid white count also suggests infection.

Sodium restriction, diuretics, and therapeutic paracentesis all help to control ascites. A portocaval shunt or peritoneal-jugular (LeVeen) shunt may be useful but will increase the risk of hepatic encephalopathy.

Liver Cancer

Hepatocellular carcinoma is an uncommon cancer associated with chronic HBV and HCV infection, as well as with cirrhosis, hemochromatosis, and aflatoxins (fungus metabolites). Metastatic cancer to the liver is 20 times more frequent than primary liver cancer and most frequently arises from breast, lung, and colon cancers. Complications include intra-abdominal hemorrhage, portal vein obstruction, **Budd-Chiari syndrome** (thrombosis of the hepatic vein causing ascites and cirrhosis), and liver failure. **Benign hepatic adenomas** are seen almost exclusively in women taking oral contraceptive pills.

Right upper-quadrant pain may be referred to the right shoulder. Other signs include weight loss, jaundice, hepatomegaly, a bruit over the liver, or a sudden worsening of ascites.

Elevated transaminases, bilirubin, and alkaline phosphatase. Patients may have elevated alpha-fetoprotein, HBsAg, or anti-HCV.

Tumors are usually seen on CT, MRI, or ultrasound. Biopsy confirms the diagnosis.

Options include partial hepatectomy, liver transplantation, and arterial chemoembolization. Prognosis is poor.

Acute Disorders

Upper Gastrointestinal Bleeding

Bleeding from the upper GI tract is most often due to peptic ulcer disease, gastritis, esophageal varices, and Mallory-Weiss tears (gastroesophageal tears due to retching). Although signs of portal hypertension seen during the examination may suggest bleeding varices, many cirrhotic patients with upper GI bleeds actually have a peptic ulcer.

Hematemesis usually indicates a rapid bleed. A "coffee ground" appearance to the vomitus means that the blood has been in the stomach long enough to be partially digested. Melena (black, tarry stool) usually reflects an upper GI source, while hematochezia (bright red blood in the feces) is usually due to a lower source but may also occur with a rapid upper GI bleed.

A guaiac test detects occult blood in the stool or vomit. Bloody aspirate from a nasogastric tube confirms an upper GI source. Upper endoscopy shows the source of bleeding in a majority of patients. Hematocrit may take 24 hours to equilibrate with the extravascular fluid and is not useful to diagnose the severity of an acute bleed. Increased heart rate and decreased blood pressure are better indicators of severity.

If the patient is not stable, fluid replacement is imperative. Most often, patients with a Mallory-Weiss tear will stop bleeding spontaneously, and only monitoring and supportive care are needed. Treatment of specific lesions is discussed under the topics of peptic ulcer disease, esophageal varices, and gastritis.

Lower Gastrointestinal Bleeding

Lower GI bleeding is defined as bleeding from a site distal to the ligament of Treitz. Chronic hematochezia (bright red blood in the feces) can originate from carcinoma, polyps, hemorrhoids, or fissures. Etiologies of heavy bleeding include diverticular disease, angiodysplasia (an abnormal mass of blood vessels in the intestinal wall), ulcerative colitis, or ischemia.

Passage of bright red blood suggests a lower GI bleed but can occasionally originate from a briskly bleeding upper GI source. Melena indicates a proximal source of blood.

Rectal examination with anoscopy or sigmoidoscopy can demonstrate most lesions; however, colonoscopy, radionuclide scan, or angiography may be necessary. Bloody aspirate from a nasogastric tube indicates an upper GI source.

Transfusion is needed less frequently than with upper GI bleeds. Some lesions, such as angiodysplasia, are treated colonoscopically. Intra-arterial vasopressin may be useful with other lesions, particularly diverticular hemorrhage. Surgery is needed if the preceding therapies are ineffective and usually consists of segmental colonic resection.

Peritonitis

Inflammation of the peritoneum is usually due to bacterial infection. **Spontaneous bacterial peritonitis** (SBP) occurs in patients with ascites from cirrhosis or nephrotic syndrome. Acute peritonitis occurs after GI perforation or an invasive procedure.

In acute peritonitis (i.e., from perforated ulcer, appendix, or diverticulum), patients experience abrupt onset of fever, severe abdominal pain, and distention. Rebound tenderness and guarding are elicited on examination. Guarding refers to the involuntary spasm of abdominal muscles, causing boardlike rigidity on examination. Rebound tenderness is pain that occurs when the palpating hand is suddenly raised, and it is due to peritoneal inflammation. Abdominal sounds are usually absent because of an ileus. Patients with SBP have a more subtle presentation, with fever, mild abdominal pain, and mental status changes due to exacerbations of hepatic encephalopathy.

Paracentesis allows examination of the peritoneal fluid. An elevated neutrophil count indicates peritonitis. The specific organism may be identified by culture. Upright abdominal films showing air under the diaphragm indicate a perforation (Figure 1-6). CT may reveal an abscess.

IV antibiotics are always indicated (third-generation cephalosporin alone for SBP and with metronidazole for acute peritonitis). Surgery is required to remove the source of infections (e.g., an abscess) or to correct a perforation.

Appendicitis

Inflammation of the appendix often has an identifiable cause, such as obstruction of the lumen by fecaliths, lymphoid hyperplasia, or fibroid bands. As distention of the appendix and compromise of blood supply develop, gangrene and perforation become increasingly likely.

Vague periumbilical abdominal pain with anorexia, nausea, and vomiting are the first symptoms; pain then localizes in the right lower quadrant. Temperature is only slightly elevated if no perforation has occurred, whereas high fever and increased pain indicate perforation. Pain over McBurney's point (one-third the distance from the right anterior superior iliac spine to the umbilicus) is typical.

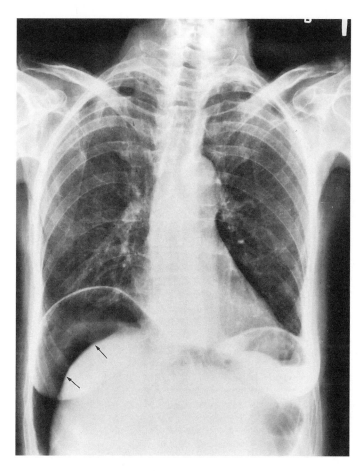

Fig. 1-6. Pneumoperitoneum. An upright chest radiograph shows air beneath the diaphragm. The liver margin is outlined by air (*arrows*). (Reprinted with permission from Daffner R: *Clinical Radiology: The Essentials,* 2nd ed. Baltimore, Williams & Wilkins, 1999, p 267.)

LABS

Leukocytosis with more than 75% neutrophils is seen in most patients.

DIAGNOSIS

A high index of clinical suspicion for appendicitis is a good idea for any case of acute abdomen. Ultrasound or CT can be diagnostic in atypical cases. Free air under the diaphragm indicates a perforation.

TREATMENT

Surgical resection is mandatory.

Intestinal Obstruction

The three most common causes of mechanical obstruction of the bowel are adhesions (particularly in patients with prior abdominal surgery or Crohn's disease), hernias, and tumors (Table 1-5). Compromise of blood flow can lead to ischemia and infarction.

GASTROENTEROLOGY

Table 1-5. Common causes of obstruction

	Duodenum	*Jejunoileum*	*Large bowel*
Neonate	Atresia Volvulus Congenital bands	Meconium ileus Volvulus Atresia Intussusception	Hirschsprung's Atresia
Adult	Pancreatic cancer	Adhesions Incarcerated hernias	Volvulus Diverticulitis Tumors

SIGNS & SYMPTOMS

Abdominal cramps, distention, and obstipation (complete lack of stool elimination) are typical. Vomiting is common with small-bowel obstruction but occurs late and is occasionally feculent with large-bowel obstruction. More severe pain, a tender abdomen, and increased distention accompany a strangulating obstruction. Scars from previous surgery, hernias, or a mass may be present on physical examination. High-pitched, hyperactive ("tinkling") bowel sounds are typical.

DIAGNOSIS

Abdominal x-ray shows proximal distention in large-bowel obstruction and ladder-like dilated loops of bowel with air-fluid levels in small-bowel obstruction (Figure 1-7).

TREATMENT

Nasogastric suction may allow small-bowel obstruction secondary to adhesions to decompress and untwist. Otherwise, a laparotomy is necessary, with surgical treatment of the source of obstruction. Rehydration of a vomiting patient is crucial.

Volvulus

Volvulus, the rotation of a bowel segment, may result in obstruction with subsequent gangrene from circulatory block. This is a common cause of bowel obstruction in elderly, bedridden patients and in newborns with disorders of intestinal rotation.

SIGNS & SYMPTOMS

Symptoms of colicky pain, abdominal distention, obstipation, and late vomiting vary depending on the location of the volvulus.

DIAGNOSIS

X-ray may show a "double bubble" sign with an air pocket on each side of the obstruction. Barium enema will show a dilated colon with a "bird's beak" at the point of the volvulus (Figure 1-8).

TREATMENT

Surgical repair is needed in pediatric patients and in adults with a cecal (right-sided) volvulus. Endoscopic decompression may be possible for sigmoid (left-sided) volvulus. Gangrenous sections must be resected.

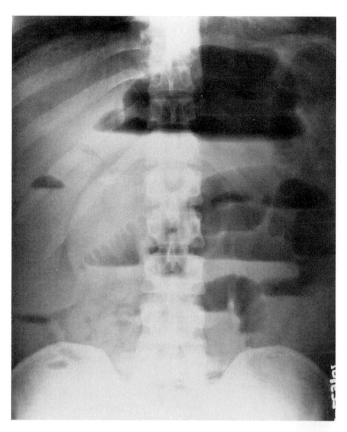

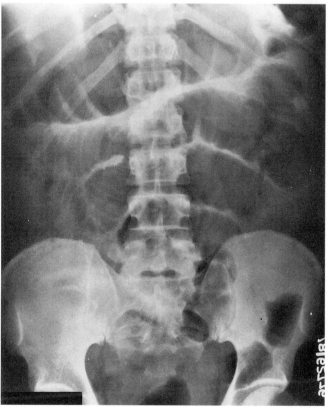

Figure 1-7. A: Small bowel obstruction, upright view. Note air-fluid levels. **B:** Small bowel obstruction, supine view. This supine view shows dilated air-filled loops of small intestine in a cascading pattern. (Reprinted with permission from Daffner R: *Clinical Radiology: The Essentials,* 2nd ed. Baltimore, Williams & Wilkins, 1999, p 257, 260.)

GASTROENTEROLOGY

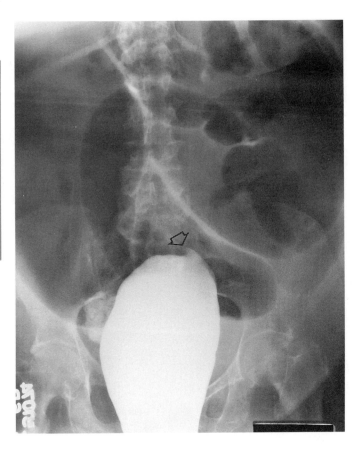

Figure 1-8. Sigmoid volvulus. Barium enema shows a massive dilation of the colon and a "bird's beak" at the site of the volvulus. (Reprinted with permission from Daffner R: *Clinical Radiology: The Essentials,* 2nd ed. Baltimore, Williams & Wilkins, 1999, p 261.)

Ileus

Ileus, a paralytic obstruction of the bowel, occurs because of loss of peristalsis. Severe infection is a common etiology, along with ischemia, vascular injury, and metabolic disorders. Postoperative ileus, resulting from anesthesia and intestinal manipulation, resolves within a few days.

Cramps, distention, vomiting, and obstipation with hypoactive or absent bowel sounds.

X-ray shows gaseous distention of affected segments. Upright abdominal films show air fluid levels.

Patients should be kept NPO until ileus resolves. Invasive treatment options include colonoscopic decompression or cecostomy.

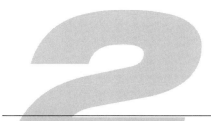

Cardiovascular Disorders

CARDIOVASCULAR

Common Symptoms of Heart Disease

Palpitations are the perception of a rapid heartbeat by the patient. Palpitations can be associated with cardiac and noncardiac conditions, including anxiety, anemia, and thyrotoxicosis. They may also be a symptom of cardiac valve disorders or arrhythmias.

Dyspnea is a sensation of difficulty breathing. Dyspnea associated with cardiac conditions usually occurs on exertion and indicates the presence of systolic dysfunction or valvular disease. **Orthopnea** (dyspnea while lying down) arises because of increased venous return to the heart, causing congestion in the lungs. Patients often sleep on a number of pillows because elevation of the head relieves the orthopnea. **Paroxysmal nocturnal dyspnea** refers to a sudden episode of difficulty breathing that awakens the patient from sleep and is relieved by sitting or standing.

Cyanosis is a bluish-gray discoloration of the skin because of a lack of oxygen. Poor oxygenation may result from decreased circulation, hypoventilation, or lung disease. Cyanosis in newborns may indicate a congenital defect. Cyanosis of the fingers and hands may be indicative of Raynaud's phenomenon, idiopathic vasoconstriction, or complex rheumatic disease.

Edema is an excessive extravascular fluid accumulation. In patients with cardiac disease, dependent edema is generally attributable to heart failure and can include dependent swelling of legs, ascites, and pulmonary edema.

Syncope (fainting) refers to a transient loss of consciousness. Generally, patients report lightheadedness, nausea, and sweating before the syncopal episode. Cardiovascular causes include arrhythmias, flow obstruction, and arteriovenous (AV) blocks. The most common etiology of syncope is vasovagal faints because of increased vagal tone. Other common causes are orthostatic hypotension and hyperventilation. It is important to differentiate syncope from seizure disorders, which are more often associated with auras and post-ictal confusion and are unlikely to start with presyncopal symptoms.

Fatigue is a sensation of tiredness, not unlike what you are experiencing now as you prepare for the Boards. It is an extremely common presenting symptom, with many possible etiologies. A good history often reveals a likely cause for fatigue, such as inadequate rest, poor nutrition, or excessive stress. However, it is important to consider endocrine disorders, anemia, rheumatic diseases, and depression. Cardiac causes of fatigue occur with overwork of the heart and may result in inadequate cardiac perfusion or heart failure.

Chest pain can be caused by cardiac disease, pleuritic pain, esophageal and gastrointestinal pain, or chest wall pain. Cardiac pain, such as that stemming from angina, heart attack, or pericardial disease, is described in more detail later in this chapter. Pleuritic pain is sharp and is aggravated by deep breathing. Esophageal and epigastric pain usually results from esophageal reflux, although chest pain may be seen in the context of gastritis, peptic ulcer disease, esophageal spasm, and pancreatitis. Chest wall pain refers to musculoskeletal discomfort and is usually benign.

Hypertension

Essential (Idiopathic) Hypertension

Hypertension is defined as resting systolic blood pressure greater than 140 mm Hg or diastolic blood pressure greater than 90 mm Hg. Of all cases, 90% to 95% are essential hypertension—that is, lacking an identifiable cause. Approximately 20% of the U.S. population has hypertension, with higher prevalence in the elderly and in African-Americans. Sequelae of uncontrolled hypertension include strokes, heart attacks, renal disease, congestive heart failure, and aortic dissection.

SIGNS & SYMPTOMS

Most patients are asymptomatic. Some report headaches, visual disturbances, and nausea or vomiting if blood pressure elevation is severe. On funduscopic examination, **arteriovenous nicking** (discontinuity in the appearance of a retinal vein due to thickened arterial walls), **cotton-wool spots** (infarction of the nerve fiber layer of the retina), retinal hemorrhages, and retinal exudates may be seen. A loud S_2 may be heard, with evidence of left ventricular enlargement on examination or ECG.

DIAGNOSIS

Blood pressure must be elevated on three separate visits to diagnose hypertension. The patient should sit quietly for approximately 5 minutes before the measurement is made. Medication should not be started after only one elevated blood pressure reading because of the possibility of "white coat" hypertension, brought on by the physician visit or by other temporary factors.

TREATMENT

Weight loss, exercise, reduction of salt and alcohol intake, smoking cessation, and stress reduction may help decrease blood pressure substantially. Classes of antihypertensive medications include diuretics, adrenergic blockers, calcium channel blockers, angiotensin-converting enzyme (ACE) inhibitors, and angiotensin II receptor blocking agents. Diuretics or beta-blockers are ordinarily used for initial therapy; however, ACE inhibitors may be especially beneficial in diabetics to prevent renal disease. ACE inhibitors and diuretics should be used in CHF, and beta-blockers and ACE inhibitors are often used after myocardial infarction (MI), the latter agents particularly in the setting of residual left ventricular systolic dysfunction (Table 2-1). Table 2-2 lists common contraindications for antihypertensive medications. It is important to determine medication compliance before making adjustments in uncontrolled hypertension, because approximately half of patients are noncompliant after 1 year.

Table 2-1. Indications for antihypertensive drug selection

Condition	Recommended drug	Reason
Diabetes mellitus type 1	ACE inhibitors	Delay progression to end-stage renal disease
Cardiac failure	ACE inhibitors	Improve mortality
	Diuretics	
Postmyocardial infarction	Beta-blockers	Improve mortality
	ACE inhibitors	

ACE, angiotensin-converting enzyme.

Table 2-2. Contraindications for hypertensive drugs

Condition	Contraindicated drugs	Reason
Asthma or COPD	Beta-blockers	May cause bronchoconstriction
Diabetes mellitus	Thiazide diuretics	Promotes impaired glucose tolerance
	Beta-blockers	May mask signs and symptoms of hypoglycemia
Cardiac failure	Calcium channel blockers	Reducing rate and contractility in an already compromised heart can cause decompensation
Pregnancy	Thiazide diuretics	Increased blood volume is normal in pregnancy and should not be reduced
	ACE inhibitors	Fetal complications
	Angiotensin II receptor blockers	
Gout	Diuretics	Increase serum uric acid levels
Depression	Beta-blockers	May exacerbate depression

ACE, angiotensin-converting enzyme; COPD, chronic obstructive pulmonary disease.

Hypertensive emergencies occur when extreme elevation of blood pressure precipitates conditions such as unstable angina, encephalopathy, or MI. Immediate blood pressure reduction with IV antihypertensives, such as diazoxide or sodium nitroprusside, is required.

Secondary Hypertension

Secondary hypertension is elevated blood pressure with an identifiable underlying cause. It constitutes only 5% to 10% of all cases of hypertension. The six major causes are listed. Most of these disorders are addressed in other chapters; therefore, this list contains only a brief summary of each disorder.

- **Estrogen** in birth control pills causes hypertension in approximately 5% of women taking oral contraceptives. Blood pressure returns to normal after discontinuation or switching to a progestin-only pill.
- Several **renal diseases** are associated with hypertension, probably because of dysfunction in the renin-angiotensin-aldosterone system. Depending on the level of residual kidney function, dialysis and antihypertensives may be necessary. Renal disease is the most common cause of secondary hypertension.
- **Renovascular hypertension,** or renal artery stenosis, is caused by a thickening of the renal artery wall. In young patients, usually women, the condition is often due to **fibromuscular hyperplasia** (an abnormal thickening of the muscular portion of the artery wall). In older patients, it is often caused by atherosclerotic changes. A renal artery bruit may be heard on examination. Treatment involves angioplasty, often with stenting, or surgery.
- **Primary hyperaldosteronism** often leads to hypertension and is usually due to adrenal adenomas. This diagnosis should be suspected in patients who are hypokalemic with high levels of urine potassium before the initiation of antihypertensive treatment. Diagnosis is confirmed with CT or MRI. Treatment involves surgical excision of the adenoma. Patients with **Cushing's syndrome** may also have hypertension because of the effects of glucocorticoid excess (see Chapter 4, Endocrine Disorders).

- **Pheochromocytoma** is an adrenal tumor that secretes epinephrine and norepinephrine. Blood pressure may undergo rapid, wide swings or may be chronically elevated. Orthostatic hypotension is often present. Diagnosis is by detection of high levels of urinary catecholamine metabolites. CT or MRI helps localize the tumor. Treatment involves surgical excision (see Chapter 4, Endocrine Disorders).
- **Coarctation of the aorta** is a congenital narrowing of the aortic arch just past the origin of the left subclavian artery. Hypertension develops in childhood and is present in the arms but absent in the legs, so blood pressure measurements of all four extremities are useful for diagnosis. Femoral pulses are weak and delayed when compared with the carotid or radial pulse. Examination or ECG may show left ventricular hypertrophy. Treatment is through surgical correction (see Chapter 8).

Arterial Diseases

Aortic Aneurysm

An aortic aneurysm is an abnormal, localized dilatation of the aorta. Most aortic aneurysms occur in the abdomen and 90% of these originate below the renal arteries. Atherosclerosis, hypertension, smoking, a family history of abdominal aneurysms, trauma, and vasculitis may all be contributing factors. Marfan's syndrome and syphilis are primary causes of thoracic aortic aneurysms but may cause abdominal aneurysms as well. The risk of rupture increases with increasing aneurysmal size. Aortic aneurysm rupture is fatal within minutes unless it is retroperitoneal, in which case local tamponade can prolong its course.

SIGNS & SYMPTOMS

Patients with abdominal aneurysms are generally asymptomatic but may rarely report a deep, boring pain in the lower back. On examination, there is a pulsating, tender mass in the abdomen. Thoracic aneurysms can be associated with dysphagia, hoarseness, dyspnea, cough, hemoptysis, and edema of the head, neck, and arms because of compression of adjacent structures. In retroperitoneal rupture, patients may complain of severe abdominal, flank, or back pain.

DIAGNOSIS

Ultrasound (abdominal or transesophageal) localizes and assesses the size of the aneurysm. Abdominal x-ray may reveal aortic calcifications. Aortography, CT, and MRI may provide additional information.

TREATMENT

Treatment depends on the size of the aneurysm. For abdominal aneurysms, surgical repair is generally recommended for asymptomatic aneurysms larger than 5 cm in diameter and for symptomatic aneurysms of any size. Smaller aneurysms are not at high risk for rupture but should be followed with periodic imaging to monitor growth. Thoracic aneurysms should be resected if greater than 6 cm or if rapidly enlarging; however, aneurysms in Marfan's syndrome should be removed at smaller sizes because of their tendency to rupture. Surgery involves resection of the aneurysmal portion and replacement with a synthetic graft, but endovascular repair with stents is gaining popularity. Acute complications of abdominal aortic aneurysm repair include MI, hemorrhage, renal insufficiency, ischemic colitis, limb ischemia, and stroke. Thoracic aneurysm repair can also result in paraplegia, due to anterior spinal artery interruption. Chronic complications include formation of graft-enteric fistulas.

Dissecting Aortic Aneurysm

Dissection of an aortic aneurysm occurs when an intimal tear progresses to separation of the layers of the wall of the aorta. Hypertension producing degenerative changes of the aortic wall causes most dissections, but congenital tissue disorders such as Marfan's syndrome may also contribute. In the Sanford classification, type A involves at least the ascending aorta and type B involves only the descending aorta.

SIGNS & SYMPTOMS

Patients report the sudden onset of a tearing or "ripping" in their chest, often radiating to the back. Physical examination may reveal weak or absent pulses but normal or increased blood pressure. If the aortic valve is disrupted, a murmur of acute aortic insufficiency may be appreciated, associated with acute heart failure.

DIAGNOSIS

Differentiation between the chest pain from a dissecting aneurysm and an MI is crucial, as their treatments differ. Although the ECG is abnormal in an MI, it is generally normal or shows only left ventricular hypertrophy in dissecting aneurysms. Chest x-ray shows a widening of the aorta (Figure 2-1). As with all aneurysms, ultrasound, CT, and aortography provide a definitive diagnosis.

TREATMENT

Emergent reduction of blood pressure with a rapid-acting antihypertensive (such as nitroprusside) and reduction of stroke output with a beta-blocker (such as propranolol) is important. Mortality from dissecting aneurysms is extremely high, and patients must be monitored in the intensive care unit. Stanford type A dissections require emergent surgical repair due to their particularly high mortality. Stanford type B dissections are generally treated medically unless complicated by rupture or occlusion.

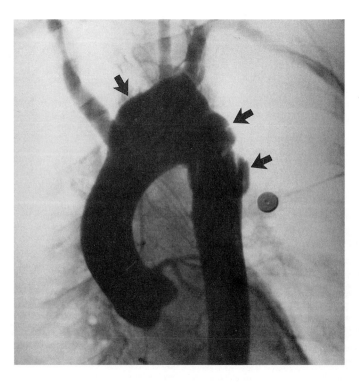

Fig. 2-1. Aortic dissection. Note the widened mediastinum and tracheal deviation to the right. (Reprinted with permission from Daffner R: *Clinical Radiology: The Essentials,* 2nd ed. Baltimore, Williams & Wilkins, 1999, p 225.)

Peripheral Arterial Vascular Disease

Peripheral arterial vascular disease refers to arterial occlusion in the extremities, usually as a result of atherosclerosis. The resulting ischemia may be acute or chronic. Chronic ischemia of the lower extremities results in **intermittent claudication,** in which an exercising muscle receives insufficient oxygenated blood. This condition may progress to complete occlusion of the vessel over time. Acute occlusion usually occurs as a result of embolization of an atherosclerotic plaque. Diabetic patients have an increased risk of developing arterial vascular disease as a result of changes in their microvascular circulation.

SIGNS & SYMPTOMS

Symptoms of peripheral ischemia classically consist of "the five Ps": **pain, pallor, pulselessness, paresthesias,** and (in late stages) **paralysis.** Associated findings are ulcerations and dry skin with poor hair and nail growth. In intermittent claudication, the patient reports reproducible, exercise-associated muscle pain and weakness that resolves completely with rest. In advanced disease, rest pain can also occur, characterized by foot pain even in the absence of exertion. It is typically nocturnal and relieved by lowering the feet, such that patients may report sleeping in chairs.

DIAGNOSIS

The preceding signs and symptoms, especially in the context of systemic atherosclerosis (e.g., a history of coronary artery disease [CAD]), suggest the diagnosis. X-rays are not helpful. Ankle systolic pressures are reduced relative to brachial systolic pressures. Doppler ultrasound is fairly accurate in assessing the extent of occlusion.

TREATMENT

Patients with intermittent claudication should begin a regimen of daily walking to increase collateral circulation. Patients at risk for developing progressive ischemia (such as diabetic patients) should be taught to perform daily foot inspection and care to detect and prevent ulceration. Primary disorders, such as diabetes, should be well controlled and smoking should be discontinued. Low-dose aspirin and pentoxifylline comprise standard medical management. Clots that develop may be evaluated angiographically and treated with angioplasty, bypass grafting, or thromboendarterectomy. Significant or prolonged ischemia may require amputation. Indications for surgery include progressive or incapacitating intermittent claudication, rest pain, or necrotic foot lesions.

Functional Arterial Vascular Disorders

Functional arterial vascular disorders are conditions resulting from excessive vascular constriction or spasm. Raynaud's phenomenon and acrocyanosis are the most frequently seen.

Raynaud's phenomenon consists of pallor and cyanosis of the fingers or toes, often followed by reddening as a result of compensatory hyperemia. It is caused by vasospasm of the digital arteries and is often precipitated by cold. Most cases of Raynaud's phenomenon are idiopathic, occurring predominantly in young women. It may also be seen in systemic lupus erythematosus (SLE) and other connective tissue disorders. Mild cases need no medical treatment, but the extremities should be kept warm. More severe cases may be treated with vasodilators and even sympathectomy.

Acrocyanosis involves pallor, cyanosis, coldness, and sweating of the hands and feet secondary to arteriolar vasoconstriction and ventilation. Aside from keeping the extremities warm, no treatment exists. Vasodilators are ineffective.

Venous Diseases

Varicose Veins

Varicose veins are superficial veins that have developed incompetent valves, resulting in elongation, dilation, tortuosity, and reversed blood flow.

SIGNS & SYMPTOMS

Varicose veins may be asymptomatic or cause warmth, fatigue, or aching pain. Symptoms resolve with leg elevation. Varicose veins may not always be visible, but they may be palpated. Symptoms do not necessarily correspond to the size of the varicosities. Complications include pigmentation (because of blood stasis), eczema, edema, and ulceration.

DIAGNOSIS

Diagnosis can be made by visual inspection and clinical presentation. Trendelenburg's test is performed by raising the affected leg above the level of the heart and quickly lowering it. Immediate distention of the leg veins indicates valvular incompetency.

TREATMENT

Nonsurgical management includes exercise to increase muscular support of the veins, compression hosiery, and leg elevation. Surgical removal of varicosities is possible but removal of the saphenous veins is discouraged, because they may be required for later bypass graft surgery. Injection sclerotherapy may be performed for both cosmetic and therapeutic reasons.

Arteriovenous Fistula

An arteriovenous (AV) fistula is an abnormal communication between an artery and a vein. It may be congenital or acquired (e.g., in the case of trauma). Superficial AV fistulas may be palpated as warm, pulsating masses, accompanied by a thrill. Other signs and symptoms include ischemia, edema, pigmentation changes, and varicosities. Embolic complications may arise. Surgery is the treatment of choice. AV fistulas in the brain or bowel wall are often associated with aneurysms and can cause life-threatening hemorrhage.

Deep Venous Thrombosis and Thrombophlebitis

Deep venous thrombosis (DVT) refers to the development of a blood clot in a vein. Thrombophlebitis refers to a secondary inflammation of the vein, resulting in pain, tenderness, and warmth. These symptoms most often occur in the lower extremities. The risk factors that predispose to the development of venous thrombi are referred to as *Virchow's triad:* injury to the endothelium of the vessel (e.g., trauma and surgery), hypercoagulable states (e.g., malignancy, estrogen use, antithrombin III deficiency), and stasis (e.g., postoperative states, extended travel). Pulmonary embolism is a major complication of deep venous thrombosis. Deep thrombophlebitis can also cause chronic venous insufficiency.

Budd-Chiari syndrome refers to obstruction of the hepatic vein, usually by thrombosis, as a consequence of the risk factors just described. Patients may develop abdominal pain, hepatosplenomegaly, ascites, and jaundice over a period of weeks to months. Treatment involves anticoagulation or surgical decompression.

Patients may be asymptomatic or may report pain, tenderness, swelling, and warmth of the affected areas. They may also note pain and soreness when walking, which is relieved with leg elevation. A "cord" (ropelike hardening of the vein) may be palpable. A positive Homan's sign (pain on simultaneous foot dorsiflexion and leg elevation) may be present, but this is an unreliable indicator of DVT.

Duplex Doppler ultrasonography is the preferred initial diagnostic test. Venography and plethysmography are also available.

Superficial thrombophlebitis may require only NSAIDs and warm compresses over the involved area. Deep venous thrombi are usually treated with leg elevation, short-term bed rest, and anticoagulation with warfarin for 3 months. Because warfarin levels take 5 to 10 days to become therapeutic (INR of 2 to 3) and because warfarin alone can cause protein C deficiency and thereby create a hypercoagulable state, heparin is used in the initial phase of treatment. Traditionally, intravenous heparin is titrated to bring the partial thromboplastin time (PTT) to twice its normal value. Subcutaneous low molecular-weight heparin, which does not require PTT monitoring, is being used with equal success, and is preferred over coumadin in pregnant patients given the contraindications of coumadin in pregnancy. Thrombolytic therapy, such as streptokinase, is effective only within the first few hours of acute thrombus formation. DVTs should be aggressively treated to prevent the severe complication of pulmonary embolism (see Chapter 3).

Prevention strategies for high-risk patients, for example, in the postoperative period include elastic stockings, pneumatic compression stockings, aspirin, and subcutaneous heparin, coumadin, or enoxaparin administration. Filters placed in large veins, such as the inferior vena cava, can catch emboli before they reach the lungs, but there is controversy as to whether these filters may increase clot formation due to the presence of a foreign body in the vein.

Vasculitis

Vasculitis refers to inflammation of the blood vessels. In addition to the etiologies in the following sections, vasculitis may occur as part of connective tissue syndromes, such as SLE, which are described in more detail in Chapter 12.

Polyarteritis Nodosa

Polyarteritis nodosa is the inflammation of small- to medium-sized muscular arteries, followed by ischemia in the tissues supplied by these arteries. Affected organs include the kidneys, heart, gastrointestinal tract, muscles, nerves, and joints. The condition is idiopathic but may be related to hepatitis B and C. Men are affected three times more often than women. Although it usually occurs in young adults, polyarteritis nodosa can strike at any age.

Common presentations include fever, abdominal pain, hypertension, hematuria, anemia, neuropathy, weight loss, and joint pain. Skin manifestations include palpable purpura, mottling, and necrotic ulcers.

Elevated WBC count, anemia, elevated erythrocyte sedimentation rate (ESR), proteinuria, and hematuria are common.

Because there are no laboratory tests specific to polyarteritis, diagnosis must be confirmed with either biopsy of necrosed areas or, if negative, visceral angiography revealing aneurysms of medium-sized vessels.

Long-term therapy with corticosteroids and other immunosuppressive agents such as cyclophosphamide may be necessary.

Giant Cell Arteritis

Also known as *temporal arteritis,* giant cell arteritis is characterized by chronic inflammation of the medium to large blood vessels, primarily the carotid and cranial arteries. Giant cell arteritis becomes more frequent (1 per 1,000) after age 50 years, and women are more likely to develop it than men. Severe sequelae, such as blindness, occur in as many as 20% of patients.

Symptoms include severe temporal or occipital headaches and visual disturbances, such as amaurosis fugax (transient blindness in one eye), blurring, and diplopia. Jaw claudication and systemic symptoms, including arthritis, fever, and weight loss, may also be present. On physical examination, the temporal artery may be swollen, tender, nodular, or pulseless, but is often normal.

Clinical presentation and elevated ESR may suggest the diagnosis, which is determined with temporal artery biopsy.

Because of the risk of blindness, treatment with high-dose prednisone should be initiated immediately if the diagnosis is suspected. Corticosteroid treatment should continue for 1–2 months. Temporal artery biopsy results are still diagnostic for 1 to 2 weeks after treatment has begun.

Inflammatory Conditions

Rheumatic Fever

Rheumatic fever is a complication that occurs 1 to 4 weeks after a throat infection with group A *Streptococcus* (*S. pyogenes*). Current theories suggest that streptococcal infections can induce the generation of autoantibodies that attack the heart valves and the joints. The mitral valve is most often affected, followed by the aortic valve, and, more rarely, the right-sided heart valves. Until recently, the incidence of rheumatic fever has been extremely low in the United States because of sanitation and antibiotic treatment of streptococcal infections, but new outbreaks have been reported, and it remains a major public health problem in developing countries. Attack rates are approximately 3% in patients with untreated exudative streptococcal pharyngitis.

A migratory arthritis, with hot, painful, swollen joints, is the most common manifestation. Endocarditis, which can result in permanent mitral or aortic disease, and pericarditis may also be present. Other manifestations include fever; subcutaneous nodules on extensor surfaces; chorea; and erythema marginatum, a transient, painless rash.

Laboratory evaluation reveals an increased sedimentation rate and an elevated WBC count. Ninety percent of patients have elevated antistreptococcal antibodies (antistreptolysin O and anti-DNAse B) EKG may show prolongation of the PR interval..

Diagnosis is made on the basis of the Jones criteria, which requires the presence of either two major criteria or one major and one minor criterion. Major criteria are carditis, erythema marginatum, subcutaneous nodules, arthritis, and Sydenham's chorea. Minor criteria include fever, arthralgia, PR prolongation, elevated ESR, evidence of a recent streptococcal infection (reflected by elevated antistreptococcal titers), and a history of rheumatic fever.

Aspirin reduces fever and joint inflammation. In severe carditis unresponsive to salicylates, a short course of corticosteroids is often therapeutic. Penicillin eradicates residual infection. If severe, cardiac damage may result in chronic rheumatic heart disease as well as heart failure. Patients with damaged heart valves should be given antibiotic prophylaxis to prevent bacterial endocarditis before receiving dental work or surgery.

Currently, prevention guidelines advocate rapid streptococcal antigen detection tests or throat cultures in all patients with pharyngitis. If the culture is positive for group A streptococci, patients should receive a 10-day course of penicillin, or erythromycin in penicillin-allergic patients. This treatment prevents rheumatic fever even if started several days after the onset of pharyngitis. Because recurrent rheumatic fever most often occurs within 5 years of the first episode, patients with a history of rheumatic fever should be readily treated with antibiotics when they develop pharyngitis.

Bacterial Endocarditis

Bacterial infection of the heart lining or valves can cause temporary or permanent damage to the heart as well as distal embolization and abscesses. This condition is seen most often in patients with pre-existing heart abnormalities (e.g., congenital defects or damage from rheumatic disease), in IV drug users, or in patients with prosthetic heart valves. Patients without these risk factors also may be affected.

Acute bacterial endocarditis (ABE) is usually caused by *Staphylococcus aureus, Streptococcus* (group A or *S. pneumoniae*), and *Neisseria gonorrhoeae.* Subacute bacterial endocarditis (SBE) is usually caused by less virulent streptococcal species, including viridans *Streptococcus* and enterococcus, and often occurs in abnormal or artificial valves after bacteremia.

Both ABE and SBE are characterized by fevers, chills, night sweats, fatigue, weight loss, and arthralgias, although the course of SBE is much more indolent than that of ABE. Physical examination is significant for new heart murmurs, petechiae over the upper half of the body, and splinter hemorrhages under the fingernails. Classic manifestations include Osler's nodes (painful, red nodules on the tips of fingers and toes), Janeway lesions (hemorrhagic lesions of the palms and soles), and Roth's spots (exudative retinal lesions). These physical signs are due to small septic emboli from a left-sided infected vegetation, which can also cause infarcts or abscesses in the brain, kidney, and other organs. Leukocytosis is common in ABE but not in SBE.

Risk factors such as artificial valves or IV drug use, combined with the preceding presentation, suggest the diagnosis. Blood cultures should be drawn to check for bacteremia, although negative cultures do not rule out the diagnosis. Transesophageal echocardiography usually shows vegetations on the valvular leaflets.

Rapid antibiotic treatment is essential, because fatality rates can be high. Empiric treatment while cultures are pending needs to cover *Staphylococcus, Streptococcus,* and enterococcus. Nafcillin or oxacillin, penicillin, and gentamycin are often used together. Antibiotics specific to the cultured organism are necessary for several weeks after the diagnosis, regardless of clinical resolution of symptoms. If valves are permanently damaged, valve replacement may be necessary.

Patients with congenital or acquired valve abnormalities or prosthetic valves who undergo dental or surgical procedures should receive prophylactic antibiotics, because these procedures often cause a transient bacteremia that may result in endocarditis.

Noninfective Endocarditis

In noninfective endocarditis, fibrin and thrombi form vegetations on the heart valves even in the absence of an infectious cause. This type of endocarditis often results from trauma, deposition of immune complexes, or hypercoagulability. One frequent type of noninfectious endocarditis is **Libman-Sacks disease,** which strikes as many as 40% of patients with SLE. Libman-Sacks disease is characterized by platelet and fibrin vegetations on the valvular leaflets. Sequelae of noninfective endocarditis include emboli and vascular obstruction.

Patients are often asymptomatic but may have audible regurgitant murmurs on examination. Arterial emboli may result in stroke or other tissue infarction.

Echocardiography may reveal vegetations on the valves. Blood cultures to rule out bacterial endocarditis will be negative. The presence of an associated disease, such as SLE, also suggests the diagnosis.

Treatment involves anticoagulation with heparin and warfarin. Infectious endocarditis must first be ruled out, because inadvertent anticoagulation of infected patients can lead to severe hemorrhage and death.

Mitral Valve Disorders

Mitral Stenosis

Mitral stenosis describes narrowing and calcification of the mitral valve, resulting in obstructed blood flow from the left atrium to the left ventricle. The continued resistance to flow results in left atrial enlargement, and further backup of this flow results in pulmonary hypertension and right ventricular hypertrophy. Rheumatic fever causes almost all cases of mitral stenosis.

Symptoms occur 10 to 20 years after the stenosis has developed, often precipitated by pregnancy or atrial fibrillation. Progressive dyspnea, orthopnea, paroxysmal nocturnal dyspnea, and fatigue are common, although patients with severe mitral stenosis can be completely asymptomatic. Auscultation reveals an "opening snap" after S_2, followed by a low-pitched, diastolic rumble.

The clinical presentation is suggestive of mitral stenosis. Depending on the advancement of disease, ECG may show left atrial enlargement and right ventricular hypertrophy. Chest x-ray may also show left atrial enlargement, as well as calcification of the mitral valve. Echocardiography confirms the diagnosis.

Symptoms of right heart failure should be treated with diuretics. Significant atrial enlargement may precipitate atrial fibrillation, which should be treated appropriately (see atrial fibrillation). Surgical valvuloplasty or valve replacement provides long-term relief.

Mitral Regurgitation

Mitral regurgitation occurs when the mitral valve becomes incompetent, resulting in systolic backflow of blood from the left ventricle into the left atrium. It often results from **mitral valve prolapse,** in which part of the mitral valve is "floppy" and falls back into the atrium. Other causes include rheumatic fever, dysfunction of the papillary muscle or chordae tendineae, left ventricle dilatation, and endocarditis.

In chronic mitral regurgitation, patients may report palpitations or dyspnea on exertion; however, many remain asymptomatic. If acute, pulmonary edema may occur. On auscultation, a harsh, blowing, holosystolic murmur is heard at the apex, radiating to the axilla. This murmur is accentuated with squatting and hand grip and decreased by exercise (Table 2-3). Mitral valve prolapse is associated with a midsystolic click, and an S_3 is often present.

CARDIOVASCULAR

Table 2-3. Physical diagnosis of systolic murmurs

	Valsalva	Standing	Squatting	Hand grip	Exercise
Mitral regurgitation	↓ or no change	↓ or no change	↑	↑	↓
Aortic stenosis	↓	↑ or no change	↓ or no change	↓ or no change	↑ or no change
Hypertrophic obstructive cardiomyopathy	↑	↑	↓	↓	↑

↑, increased; ↓, decreased.

Chest x-ray shows left atrial enlargement and left ventricular hypertrophy. Echocardiography provides the definitive diagnosis.

Valve repair is indicated in most acute mitral regurgitation and in severe chronic disease. Because mitral valve abnormalities are associated with endocarditis, prophylactic antibiotics should be given for procedures that might produce bacteremia (e.g., surgery, dental visits).

Aortic Valve Disorders

Aortic Stenosis

Aortic stenosis describes narrowing of the aortic outflow tract, resulting in obstructed blood flow from the left ventricle to the aorta and systemic circulation. Aortic stenosis usually results from congenital bicuspid aortic valves, present in 1% of the population, which undergo progressive fibrosis and calcification. Other causes include aortic valve sclerosis and calcification in the elderly and rheumatic heart disease. Aortic stenosis should be differentiated from hypertrophic obstructive cardiomyopathy (HOCM; see Hypertrophic Cardiomyopathy later in this chapter), a form of hypertrophic cardiomyopathy in which the aortic outflow tract is dynamically obstructed during systole by a hypertrophied septum.

The classic triad of symptoms in severe cases is angina, dyspnea on exertion, and syncope. The patient's pulse is often weak and prolonged, and a crescendo-decrescendo systolic ejection murmur is frequently heard at the right upper sternal border, radiating to the carotid arteries. A palpable left ventricular heave or thrill, a weak or absent aortic S_2, or reversed splitting of the S_2 with respiration may be present.

Valsalva decreases the murmur in aortic stenosis but increases it in HOCM (see Table 2-3). ECG indicates left ventricular hypertrophy and may show T wave inversion. Chest x-ray may reveal a calcified aortic valve and a dilated ascending aorta. Doppler echocardiography can estimate the aortic valve gradient and can assess cardiac function, but it can be inaccurate in severe disease. Cardiac catheterization provides the definitive diagnosis.

Beta-blockers can help slow heart rate and improve coronary flow. Valve replacement is indicated if symptoms are present, or if aortic stenosis is severe or left ventricular function is declining. Stenosis often recurs after valvuloplasty.

Aortic Regurgitation

Aortic regurgitation occurs when the aortic valve becomes incompetent, resulting in diastolic backflow of blood from the aorta into the left ventricle. In children, the most common cause is a congenital ventricular septal defect with associated aortic valve prolapse. In adults, the common causes of mild aortic regurgitation include a congenitally bicuspid aortic valve, infective endocarditis, and hypertension. Rheumatic heart disease, tertiary syphilis, and aortic dissection can also cause aortic regurgitation.

If chronic and progressive, dyspnea on exertion, angina, and orthopnea may be present, although most patients remain asymptomatic for many years. If acute in onset, sudden dyspnea is common secondary to acute left ventricular failure and pulmonary edema. On physical examination, a "water hammer" pulse may be noted, characterized by a rapid upstroke and downstroke. This pulse may be heard as a "pistol shot" over the femoral arteries. A widened pulse pressure (difference between the systolic and the diastolic blood pressures) may also be present. A pulsatile whitening of the fingernails may be elicited under slight pressure (Quincke's sign).

On auscultation, a diastolic decrescendo murmur may be heard best at the right second intercostal space. An additional late diastolic rumble (Austin Flint murmur) may be noted at the apex, as the blood flowing through the incompetent aortic valve strikes the mitral valve.

Chest x-ray usually reveals an enlarged left ventricle with a dilated aorta. ECG tracings are usually consistent with left ventricular hypertrophy. Doppler echocardiography can diagnose and evaluate the severity of regurgitation. Cardiac catheterization is often used to assess severity as well as for preoperative evaluation of the aortic root and coronary arteries.

Medical management consists of afterload reduction with ACE inhibitors, calcium channel blockers, or nitrates. Valve replacement or repair is indicated if symptoms are present or if left ventricular dysfunction is severe or progressive.

Arrhythmias

A normal ECG is shown in Figure 2-2 for reference. Antiarrhythmic pharmacology is shown in Table 2-4.

Paroxysmal (Supraventricular) Tachycardia

Supraventricular tachycardia (SVT) refers to a rapid arrhythmia arising from the atria. It occurs most often in young patients with normal hearts and is caused by a reentry rhythm,

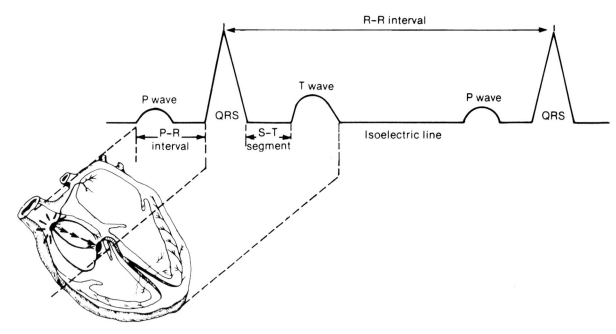

Fig. 2-2. A normal electrocardiogram. The P wave corresponds to atrial depolarization, and the QRS complex corresponds to ventricular depolarization. The T wave corresponds to ventricular repolarization. (Reprinted with permission from Caroline N: *Emergency Care in the Streets,* 5th ed. Boston: Little, Brown, 1995, p 530.)

Table 2-4. Antiarrhythmic pharmacology

	Agents	Action	Some clinical indications
Class I		Sodium channel blockers	
Ia	Quinidine	Prolong AP duration	SVT, VT, VF prophylaxis,
	Procainamide		symptomatic PVCs
	Disopyramide		
	Moricizine		
Ib	Lidocaine	Shorten AP duration	VT, VF, prophylaxis,
	Mexiletine		symptomatic PVCs
	Phenytoin		
Ic	Flecainide		
	Propafenone	No effect on AP duration	VT, VF, refractory SVT
Class II	Esmolol	Beta-blockers	SVT, may prevent VF
	Propranolol		
	Acebutolol		
Class III	Amiodarone (also class I properties)	Potassium channel blockers	Amiodarone: SVT, refractory VT, VT prophylaxis, VF
	Sotalol		Sotalol: VT
	Bretylium		Bretylium: VT, VF
	Ibutilide		Ibutilide: a-flutter, a-fibrillation
Class IV	Verapamil	Calcium channel blockers	SVT
	Diltiazem		
Miscellaneous	Adenosine	Na/K ATPase inhibitor	SVT
	Digoxin		

AP, action potential; PVC, premature ventricular contraction; SVT, supraventricular tachycardia; VF, ventricular fibrillation; VT, ventricular tachycardia.

in which an impulse is repeatedly sent back to the atria through an abnormal signaling loop. In **AV nodal reentry,** the most common cause of SVT, slow and fast conduction pathways exist within the AV node, and atrial contraction is repeatedly triggered by reentry of an impulse through the AV node. In **AV reentry** (also known as Wolff-Parkinson-White), conduction of the reentrant signal to the atria occurs through an accessory pathway between the atria and the ventricles. Although AV nodal reentry tachycardia (AVNRT) is a fairly benign condition, AV reentry tachycardia (AVRT) can precipitate ventricular fibrillation in a patient with atrial fibrillation.

Attacks are characterized by sudden onset and resolution, but they may last for several hours. Heart rate is fixed and regular, occurring between 150 to 250 beats per minute. Patients may be asymptomatic or may experience mild chest pain, shortness of breath, and the sensation of a racing heartbeat.

ECG shows tachycardia and a characteristic pattern of P waves hidden in T waves.

Carotid sinus massage or the Valsalva maneuver may stop the paroxysmal (supraventricular) tachycardia by stimulating the vagus and delaying atrioventricular conduction. Drugs, such as adenosine, calcium channel blockers, digoxin, or beta-blockers, may help as well, but these AV node blocking agents are generally contraindicated in the Wolff-Parkinson-White syndrome (a wide complex AVRT), as they can precipitate ventricular fibrillation in this setting. Accessory pathways can be surgically ablated.

Atrial Flutter

Atrial flutter is caused by the rapid firing of an ectopic focus in the atria. The resulting atrial rate is typically 300 beats per minute and regular. Most impulses are blocked at the AV node, so that the ventricular rate is a fraction of the atrial rate (e.g., 2 to 1 conduction will result in a ventricular rate of 150 beats per minute). Atrial flutter is usually associated with pre-existing heart disease, including CAD, valvular disease, and pericardial disease.

Patients are usually asymptomatic but may experience palpitations, syncope, and lightheadedness at higher heart rates.

ECG tracing shows a characteristic "sawtooth" appearance, made up of identical P waves generated by the ectopic atrial focus (Figure 2-3). The figure shows 4 to 1 ventricular conduction.

Treatment involves slowing of the ventricular firing rate, if necessary, with digoxin, beta-blockers, and calcium channel blockers and converting to sinus rhythm with chemical or electrical cardioversion.

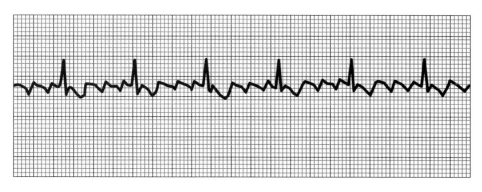

Fig. 2-3. Atrial flutter. (Reprinted with permission from Caroline N: *Emergency Care in the Streets,* 5th ed. Boston: Little, Brown, 1995, p 541.)

Atrial Fibrillation

Atrial fibrillation occurs when atrial firing from multiple atrial foci is rapid and disorderly. The irregular impulses reaching the AV node result in sporadic ventricular contraction. Patients with a rapid ventricular response are at risk for MI and heart failure. Because the atria do not contract efficiently, blood stasis occurs, promoting the formation of atrial thrombi. The thrombi can then be a source of emboli to the lungs, brain, or other organs. Atrial fibrillation is associated with coronary artery disease, hypertensive heart disease, rheumatic valvular disease, mitral valve prolapse, pericarditis, pulmonary disease, and hyperthyroidism.

SIGNS & SYMPTOMS

Patients are usually symptomatic and experience palpitations and chest discomfort. Shortness of breath, lightheadedness or syncope, and fatigue are also common. The classic physical finding is an irregularly irregular pulse.

DIAGNOSIS

ECG tracing reveals an irregular baseline appearance with absent P waves (Figure 2-4) and an irregularly irregular ventricular rhythm. Echocardiogram may reveal a thrombus.

TREATMENT

Treatment involves achieving rate control, restoring sinus rhythm if possible, preventing emboli, and treating the underlying disorder. Control of the ventricular rate is achieved with digoxin, calcium channel blockers, and beta-blockers followed by cardioversion (electrical or chemical) if necessary. If there is evidence of thrombus formation or if the atrial fibrillation is more than 2 days old, anticoagulation is required for 3 to 4 weeks before cardioversion and for several weeks thereafter. Chemical cardioversion with amiodarone, ibutilide, procainamide, or sotalol may be attempted before electrical conversion. Lifelong anticoagulation with aspirin or warfarin and rate control agents may be indicated for patients with intractable atrial fibrillation, especially in patients with concomitant cardiac disease, hypertension, or diabetes.

Premature Ventricular Contraction

Premature ventricular contractions (PVCs) are ectopic beats arising from ventricular foci. PVCs are quite common and may be benign in the absence of pre-existing heart disease. However, in patients with known cardiac disease, the presence of PVCs is associated with an increased rate of sudden death. Noncardiac causes of PVCs include hyperthyroidism, electrolyte abnormalities, hypoxia, stress, and (our favorite) caffeine. Arrhythmias in which every second or third beat is premature are known as *bigeminy* and *trigeminy,* respectively.

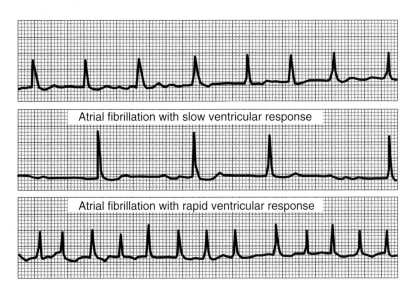

Fig. 2-4. Atrial fibrillation. (Reprinted with permission from Caroline N: *Emergency Care in the Streets,* 5th ed. Boston: Little, Brown, 1995, p 542.)

Patients may be asymptomatic or may experience palpitations or skipped beats. On examination, extra or skipped beats may be noted.

ECG shows wide QRS complexes that occur early, are not preceded by a P wave, and are followed by a compensatory pause (Figure 2-5).

No treatment is needed if the patient is asymptomatic and has no cardiac disease. Noncardiac etiologies should be identified and treated. Patients who are symptomatic or have cardiac disease may benefit from beta-blockers or antiarrhythmics.

Bradycardia

Sinus bradycardia is present when heart rate falls below 50 beats per minute. While this can occur in healthy individuals via increased vagal tone, it can also occur in the setting of sino-atrial node disease. It occurs commonly in the elderly and in patients with a history of heart disease. Patients may present with generalized weakness, and, if severe, alterations in mental status or syncope. Sinus bradycardia predisposes to the development of ectopic rhythms. Cardiac pacing is definitive treatment.

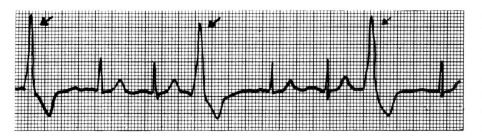

Fig. 2-5. Premature ventricular contractions in trigeminy. (Reprinted with permission from Caroline N: *Emergency Care in the Streets,* 5th ed. Boston: Little, Brown, 1995, p 550.)

CARDIOVASCULAR

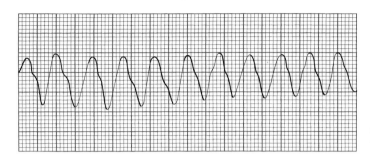

Fig. 2-6. Ventricular tachycardia. (Reprinted with permission from Thaler M: *The Only EKG Book You'll Ever Need,* 3rd ed. Philadelphia: Lippincott Williams & Wilkins, 1999, p 132.)

Atrioventricular junctional rhythms often occur in severe sinus bradycardia or in atrioventricular node conduction delay. The heart rate is usually between 40 to 60 beats/min and increases with exercise. In junctional rhythms, cannon A waves may be present, as the atria contract onto closed tricuspid (and mitral) valves. The ECG will show atrioventricular dissociation or the absence of P waves.

Ventricular Tachycardia

Ventricular tachycardia is defined as three or more consecutive PVCs and usually occurs at a rate of 160–240 beats per minute. It is often associated with MI or other underlying cardiac diseases. Ventricular tachycardia is sustained if it lasts more than thirty seconds. **Torsades de pointes** is a form of ventricular tachycardia with varying QRS morphology, axis, and amplitude. It carries a very poor prognosis.

SIGNS & SYMPTOMS

As with PVCs, patients may be asymptomatic or experience skipped or extra beats, which also may be noted on physical examination. Syncope and presyncopal symptoms may also occur.

DIAGNOSIS

ECG shows a series of wide QRSs in a regular, rapid rhythm, often accompanied by the presence of independent P waves (Figure 2-6). In torsades de pointes, QRS morphology, axis, and amplitude varies, and the QRS complexes appear to spin around the baseline.

TREATMENT

In acute ventricular tachycardia, drug treatment includes lidocaine and other antiarrhythmics. Persistent ventricular tachycardia in an unstable patient requires cardioversion. In patients with chronic recurrent ventricular tachycardia, options include antiarrhythmic agents, an implantable cardiac defibrillator, and, in some cases, ablation. In torsades de pointes, agents that prolong the QT interval (such

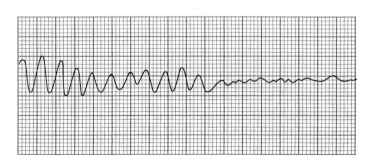

Fig. 2-7. Ventricular tachycardia degenerating into ventricular fibrillation. (Reprinted with permission from Thaler M: *The Only EKG Book You'll Ever Need,* 3rd ed. Philadelphia: Lippincott Williams & Wilkins, 1999, p 133.)

as Group Ic and III agents, refer to Table 2-4) are contraindicated. Treatment involves beta-blockers, magnesium, or ventricular or atrial pacing.

Accelerated Idioventricular Rhythm

Accelerated idioventricular rhythm is distinct from ventricular tachycardia. Although wide complex, it occurs at a rate of 60–120 beats per minute and is not sudden in onset. It often occurs in the setting of MI and coronary thrombolysis, and it carries a lower risk than ventricular tachycardia of progression to ventricular fibrillation. No treatment is required if the patient is hemodynamically stable.

Ventricular Fibrillation

In ventricular fibrillation, a lack of ordered ventricular contraction results in an absence of cardiac output; it is rapidly fatal. This condition is usually seen after a severe, acute MI, but it can also develop spontaneously, often after an episode of ventricular tachycardia, causing most cases of **sudden cardiac death.** Most patients with sudden cardiac death have coronary artery disease.

SIGNS & SYMPTOMS

Lack of cardiac output causes the patient to lose consciousness. No pulses are appreciated on examination.

DIAGNOSIS

Definitive diagnosis requires ECG, which reveals a totally erratic tracing with no identifiable P or QRS waves (Figure 2-7).

TREATMENT

Call for the code team and begin cardiopulmonary resuscitation immediately. Electrical defibrillation is usually necessary. Chemical cardioversion with epinephrine or lidocaine may be attempted simultaneously. If patients survive an episode of sudden cardiac death, recurrences are frequent, and an implantable defibrillator is indicated.

Disorders of Lipid Metabolism

Serum Lipids

Cholesterol and triglycerides are carried in the blood by lipoprotein complexes. An elevated level of low-density lipoproteins (LDLs) is a risk factor for atherosclerosis and CAD, whereas an elevated level of high-density lipoproteins (HDLs) is protective against atherosclerosis. The risk associated with high triglycerides is debated. Serum lipid levels can be adversely affected by behavioral factors (high-fat diet, smoking, obesity, and heavy alcohol intake), endocrine abnormalities (diabetes, hypothyroidism, Cushing's syndrome), medications (diuretics, beta-blockers, oral contraceptives), and genetic disorders (see following sections).

CARDIOVASCULAR

Primary Hypercholesterolemia

Familial hypercholesterolemia and **familial defective apoprotein B** are both common autosomal-dominant diseases involving defective removal of LDLs from plasma. In familial hypercholesterolemia, the receptor involved in removing LDL from the blood is abnormal, whereas in familial defective apoprotein B, a protein component of LDL is malformed, causing it to be poorly recognized by the receptor. Homozygotes, although rare, show signs of CAD by adolescence. Women are less likely to show clinical disease, perhaps because of estrogen status. Other risk factors for atherosclerosis, such as smoking and hypertension, are more likely to cause atherosclerosis in patients with primary hypercholesterolemia, independent of gender.

The classic clinical picture is CAD or an MI in a young man (average age of first MI is 41 years). Lipid deposits in the tendons (xanthomas) and eyelids (xanthelasma) are pathognomonic. Xanthomas are found most commonly in the Achilles tendon or the extensor tendons of the hand. Homozygotes may have xanthomas in childhood. Corneal arcus may occur.

Heterozygotes have plasma cholesterol of 300 to 600 mg/dL. Homozygotes have cholesterol levels of 600 to 1,200 mg/dL. Triglyceride level is normal or slightly increased.

Smoking cessation, a low-fat and low-cholesterol diet, and cholesterol-lowering medication (bile acid-binding resins, niacin, or HMG-CoA reductase inhibitors) may control effects of disease. Screening family members is advisable.

Primary Hypertriglyceridemia

Familial hypertriglyceridemia is a common autosomal-dominant trait leading to enhanced hepatic triglyceride synthesis. Patients are not predisposed to CAD but may be more likely to develop pancreatitis. Serum triglycerides are elevated, with a normal LDL count. Serum may appear milky if triglycerides are very high. These patients are unusually sensitive to other factors causing hypertriglyceridemia, such as alcohol, obesity, and certain medications (estrogen, diuretics, beta-blockers, and glucocorticoids).

Primary Hyperlipidemia

Familial combined hyperlipidemia is an autosomal-dominant trait. Affected individuals may have elevated cholesterol, elevated triglycerides, or both, at different times. CAD occurs early, as with familial hypercholesterolemia. There are no characteristic xanthomas. Diagnosis depends on examining family members.

Familial dysbetalipoproteinemia is a relatively rare disorder of the catabolism of lipoprotein remnants. Patients tend to have palmar or tuberous xanthomas and an increased risk of both peripheral vascular disease and CAD. Both cholesterol and triglycerides are elevated. Diagnosis can be established by using electrophoresis to demonstrate abnormalities of very low-density lipoprotein.

Managing Hypercholesterolemia

In 2001, the National Cholesterol Education Program issued its third set of cholesterol treatment guidelines. They recommend cholesterol screening using total cholesterol, LDL, HDL, and triglycerides, measured in a fasting state. After determining cholesterol levels, the next step is to count risk factors. The five risk factors are:

- Age (men >45 years; women >55 years)
- Low HDL cholesterol (<40 mg/dL)
- Cigarette smoking
- Hypertension (blood pressure >140/90 or on antihypertensives)
- Family history of premature coronary heart disease (CHD in male first-degree relative <55 years or female first-degree relative <65 years)

Having high HDL (>60 mg/dL) cancels one other risk factor. The decision to initiate lifestyle changes or medications to lower LDL depends on the presence of CHD or diabetes, the number of risk factors, and the LDL levels (Table 2-5). Diabetes is now considered a CHD equivalent, and high cholesterol in the setting of diabetes is treated accordingly.

Lifestyle changes include a diet low in saturated fat with total fat contributing 25–35% of calories, increased physical exercise, and weight loss. A 3-month trial of lifestyle changes is recommended before initiating drug therapy. See Table 2-6 for medication choices.

Table 2-5. Recommendations for initiating treatment in individuals with high cholesterol

Risk category	LDL goal	LDL level at which to initiate lifestyle changes	LDL level at which to consider medications
CHD or diabetes	<100 mg/dL	≥100 mg/dL	≥130 mg/dL
Two or more risk factors	<130 mg/dL	≥130 mg/dL	≥130–160 mg/dL
Zero or one risk factor	<160 mg/dL	≥160 md/dL	≥190 mg/dL

Adapted from Executive Summary of the Third Report of the NCEP Expert Panel on Detection, Evaluation and Treatment of High Blood Cholesterol in Adults (Adult Treatment Panel III) JAMA 2001, 285:2486–2497.

Table 2-6. Medications used for treating hyperlipidemia

Agent	Cost	Effect on LDL	Effect on HDL	Effect on triglycerides
Bile acid sequestrants (cholestyramine, colestipol, colesevelam)	$$			none
Fibric acids (gemfibrozil, fenofibrate)	$$$			
Nicotinic acid	$			
Statins (lovastatin, pravastatin, simvastatin, fluvastatin, atorvastatin)	$$$$			

Adapted from Safeer RS, Lacivita CL. Choosing drug therapy for patients with hyperlipidemia. Am Fam Physician 2000:61:3374–3375.

CARDIOVASCULAR

Ischemic Disease

Atherosclerosis and Coronary Artery Disease

Atherosclerosis describes the degeneration of arteries by intimal plaques, which are made up of extracellular lipid and smooth muscle. These plaques can calcify and rupture and can lead to narrowing occlusion or aneurysm. Atherosclerosis is the leading cause of CAD in the United States, and CAD is currently the leading cause of death in the United States. However, incidence of CAD has been declining since the 1960s, presumably because of better hypertension diagnosis and control. Risk factors for CAD include male gender, advanced age, family history of premature CAD, hypertension, smoking, high LDL cholesterol, low HDL cholesterol, diabetes, obesity, sedentary lifestyle, elevated serum homocysteine, and low estrogen levels in women.

Atherosclerosis can manifest in a number of ways, most often through ischemia. These presentations include angina, MI, intermittent claudication, stroke, and mesenteric ischemia. On examination, patients may have high blood pressure, hypertensive retinal changes, tendon xanthomas (yellowish, nodular fatty depositions on tendons), xanthelasma (yellow fatty depositions on eyelids), and S_3 or S_4 heart sounds.

An exercise stress test (ECG performed while patient is on a treadmill) showing ST wave segment changes or a Persantine-thallium scan showing an area of decreased circulation indicates CAD. Angiography is the gold standard; however, this test is invasive and may only be indicated if surgical intervention is an option.

Reduce precipitating risk factors, including smoking, hypertension, hyperglycemia, and hyperlipidemia. Angioplasty or bypass surgery may be indicated if the condition is severe.

Angina Pectoris

Angina pectoris refers to chest discomfort on exertion that arises from temporary myocardial ischemia. The most common cause of angina is CAD. Other causes include arterial vasospasm, chronic valvular disorders, paroxysmal tachycardias with rapid ventricular rates, and increased metabolic demand (e.g., hyperthyroidism, anemia). Note that myocardial ischemia can be clinically silent (e.g., in diabetes mellitus).

The classic presentation involves substernal pain or pressure that may radiate to the left shoulder, arm, back, or jaw, usually triggered by physical activity or stress and lasting a few minutes, with resolution of symptoms following rest or the use of nitroglycerin.

The preceding symptoms suggest the diagnosis. Exercise stress testing is the test of choice to assess ischemia during stress. Dipyridamole USP (Persantine)-thallium radionuclide scanning is an alternative if exercise testing is contraindicated, and provides more information on cardiac function. Other tools include radionuclide angiography and echocardiography to image left ventricular function, and ambulatory ECG monitoring. Coronary angiography, which can demonstrate obstruction or narrowing of coronary vessels, is rarely indicated for diagnosis alone.

Nitroglycerin, administered sublingually, is the immediate treatment of choice for an anginal attack. Nitroglycerin before exertion, long-acting nitrates, beta-blockers, and calcium channel blockers are the preferred forms of chronic therapy. Antiplatelet drugs, such as aspirin, reduce the incidence of more severe coronary events such as unstable angina and MI. Severe angina may require angioplasty or coronary artery bypass grafting for more long-term relief. Risk factor reduction should be emphasized.

Coronary Insufficiency

Coronary insufficiency, also known as **unstable angina,** describes a change in the status of previously established angina, frequently a result of plaque rupture, ulceration, or hemorrhage with subsequent thrombosis. About one-third of unstable angina patients will progress to MI or sudden death within 3 months; therefore, unstable angina is an emergent medical condition that may require intensive care.

Patients experience anginal attacks of severe chest pain and pressure that are longer or more severe than their previous attacks of angina, occur with less exertion or at rest, and are less responsive to medication. Radiation of pain may occur, as in angina pectoris.

ECG changes often occur during episodes of angina, with ST segment depression or elevation, and T-wave flattening or inversion. Patients with uncontrolled unstable angina should not undergo stress testing. Angiography may be helpful in assessing the specific location of coronary occlusion.

Heparin and aspirin therapy, oxygen, nitrates, and beta-blockers are part of the initial treatment regimen. Calcium channel blockers may be used if these measures do not improve symptoms or if nitrates or beta-blockers are contraindicated. If these measures do not resolve the patient's pain, early coronary angiography and revascularization by percutaneous transluminal coronary angioplasty (PTCA) or coronary artery bypass grafting (CABG) is indicated. Recurrent unstable angina, MI, and sudden death can follow episodes of unstable angina. Therefore, if the patient is stabilized with medical measures, coronary angiography is used to risk stratify patients. Appropriate patients may benefit from angioplasty or CABG.

Myocardial Infarction

Commonly known as a heart attack, myocardial infarction (MI) refers to ischemia and necrosis of the myocardium because of insufficient blood supply. As with angina pectoris and unstable angina, the most common etiology is atherosclerosis. MI is usually caused by the acute development of a thrombus in the coronary arteries at the site of an atherosclerotic lesion. Sudden death after MI is common, and approximately 20% of patients die before reaching the hospital.

CARDIOVASCULAR

SIGNS & SYMPTOMS

Many patients experience ischemic symptoms in the weeks before an MI, including angina, dyspnea, dyspepsia, and fatigue. Onset of the MI is usually characterized by prolonged, severe, substernal pressure or pain, with radiation to the left arm, back, or jaw. Up to 20% of MIs may be "silent," with little or no discomfort. Silent MIs often occur in diabetic patients. Symptoms of left-sided heart failure, such as dyspnea, orthopnea, cough, and wheezing, may develop. Nausea, vomiting, lightheadedness, and profuse sweating are also common.

On physical examination, the patient is usually pale and diaphoretic and may be cyanotic, with cool skin and a weak pulse. Heart sounds may be distant, and an S_4 is almost always present. A blowing systolic murmur, indicating papillary muscle necrosis, may be heard.

LABS

Levels of creatinine phosphokinase of myocardial origin (CPK-MB) begin rising 2 to 12 hours after the MI, peak after 12 to 40 hours, and decrease after 24 to 72 hours. The more cardiac-specific troponin I rises within several hours and can stay elevated for 5 to 7 days. Serum lactic dehydrogenase (LDH) levels also rise, peaking 3 to 6 days after the MI.

DIAGNOSIS

ECG changes can provide a definitive diagnosis for transmural infarcts (involving the entire thickness of the myocardium), which are associated with the development of abnormal Q waves (and are called Q wave infarctions). Nontransmural infarcts (non-Q wave infarctions) cause elevated ST segments and abnormal T waves (Figure 2-8). Serial cardiac enzyme measurements demonstrate the development of cardiac necrosis. Chest x-ray signs of CHF often lag behind the clinical findings. Echocardiography can identify wall-motion abnormalities.

TREATMENT

If the patient presents within 12 hours of the onset of the event (the earlier the better), thrombolytic therapy (e.g., t-PA, reteplase, streptokinase, and anistreplase) has been shown to reduce mortality. It should obviously not be given to patients with other risk factors for serious bleeding. Immediate cardiac catheterization and angioplasty is sometimes used as an alternative to thrombolysis and is beneficial to patients with cardiogenic shock, but it is only available at specialized centers.

Aspirin should be chewed immediately and has proven clinical benefit. Adequate arterial P_{O_2} should be maintained with oxygen therapy. Cardiac work can be reduced with beta-blockers, which

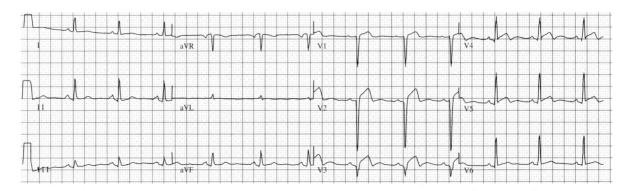

Fig. 2-8. Acute anterior myocardial infarction. Note Q waves in leads II and III and ST segment elevation in V_1–V_5.

lower heart rate. Nitroglycerin decreases cardiac work by decreasing preload and often relieves ischemic pain. If residual pain remains, IV morphine should be used. Antiarrhythmics (typically lidocaine) to prevent ventricular fibrillation are only indicated if the patient has frequent PVCs or nonsustained ventricular tachycardia. Subsequent to an MI, chronic aspirin therapy and beta-blockers each reduce mortality by approximately 25%. ACE inhibitors also have significant proven benefit. Only in non-Q wave infarction have calcium channel blockers shown any benefit.

There are a variety of possible complications following an MI. Infarct extension, post-infarction angina, SVT, sinus bradycardia, and ventricular arrhythmias are common. Myocardial dysfunction, papillary muscle necrosis, septal or free wall rupture, and left ventricular aneurysm can also occur. The formation and embolization of mural thrombi are common in large anterior infarctions.

PREVENTION

Primary prevention of MIs involves managing risk factors: quitting smoking, losing weight, avoiding a sedentary lifestyle, reducing cholesterol, and controlling hypertension and diabetes.

Acute Myocarditis

Acute myocarditis involves inflammation of the myocardium. It is most often due to infections, but a number of other causes have been identified, including toxins, drugs, and endocrine abnormalities. Myocarditis may resolve spontaneously or progress to dilated cardiomyopathy. Viral infections, usually Coxsackie viruses, are the most common cause. Other infectious agents include bacteria, rickettsiae, fungi, and parasites, with *Trypanosoma cruzi* (Chagas' disease) a common cause in Central and South America. Drug and toxin causes include doxorubicin, cocaine, antimony-containing compounds, chloroquine, phenothiazines, radiation, and hypersensitivity reactions to salicylates, sulfonamides, and penicillins.

**SIGNS &
SYMPTOMS**

Patients often present with symptoms of heart failure days to weeks after an upper respiratory infection or an acute febrile illness. Complaints of pleuritic chest pain are common.

LABS

ECG shows nonspecific ST-T changes and conduction abnormalities. Cardiomegaly is common on chest x-ray.

DIAGNOSIS

Echocardiography can assess cardiomegaly and cardiac function. Paired viral titers and serologic tests for other infectious causes can be useful. Endomyocardial biopsy can be informative but may be insensitive.

TREATMENT

If an infectious cause is identified, treatment is directed against it. Toxic agents are withdrawn.

Cardiomyopathies

Cardiomyopathies involve structural or functional abnormalities of the ventricular myocardium.

Dilated Cardiomyopathy

Dilated (congested) cardiomyopathy involves left or biventricular dysfunction with subsequent ventricular dilation and heart failure.

It can result from myocarditis, alcohol use, doxorubicin, delivery, thyroid dysfunction, pheochromocytoma, and hemochromatosis. Dilated cardiomyopathy has a poor prognosis, with 70% of patients dying within 5 years.

Patients with dilated cardiomyopathy may show signs and symptoms of both left-sided and right-sided heart failure, including chronic dyspnea, fatigue, neck vein distention, inspiratory rales, and an S_3 gallop. Ventricular dilation may cause a murmur of mitral regurgitation.

The presentation suggests congestive heart failure. ECG shows sinus tachycardia with ST-T changes and conduction abnormalities. The chest x-ray shows cardiomegaly and pulmonary congestion. Echocardiography demonstrates left ventricular dilation and rules out contributing valvular disorders.

Underlying disorders, such as chronic alcohol abuse, should be treated. Because of the risk of mural thrombus formation, prophylactic anticoagulants may be indicated. Otherwise, treatment is the same as for congestive heart failure.

Hypertrophic Cardiomyopathy

Hypertrophic cardiomyopathy refers to an inherited or acquired ventricular hypertrophy that develops under normal afterload. Causes of acquired hypertrophic cardiomyopathy include hemochromatosis and sarcoidosis. The stiff, noncompliant ventricle cannot readily be filled. In **hypertrophic obstructive cardiomyopathy** (HOCM), also known as **idiopathic hypertrophic subaortic stenosis** (IHSS), the left ventricular outflow tract is dynamically obstructed during systole by a bulging septum. This obstruction is worsened by increased contractility or decreased left ventricular filling. These patients are at increased risk for atrial and ventricular arrhythmias and sudden death.

Patients may report chest pain, exertional syncope, palpitations, and dyspnea. An S_4 and a sustained apical impulse suggest hypertrophy and are apparent on examination. If ventricular outflow is obstructed, a systolic murmur may be heard that increases with standing and the Valsalva maneuver (in contrast to aortic stenosis) and diminishes with squatting (see Table 2-2).

ECG changes demonstrate left ventricular hypertrophy. Echocardiography is diagnostic, revealing asymmetric left ventricular and septal hypertrophy. Doppler ultrasound can demonstrate a dynamic gradient across the aortic valve. Cardiomegaly is not observed on x-ray. Atrial fibrillation and ventricular arrhythmias may be detected.

TREATMENT

Patients with hypertrophic cardiomyopathies have a poor prognosis, with a 20% mortality after 5 years. Beta-blockers and verapamil can both increase cardiac compliance, improving diastolic ventricular function. Removal of septal muscle is only occasionally useful. Implantable defibrillators may help prevent sudden death in patients with ventricular arrhythmias.

CARDIOVASCULAR

Heart Failure

Congestive Heart Failure

The term heart failure describes a clinical syndrome that can arise from many different conditions resulting in the inability of the heart to meet the body's circulatory needs. Common conditions that may result in heart failure include valvular heart disease, ischemic heart disease, and myocardial heart disease. Heart failure can be separated into systolic and diastolic dysfunction, and into left-sided and right-sided failure.

In **systolic dysfunction,** cardiac function is inadequate for tissue demands, usually due to depressed myocardial contractility (e.g., MI) but also due to elevated preload (e.g., valvular regurgitation), elevated afterload (e.g., aortic stenosis), or inappropriately slow or fast heart rate. High output states, such as severe anemia, thyrotoxicosis, beriberi, and pregnancy, can also cause systolic heart failure.

In **diastolic dysfunction,** decreased ventricular filling due to reduced ventricular compliance leads to elevated diastolic pressures and eventually reduced cardiac output. Hypertrophy and restrictive cardiomyopathy both can cause diastolic dysfunction.

In **left-sided heart failure,** the left side of the heart is unable to supply the needed cardiac output. Blood backs up into the lungs, and pulmonary edema and even pulmonary hypertension can develop. Chronic left heart failure can result in left ventricular hypertrophy. Conditions that precipitate left-sided failure include CAD, hypertension, aortic valve disease, and congenital defects.

In **right-sided heart failure,** right-sided compromise results in right ventricular hypertrophy and backup of blood into the venous system. The most common cause of right heart failure is left heart failure. Other causes include pulmonary hypertension (caused by factors other than left heart failure), valvular disorders, pulmonary emboli, and atrial septal defects.

SIGNS & SYMPTOMS

Clinical manifestations of left-sided failure include fatigue, dyspnea on exertion, paroxysmal nocturnal dyspnea, orthopnea, and cough, which may be productive of whitish sputum. The development of acute pulmonary edema is a medical emergency and is addressed in more detail in Chapter 3. Right-sided failure results in fatigue, neck vein distention, liver enlargement, and peripheral edema. Late-stage symptoms can include ascites, pleural effusions, and severe pitting edema of the lower extremities.

Auscultation may reveal an S_3, an early diastolic sound that occurs with rapid filling of the ventricles, and suggests ventricular volume overload. An S_4, a late diastolic sound caused by a noncompliant ventricle, may be heard when there is abnormal relaxation of the hypertrophied ventricle. Both S_3 and S_4 can be heard in normal patients as well as in other medical conditions and are not specific to heart failure; however, an S_3 is the most reliable predictor of heart failure.

CARDIOVASCULAR

Diagnosis may be evident from physical findings, as well as from the presence of a precipitating medical condition. Chest x-ray shows increased vascular congestion and cardiac enlargement (Figure 2-9). Kerley's B lines may be present and reflect thickening of the interlobular septa of the lungs from persistent edema. There are no specific ECG findings, but abnormal tracings may reflect the underlying cardiac source. Echocardiogram can assess the size and function of the ventricles and atria, pericardial effusion, valve abnormalities, wall motion abnormalities, and shunts.

Treatment of the underlying disorder may be possible for valvular disorders or noncardiac disorders such as thyrotoxicosis, myxedema, or severe anemia. Intravascular volume should be decreased with salt restriction and diuretics. ACE inhibitors reduce preload by vasodilation and increase cardiac output by afterload reduction. They have been shown to delay progression and improve survival in heart failure. Beta-blockers and spironolactone are also beneficial in CHF. Other vasodilators (nitrates and hydralazine, alpha-adrenergic blockers) and digoxin are also useful.

Cor Pulmonale

Cor pulmonale refers to hypertrophy of the right ventricle and eventual right-sided heart failure that results from a reduction of the effective pulmonary vascular bed or pulmonary vasoconstriction. The most common underlying pulmonary disorder is chronic obstructive pulmonary disease (COPD).

Dyspnea on exertion and cough are the most common symptoms. Signs and symptoms of right-sided heart failure, such as a right-ventricular heave and gallop, distended neck veins, hepatic engorgement, ascites, and edema, may be noted in later stages. Clubbing of the fingernail beds is a sign of long-standing pulmonary disease and often is accompanied by cyanosis.

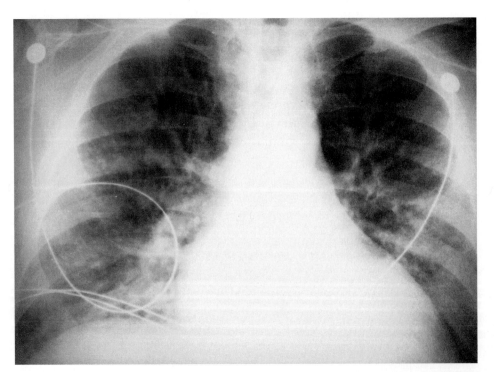

Fig. 2-9. Pulmonary edema in a patient with CHF. Note the enlarged cardiac silhouette, engorged pulmonary veins, and patchy densities. (Reprinted with permission from Daffner R: *Clinical Radiology: The Essentials,* 2nd ed. Baltimore: Williams & Wilkins, p 222.)

CARDIOVASCULAR

The preceding signs and symptoms in the context of a likely history (e.g., smoking) and a low arterial saturation (<90) should suggest the diagnosis. Pulmonary function tests diagnose the underlying lung disease. ECG tracings show right axis deviation and peaked P waves. Chest x-ray may show signs of right heart enlargement.

Treatment is directed at the underlying lung disorder. Continuous oxygen supplementation to reverse hypoxia improves survival in patients with COPD. Salt and fluid restriction and diuretics relieve symptoms and may improve gas exchange.

Pericardial Diseases

Acute Pericarditis

Acute pericarditis is any acute inflammation of the pericardium. It most often follows upper respiratory tract viral infections. It can occur after MIs (Dressler's syndrome) and may be seen in the settings of collagen vascular diseases such as SLE; tubercular, streptococcal, and staphylococcal infections; drug use, including isoniazid and hydralazine; and pericardial metastasis, especially from the breast or the lung; and uremia.

Inspiratory substernal chest pain is the most common symptom. Postural changes (e.g., sitting) may relieve pain. A friction rub (a scratchy, leathery sound present throughout diastole and systole) is the characteristic sign of acute pericarditis. Fever and leukocytosis are common. Pulsus paradoxus, an exaggerated drop in systolic blood pressure with inspiration, is also present.

The friction rub suggests the diagnosis. Echocardiography shows pericardial effusion. ECG findings often include diffuse ST segment elevation in all leads or T-wave inversion. Chest x-ray may show an enlarged cardiac silhouette.

Treatment of a known underlying disorder can be curative. NSAIDs decrease pericardial inflammation and associated chest pain, and steroids are used in intractable cases. Uremic pericarditis improves with dialysis.

Chronic Constrictive Pericarditis

Chronic constrictive pericarditis arises as a reactive, diffuse thickening of the pericardium after pericardial inflammation. Pericardial changes restrict diastolic filling, elevating venous pressures and decreasing cardiac output. Any cause of acute pericarditis can lead to chronic constrictive pericarditis, but radiation and cardiac surgery are common etiologies.

Patients usually present with a history of dyspnea on exertion and orthopnea. They may have signs of right-sided failure, such as jugular venous distention, ascites, and edema. Kussmaul's sign (increasing neck vein distention with inspiration) is present. Atrial fibrillation is common.

CARDIOVASCULAR

Chest x-ray shows pericardial calcifications in 50% of patients. Cardiac catheterization is most diagnostic, showing equal diastolic pressures in all four chambers. Echocardiography, CT scan, or MRI can identify pericardial thickening.

Surgical removal of the pericardium is curative but carries a high mortality rate.

Pericardial Effusion

Pericardial effusion involves an accumulation of fluid in the pericardial space and occurs in the setting of pericarditis. In acute pericarditis, the fluid is transudative, but in neoplasms or fibrosis the fluid is exudative. If filling occurs rapidly, the fluid compresses the heart and causes tamponade (see next section).

Patients with pericardial effusion may be asymptomatic, especially if fluid accumulates slowly; however, if ventricular filling is limited, patients may present with symptoms of congestive heart failure. Pain is often present but is typically absent in uremic or neoplastic pericarditis. On examination, heart sounds are distant and a friction rub may be audible.

Chest x-ray shows symmetric enlargement of the cardiac silhouette. ECG shows low QRS voltage. Echocardiography demonstrates the pericardial fluid and is diagnostic. Fluid removed from the pericardial sac by pericardiocentesis and biopsy specimens can be evaluated for infectious causes (e.g., tuberculosis), collagen vascular diseases, and cancer.

The underlying disorder should be treated. As in acute pericarditis, NSAIDs decrease pericardial inflammation. Fluid can be aspirated for symptom relief.

Cardiac Tamponade

Cardiac tamponade occurs when pericardial fluid compresses the heart and drastically reduces cardiac output. This is a life-threatening condition.

Patients present with dyspnea, tachypnea, tachycardia, and a narrow pulse pressure. Pulsus paradoxus and neck vein distention may be noted. Kussmaul's sign is absent.

Chest x-ray may show an enlarged heart. ECG shows low QRS voltage and, rarely, electrical alternans, an alternating variation in the amplitude of ECG waves. Echocardiography demonstrates the pericardial effusion.

TREATMENT

Removal of fluid by emergent pericardiocentesis restores cardiac output.

Cardiogenic Shock

Cardiogenic shock occurs when cardiac output is not sufficient to maintain a normal blood pressure. It may result from any pathologic state that compromises cardiac output, including MI, tamponade, and pulmonary embolism.

SIGNS & SYMPTOMS

The patient is frequently sleepy or confused, with cold, moist extremities that are typically pale and cyanotic. On examination, the patient's pulse is weak and rapid, and systolic blood pressure is less than 90 mm Hg. Tachypnea, engorged neck veins, and signs of pulmonary congestion are often present.

DIAGNOSIS

The clinical presentation, particularly in a patient with a known underlying disorder, suggests a diagnosis. Neck vein engorgement and pulmonary congestion suggest cardiogenic shock over other types of shock.

TREATMENT

Treatment of the underlying cause may reverse cardiogenic shock. If intravascular hypovolemia is present, fluid boluses should be given. Oxygen and ventilatory assistance, if necessary, are important initial steps. Dopamine will reverse profound hypotension and preserve kidney function. Catheterization permits monitoring of the central venous pressure. If inotropic agents are insufficient, intra-aortic balloon counter pulsation should be attempted.

Life Support

Life support is divided into basic and advanced interventions.

Basic life support can be done immediately, using the ABC mnemonic:

A: Airway is opened by a head tilt and chin lift, but this procedure is contraindicated in spinal injury. In that setting, a jaw thrust alone is appropriate.

B: Breathing is restored by mouth-to-mouth resuscitation.

C: Circulation is restored by external cardiac compression.

Complications of basic life support techniques include rib fractures and liver and spleen lacerations.

Advanced cardiac life support adds a "D" to the list:

D: Definitive treatment consists of
- Defibrillation
- Drugs (e.g., lidocaine and epinephrine)
- Diagnostic aids (ECG, echocardiography)

Cardiovascular Treatment Issues

Dietary Measures

Diet plays a large role in the development of heart disease. Initial treatment for most acquired heart diseases involves dietary restrictions. In general, salt intake should be maintained between 1 and 3 g per day, cholesterol intake less than 300 mg per day, and fat intake less than 30% of total calories. Because most dietary modifications require the development of new, lifelong habits, however, the success of dietary treatment measures is quite variable and depends primarily on patient motivation.

Medication

Only approximately half of patients who take antihypertensive medications are compliant after 1 year, and rates are similar for other cardiac medications. Lack of compliance should be considered when there is insufficient improvement in the patient's condition. If necessary, compliance can be checked with pill counts and blood tests. Other issues that may affect compliance are the cost of the drug, the dosing schedule (the more often it needs to be taken, the lower the compliance), and possible side effects.

Special Concerns of the Elderly

Many patients with chronic cardiac conditions are elderly and require special attention. Falls are a major concern in the elderly, so drugs with side effects such as orthostatic hypotension and sedation should be monitored. The patient's state of hydration and visual acuity are also important considerations. Because many elderly patients have more than one chronic condition, polypharmacy may become a major concern and should be monitored carefully to reduce side effects. Table 2-7 discusses strategies for medical visits with elderly patients. A list of common drug reactions in the elderly is presented in Table 2-8.

Table 2-7. Strategies for medical visits with the elderly

1. Review all medications. Ask the patient to bring all pill bottles to each medical visit.
2. Question patients regarding their use of over-the-counter drugs. More than 75% of older patients are frequent users, and they may be unaware of potential interactions with their prescription medications.
3. Assess the benefits and side effects of each medication and reduce their total number or dosage if possible.
4. Try to select medications that are not centrally acting, do not cause postural hypotension, and have shorter durations of action.
5. Ensure that the patient's symptoms are not caused by medications.
6. Initiate medications at dosages lower than the usual adult dosage because metabolism and clearance rates are generally lower in the elderly. Serum albumin levels are also decreased, so albumin-bound drugs may reach toxic concentrations at lower doses.

Table 2-8. Cardiac medications and their drug reactions in the elderly

Drug type	Side effect
Antihypertensives	Postural hypotension
Digitalis	Toxicity, depression, confusion, anorexia (can occur even at therapeutic levels), nausea, vomiting
Anticoagulants	Increased risk of bleeding after minor falls
Diuretics	Dehydration (do not routinely give for ankle edema; use compression stockings)

CARDIOVASCULAR

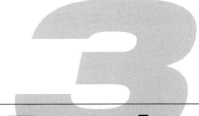

Respiratory Disorders

RESPIRATORY

Upper Respiratory Infections

Viral Rhinitis

Viral rhinitis is also known as "the common cold." Symptoms result from inflammation of the upper airways, including the nose, sinuses, throat, and often the bronchi. Associated viruses include rhinoviruses, influenza, parainfluenza, and adenoviruses.

Patients report nasal or throat irritation, followed by sneezing, rhinorrhea (runny nose), and malaise. A dry cough may persist for 1 to 2 weeks. Bacterial complications, such as sinusitis, otitis media, and bronchitis, may develop.

Clinical signs and symptoms are adequate for diagnosis. A throat culture may be performed if streptococcal pharyngitis is suspected.

Rest, analgesics, antihistamines, and decongestants may be helpful. Aspirin should not be given to children as it is associated with an increased risk of **Reye's syndrome** (a highly fatal encephalopathy discussed in Chapter 13). Antibiotics are not helpful and may place the patient at risk for drug reactions and for future bacterial resistance.

Thrush

Also known as *oral candidiasis,* thrush occurs predominantly in individuals with increased susceptibility to infection, including infants, the chronically ill, the immunocompromised, corticosteroid users, and those receiving antibiotics. It is caused by the fungus *Candida albicans* and is usually benign in children. In adults, it may suggest the presence of an underlying immunocompromised state, such as AIDS.

The typical lesion is a creamy-white, exudative patch with an erythematous base on the tongue or buccal mucosa. The patches can be scraped off, leaving a sensitive, bleeding surface.

Gram's stain or KOH mount shows typical yeasts and pseudohyphae.

Antifungals, such as nystatin or clotrimazole, may be administered as lozenges. Because of high relapse rates, AIDS patients often require continuous prophylaxis with oral fluconazole.

Influenza

Known as "the flu," influenza is caused by specific influenza viruses. Significant mortality is associated with the development of influenza in elderly and chronically ill patients.

Generalized malaise, arthralgias, myalgias, and headache are early symptoms, ordinarily followed by a sore throat, a runny nose, and a nonproductive cough. High fevers are common. Symptoms typically last for several days but may persist for weeks. Sequelae include severe hemorrhagic bronchitis and pneumonia.

Clinical signs and symptoms are generally sufficient. A definitive diagnosis with serologic tests and viral culture is rarely necessary.

Rest and symptomatic treatment are generally adequate. Amantadine may be helpful in the early stages of influenza A and is given to elderly patients or patients with chronic infections.

Influenza vaccinations are developed annually based on the predominant viral strains. They are recommended for people age 50 years and older, health care workers, and people with chronic respiratory or cardiovascular diseases (see Chapter 9).

Streptococcal Pharyngitis

Also known as "strep throat," a streptococcal pharyngitis infection is caused by group A beta-hemolytic streptococci, usually *Streptococcus pyogenes.*

Fever, sore throat, and a beefy, red pharynx with tonsillar exudate are characteristic but are not specific to streptococcal infections. Tender cervical lymph nodes may be present. In young children, rhinorrhea may be the sole manifestation.

Rapid strep antigen detection tests and streptococcal culture establish the diagnosis.

Spontaneous resolution will occur in approximately 10 days; however, untreated streptococcal infections may have severe sequelae, including rheumatic fever and acute glomerulonephritis. Penicillin significantly reduces this risk and should be given even if symptoms appear to be resolving.

RESPIRATORY

Tonsillitis

Tonsillitis is an acute inflammation of the palatine tonsils that usually occurs as a result of streptococcal or viral infection.

Sore throat, pain with swallowing, and referred pain to the ears are common. Patients may also have high fever, malaise, headache, and vomiting. Young children may not report sore throat but are often unable to swallow food because of discomfort and obstruction. Examination reveals red, swollen tonsils with a purulent exudate. A white, thin membrane that peels away without bleeding may be present on the tonsillar surface.

The preceding history and symptoms are diagnostic. Streptococcus may be found on culture.

Although treatment is primarily symptomatic, penicillin should be given for streptococcal infections. Recurrent episodes of acute tonsillitis may require tonsillectomy.

Peritonsillar Abscess

The formation of an abscess near the palatine tonsils is rare in children but more common in young adults. The most common organism is group A beta-hemolytic *Streptococcus,* but anaerobes, such as *Bacteroides,* may also be present.

Patients experience fever, severe pain on swallowing, trismus (muscle spasm resulting in difficulty opening the mouth), and a "hot potato" voice. The head may be tilted toward the affected side, and the uvula may be displaced to the opposite side. On examination, the palate is erythematous and the tonsils may appear asymmetric.

The preceding symptoms and visualization of the abscess suggest the diagnosis.

IV penicillin is administered over 24 to 48 hours. Incision and drainage are usually necessary. Because these abscesses tend to recur, tonsillectomy is often indicated after the acute infection has resolved.

Sinusitis

Infection of the paranasal sinuses is typically precipitated by allergic rhinitis or viral URIs, which cause mucosal swelling that obstructs sinus drainage. Infection is commonly due to

Streptococcus pneumoniae and *Haemophilus influenzae.* The maxillary and frontal sinuses are frequently involved.

Pain over the involved sinuses is characteristic. Nasal membranes are red and swollen, with yellow or green purulent discharge. Inability to transilluminate the sinuses indicates local fluid accumulation. Maxillary toothache may be present.

The history and physical examination suggest the diagnosis. X-rays show air-fluid levels or opacification of the sinuses but are generally necessary to confirm the diagnosis only if empiric antibiotic therapy fails. CT scan is the gold standard and may aid diagnosis in difficult cases.

Antibiotics are necessary for at least 2 weeks. Nasal vasoconstrictors and decongestants may promote sinus drainage. Recurrent or chronic sinusitis may require surgery to improve drainage.

Lower Respiratory Infections

Definitions

Bronchospasm. This spasmodic muscular contraction of the bronchi usually occurs in the context of asthma; however, occupational dust exposure, acute allergic reactions, and water inhalation may all result in bronchospasm in the absence of asthma.

Wheezing. Described as a whistling sound in the lungs during respiration, wheezing is most commonly caused by asthma. Other causes include foreign body obstruction (known as an "asthmatoid wheeze"), chronic obstructive pulmonary disease (COPD), chronic heart failure, and inflammation, as seen in pneumonia and bronchitis.

Pleurisy. Also known as pleuritis, pleurisy is a general term describing inflammation of the pleural lining. Multiple causes, including infectious diseases (e.g., pneumonia), neoplasms (e.g., metastatic cancer), and connective tissue disorders (e.g., systemic lupus erythematosus) may be involved. Pain resulting from pleurisy may be referred to the shoulder as a result of diaphragmatic irritation.

Acute Bronchitis

Acute bronchitis, inflammation of the trachea and bronchi, often arises after an acute viral or bacterial URI, but it may also occur in an occupational setting after exposure to dust or respiratory irritants. In nonsmokers, the most common bacterial etiology is *Mycoplasma pneumoniae.* In smokers, acute bacterial exacerbations of chronic bronchitis are caused by *S. pneumoniae* and *H. influenzae.*

A persistent cough after a URI is initially nonproductive, but with bronchitis it becomes productive of small amounts of sputum. Purulent sputum suggests a bacterial etiology. Fever and sore throat are also common symptoms.

Symptoms suggestive of bronchitis are adequate for diagnosis. On examination, scattered rhonchi (moist, gurgling noises from the larger bronchi) and wheezing may be noted. Chest x-ray may be necessary to rule out pneumonia.

Most cases are viral and require only rest, fluids, and analgesics. Bacterial cases may be treated with antibiotics, but this is controversial.

Bronchiectasis

Bronchiectasis is a chronic destructive process that results in dilation of the bronchial tree. Bronchiectasis commonly occurs in patients with cystic fibrosis, immunodeficiencies, lung infection, and foreign body aspiration.

Classic symptoms include cough productive of large quantities of sputum, dyspnea, and hemoptysis. Recurrent URIs and episodes of pneumonia are common. Chest examination is significant for moist rales and rhonchi over the affected areas. Clubbing of the fingers may be present.

Chest x-ray may show increased bronchial markings, "honeycombing," and areas of atelectasis. Sputum cultures should be obtained.

Treatment consists of antibiotics, bronchodilators, postural drainage, and chest percussion, as well as further treatment of underlying conditions. Surgical resection is useful in patients with recurrent pneumonia who fail medical therapy.

Viral Pneumonia

The most common pneumonia seen in children, viral pneumonia is associated with a number of pathogens, including influenza viruses, parainfluenza virus, respiratory syncytial virus, and adenoviruses. Cytomegalovirus may be seen in immunocompromised patients.

Nonspecific symptoms, such as fever, headaches, and myalgias, arise first, followed by a usually nonproductive cough. On examination, rales or pleural effusions may be present.

Chest x-ray shows patchy infiltrates. WBC count is normal or slightly elevated. Specific identification of the causative virus is not necessary, except in suspected outbreaks.

Supportive care is sufficient, and symptoms usually resolve within a few weeks. Amantadine may be helpful in early treatment of influenza A pneumonia.

Annual influenza vaccinations are recommended for persons age 50 years and older and in those with chronic respiratory or cardiovascular diseases. The vaccine is a heat-killed virus that is noninfectious and can be administered during pregnancy.

Pneumococcal Pneumonia

Caused by *S. pneumoniae,* pneumococcal pneumonia is the most common bacterial pneumonia seen in adults. It is an important cause of community-acquired pneumonia (occurring at home as opposed to in an institution or hospital). Approximately half of normal adults harbor *S. pneumoniae* without accompanying symptoms. Those who develop pneumococcal pneumonia tend to have other underlying medical conditions (e.g., diabetes and cardiopulmonary disease).

Sudden onset of high fever, chills, cough, and pleuritic pain are characteristic. The cough is typically productive of a red-brown "rusty" colored sputum that becomes yellow during resolution of the illness. Physical examination findings include rales, decreased breath sounds, dullness to percussion, and tactile fremitus (vibrations felt over areas of consolidation in the lung when the patient speaks).

Gram's stain of sputum reveals gram-positive diplococci and neutrophils. Chest x-ray typically shows lobar consolidation or patchy infiltrates, sometimes accompanied by a small pleural effusion (Figure 3-1).

Penicillin is the drug of choice for sensitive organisms, although penicillin-resistant *S. pneumoniae* is increasing in prevalence. Cephalosporins or vancomycin are used for resistant strains. Macrolides are a good empiric therapy for community-acquired pneumonias because *H. influenzae* is also sensitive.

Pneumococcal vaccine (Pneumovax) is recommended for patients age 65 years and older or for patients with chronic disease (see Chapter 9).

RESPIRATORY

RESPIRATORY

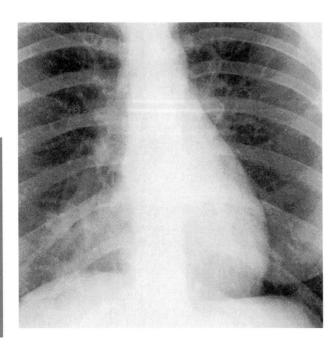

Fig. 3-1. Pneumococcal pneumonia. The right heart border is blurred due to a middle lobe consolidation. (Reprinted with permission from Khan M and Lynch J (eds.): *Pulmonary Disease, Diagnosis, and Therapy: A Practical Approach,* 1st ed. Philadelphia, Lippincott Williams & Wilkins, 1997, p 30.)

Haemophilus influenzae Pneumonia

H. influenzae is a community-acquired bacteria that causes pneumonia primarily in patients with COPD.

As in pneumococcal pneumonia, fever, chills, cough, and pleuritic pain are seen; however, onset is generally slower. If pleural effusions develop, physical examination will reveal decreased breath sounds and mild dullness to percussion.

Because *H. influenzae* is commonly seen in the upper respiratory tract of healthy people, Gram's stain of the sputum is not diagnostic unless it shows large numbers of small gram-negative coccobacilli. Diagnosis may be established by culture of sputum, pleural fluid, or blood. Chest x-ray shows patchy bronchial infiltration or lobar consolidation.

Ampicillin is the drug of choice, but resistant strains require cephalosporins or trimethoprim-sulfamethoxazole.

The *H. influenzae* vaccine protects against pneumonia caused by type b but not other strains of *H. influenzae*. The vaccine is given to children ages 2 months to 5 years.

Klebsiella and Gram-negative Pneumonias

Gram-negative pneumonias, seen primarily in alcoholics, are often caused by aspiration. In the community, the immunocompromised, the elderly, and infants are also at increased risk, but these pneumonias are more commonly nosocomial rather than community-acquired. Gram-negative bacteria that may be involved include *Klebsiella, Escherichia coli,* and Enterobacteriaceae.

The course of illness is generally rapid. In *Klebsiella* pneumonia, typical pneumonia symptoms are present and often include a cough productive of reddish "currant jelly" sputum.

Gram's stain of the patient's sputum shows multiple encapsulated gram-negative bacilli in the case of *E. coli* infection. Blood and sputum cultures should be performed. Chest x-ray shows involvement of multiple lobes, especially the right upper lobe, with possible abscess formation.

Combinations of cephalosporins and aminoglycosides are recommended, but mortality rates may approach 50% in spite of treatment.

Staphylococcal Pneumonia

Staphylococcal pneumonia is seen in both community and hospital settings and may follow URIs. Infants, the immunocompromised, and the elderly are at increased risk. Staphylococcal pneumonia may develop by hematogenous spread of a distant staphylococcal infection, such as endocarditis.

Symptoms resemble pneumococcal pneumonia and include fever, chills, productive cough, and pleuritic pain. Pink ("salmon-colored") sputum may be seen.

Sputum Gram's stain shows gram-positive cocci in grape-like clusters. Chest x-ray shows patchy bronchial infiltration; in infants, pneumatoceles (benign, thin-walled, air-filled cysts) are pathognomonic for staphylococcal pneumonia.

Beta-lactamase–resistant penicillins, such as nafcillin, are recommended. Rates of methicillin-resistant infection continue to increase, in which case vancomycin is the antibiotic of choice. Mortality rates of staphylococcal pneumonia approach 40%, but this rate may be partially attributable to concurrent illnesses.

Mycoplasma Pneumonia

Mycoplasma pneumonia is a community-acquired pneumonia that tends to occur among young people in close contact (e.g., in schools and the military). It is the most common pneumonia seen in teens and young adults. Its clinical and laboratory differences from pneumococcal pneumonia have led to its description as an "atypical" pneumonia.

RESPIRATORY

Gradual onset with a nonproductive cough, fever, headache, and myalgia is typical. Cervical lymphadenopathy and small amounts of whitish sputum may also be seen. On physical examination, fine rales may be heard. Severe symptoms are rare.

Because *Mycoplasma* has no cell wall, it is not visible on Gram's stain. *Mycoplasma* cultures are difficult and require 7 to 10 days for growth. Serum complement fixation antibodies are more sensitive. Chest x-ray is variable and may show patchy infiltrates, especially in the lower lobes, that often appear much more severe than symptoms suggest. A cold agglutinin test may be positive.

Antibiotics, such as erythromycin and azithromycin, are helpful, although many cases will resolve spontaneously.

Pseudomonas Pneumonia

Seen primarily in chronically ill and immunocompromised patients, *Pseudomonas* pneumonia is usually a hospital-acquired pneumonia associated with ventilator use. Patients with cystic fibrosis are also at increased risk for developing this type of pneumonia.

Symptoms are similar to those seen in other gram-negative pneumonias and include rapid onset and a productive cough.

A likely history of nosocomial infection and typical symptoms of *Pseudomonas* pneumonia suggest the diagnosis. Cultures are definitive.

Because resistant strains develop rapidly, treatment should be based on specific sensitivities. Currently, an antipseudomonal penicillin combined with an aminoglycoside is recommended.

Legionella Pneumonia

Caused by *Legionella pneumophila*, *Legionella* pneumonia may develop in both community and hospital settings. Similar to *Mycoplasma* pneumonia, *Legionella* pneumonia is considered an atypical pneumonia because of both difficulty in diagnosis with routine laboratory techniques and clinical differences from pneumococcal pneumonia. *Legionella* is typically seen in middle-aged men, often in association with smoking, alcohol use, and immunosuppression. Outbreaks of *Legionella* are associated with aerosolized water, such as in air conditioners.

An incubation period of 2 to 10 days is followed by a cough productive of scanty nonpurulent sputum. A febrile illness, with myalgia and fatigue, is common and is often seen with GI symptoms such as nausea and diarrhea. CNS symptoms, such as confusion and ataxia, also may be present. Respiratory failure occurs in 20%–40% of patients.

Gram's stain shows neutrophils but no bacteria. The definitive diagnosis can be made with fluorescent antibody tests of sputum and serum antibody titers during the convalescence phase. Chest x-ray reveals patchy infiltrates and possible lobar consolidation and pleural effusion. WBC counts may be mildly elevated.

Azithromycin or a fluoroquinolone is the treatment of choice.

Tuberculosis

Tuberculosis (TB) is caused by *Mycobacterium tuberculosis.* Its incidence in the United States had been declining for 40 years, but the past 15 years have shown a steady increase. Socioeconomic changes and the HIV epidemic are both responsible for this increase. Most cases arise from reactivation of dormant mycobacteria, usually in the upper lobes of the lung. Extrapulmonary manifestations include meningitis, pericarditis, and bone invasion (known as **Pott's disease**). **Miliary TB** refers to widespread dissemination of TB infection to multiple organs; "miliary" refers to the millet seed–like appearance of the lesions.

Symptoms include a cough productive of blood-tinged sputum, weight loss, night sweats, chest pain, dyspnea, anorexia, and manifestations of extrapulmonary disease. Patients with dormant infection are asymptomatic.

Acid-fast staining of sputum may confirm mycobacterial infection, and the presence of *M. tuberculosis* is confirmed by culture. Patients may have a positive tuberculin skin test (purified protein derivative, or PPD), although false-negatives are common. Chest x-ray may show a **Ghon complex,** consisting of a calcified tubercular granuloma in the lung combined with a calcified regional lymph node. Primary lesions typically occur in the lower lobes, while reactivation lesions tend to occur in the lung apices.

Respiratory isolation is important for patients with active disease, and the local health department must be notified. At least four antituberculin drugs must be used initially because of the high rates of resistance, and prolonged treatment is necessary. Good choices include isoniazid (INH), rifampin, pyrazinamide, and ethambutol or streptomycin. Susceptibility testing should be performed, and therapy may then be adjusted.

PPD is a useful screening method for exposure to TB. Induration of 15 mm in nonimmunocompromised patients indicates infection, whereas 10 mm in patients with predisposing conditions and 5 mm in patients with HIV are considered to be positive.

Prophylactic INH therapy is recommended for certain groups of PPD-positive patients. These include new PPD converters, especially if younger than 35 years, HIV-positive individuals, and close contacts of people with newly diagnosed, infectious tuberculosis.

Tobacco Use

Smoking-associated Disease

Cigarette smoking has been identified as the single biggest cause of preventable morbidity and mortality in the United States. The majority of smoking-related deaths falls into three categories: atherosclerotic disease, cancer, and respiratory diseases.

Atherosclerotic disease is manifested in a number of ways, most of which have been strongly associated with cigarette smoking. The incidence of coronary heart disease, including angina and myocardial infarction, as well as strokes and peripheral vascular disease (e.g., intermittent claudication), are all significantly increased in smokers.

Numerous **neoplastic diseases** have also been associated with smoking. In addition to the most commonly known cancers, such as lung, oral, and laryngeal cancers, other smoking-related cancers include esophageal, stomach, pancreatic, bladder, kidney, and cervical cancers.

The primary **respiratory illness** seen in smokers is COPD, which consists of emphysema and chronic bronchitis. Smokers are also more likely to develop upper respiratory infections and pneumonia than nonsmokers, and they may experience more recurrences of TB as well.

Other smoking-related disorders include **GI disease** (e.g., peptic ulcer disease, gastritis, and esophageal reflux) and **complications of pregnancy,** including intrauterine growth retardation, stillbirth, and spontaneous abortion. Passive smoke exposure has also been associated with an increased risk of lung cancer, and passive exposure in children causes an increased incidence of URIs and asthma.

Currently, prevalence rates of smoking are decreasing in all age groups in the United States; however, for some age groups, rates are rising in specific ethnic groups, such as Asians. Smoking prevalence is also rising around the world. Changes in cigarette tar content have not been shown to reduce the risks of smoking. Smokeless tobacco has been promoted as an alternative to smoking but is associated with a greatly increased risk of oral cancer.

Smoking Cessation

Although a majority of smokers would like to quit, more than 70% of those who attempt to quit relapse. It is estimated that only 1% of smokers will quit spontaneously, without help; that 3% will quit on the advice of a physician; and that 5% to 30% of smokers who participate in formal intervention programs will quit. More intensive programs are more successful.

The National Cancer Institute recommends the "four A's" for physicians promoting smoking cessation:

1. Ask about a smoking habit.
2. Advise smokers to quit.
3. Assist the patient in quitting and remaining cigarette free.
4. Arrange follow-up visits to support nonsmoking behavior.

Physician assistance may involve education, self-help material, referral to smoking-cessation programs, and nicotine replacement therapy. Nicotine replacement, via nicotine gum or a transdermal nicotine patch, has been shown to be effective in enhancing quit rates, as has the antidepressant bupropion.

Chronic Obstructive Pulmonary Disease

Emphysema

Emphysema is seen almost exclusively in smokers. Chronic inflammation caused by smoking results in continual release of proteolytic enzymes from neutrophils and macrophages. These enzymes destroy the alveoli and damage the small airways, causing panacinar airspace enlargement and often leading to a reduction in the capillary bed.

One rare form of emphysema is seen in patients with congenital **deficiency of alpha$_1$-antitrypsin.** In this disorder, the individual is unable to neutralize the proteases that are released into the lung by neutrophils and macrophages, resulting in destruction of the alveolar walls. These patients typically develop emphysema by their 30s or 40s, independent of cigarette use. They are also at high risk for liver disease.

The incidence of COPD is increasing, particularly among women. However, it is expected to decrease eventually, following the downward trend in the incidence of smoking.

SIGNS & SYMPTOMS

Physical findings typically include a barrel-chested appearance, prolonged expiration, and pursed-lip breathing. On examination, decreased heart and breath sounds accompanied by rhonchi may be present. Exacerbations present with increased cough and sputum and worsening dyspnea.

DIAGNOSIS

Changes in pulmonary function tests (PFTs, see box) and changes on x-ray establish the diagnosis. PFTs typically show a severely reduced forced expiratory volume (FEV$_1$—the amount of air that can be forced out of the lung in one second) and a reduced forced vital capacity (FVC—the maximum amount of air that can be expired after a full inspiratory effort). The FEV$_1$-to-FVC ratio in COPD patients commonly falls to less than 60% of normal values. In emphysema, these changes are due to the loss of elasticity of the airways (causing them to collapse on expiration) and subsequent air trapping. Chest x-ray reveals lung hyperinflation, a depressed diaphragm, and decreased vascular markings. Bullae (small fluid-filled vesicles) may be noted, although they are not specific to emphysema.

TREATMENT

Smoking cessation is essential in these patients. Patients are treated for their symptoms with antibiotics for bronchial infections and inhalers for improved airway tone. Appropriate immunizations are critical. Patients with COPD should not receive sedatives or hypnotics, as these drugs may reduce respiratory drive. Patients with alpha$_1$-antitrypsin deficiency may receive enzyme replacement therapy, but there are few data supporting the clinical efficacy of this therapy. In severe illness, lung transplantation may be considered.

RESPIRATORY

Pulmonary Function Tests

Pulmonary function tests are used to help differentiate between obstructive pulmonary disease (asthma, emphysema, chronic bronchitis) and restrictive pulmonary disease (chest wall disorders, neuromuscular disease, pleural and interstitial disease). PFTs also give information about severity of disease and response to therapy.

The following measurements are common and are illustrated in Figure 3-2:

Tidal volume: Amount of air moved when the patient is breathing quietly.

Total lung capacity: The total volume of air in the lungs after full inspiration.

FVC: Amount of air that can be expired after a full inspiration.

Residual volume: Amount of air remaining in the lungs after full expiration.

FEV_1: The volume of air that can be expired from the lung in the first second of expiration following a maximal inspiratory effort.

$FEV_1(\%)$ = FEV_1 to FVC: The percent of FVC expired in the first second. $FEV_1(\%)$ is decreased in obstructive disease but normal or increased in restrictive disease.

Diffusion capacity: This test assesses adequacy of the alveolar-capillary membrane by measuring how well carbon monoxide diffuses. In obstructive disease, decreased diffusion capacity is caused by emphysema. In restrictive disease, it is caused by interstitial lung disease.

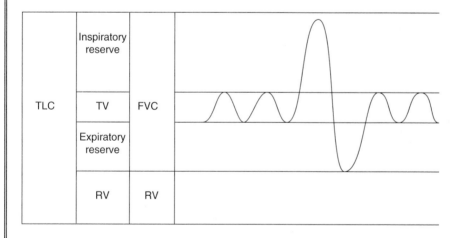

Fig. 3-2. Lung volumes assessed in pulmonary function testing. FVC, forced vital capacity; RV, residual volume; TLC, total lung capacity; TV, tidal volume.

Chronic Bronchitis

Chronic bronchitis is almost always associated with smoking. Exacerbations of chronic disease are commonly caused by *S. pneumoniae* and *H. influenzae.* A less common type of chronic bronchitis is seen in chronic asthmatics, in whom the symptoms of bronchitis do not resolve despite maximal asthmatic therapy.

The patient presents with a productive cough, mild wheezing, recurrent respiratory infections, and progressive shortness of breath.

Diagnosis requires the presence of a cough productive of bronchial mucus secretion for 3 months per year for more than 2 years. The preceding signs and symptoms in a person at risk for developing the condition (e.g., a smoker or asthmatic) are suggestive.

Smoking cessation typically causes reversal of all symptoms. Recurrent URIs are treated with broad-spectrum antibiotics, such as trimethoprim-sulfamethoxazole, clarithromycin, or amoxicillin with clavulanic acid. Bronchial dilators and corticosteroids are helpful in patients with exacerbations.

Respiratory Tract Neoplasms

Laryngeal Carcinoma

Laryngeal carcinoma is typically squamous cell in origin and is highly associated with smoking and alcohol use.

The primary symptom is hoarseness, usually present for several weeks and often worsening gradually over time. Difficulty in swallowing may also be noted.

Laryngoscopy should be performed on any patient reporting hoarseness lasting more than 2 weeks. A number of benign laryngeal tumors may cause a similar presentation. Biopsy will reveal the presence of malignancy.

Radiation and surgery. Complete laryngectomy may be necessary in advanced cases. Rehabilitation after surgery may include training in "esophageal speech," which allows the individual to form words by expelling air from the esophagus.

Lung Cancer

Lung cancer is currently the most common cancer and the leading cause of cancer death in both men and women in the United States. Cigarette smoking is responsible for as many as 90% of cases, but occupational exposures (such as asbestos) have also been implicated.

Four major types of lung cancer include squamous cell carcinoma (accounting for 25% to 35% of cases), adenocarcinoma (25% to 35% of cases), small cell ("oat cell") carcinoma (20% to 25% of cases), and large cell carcinoma (5% to 15% of cases). Small cell carcinoma, the type most strongly associated with smoking, sometimes produces hormones, resulting in paraneoplastic syndromes (see Chapter 4).

The lung is also a common site for bloodborne metastases of other primary cancers. Of incidentally found solitary pulmonary nodules, 10% are metastatic. The most common primary cancer sites associated with lung metastases are the breast, colon, prostate, and cervix.

SIGNS & SYMPTOMS

The typical history consists of cough with bloody sputum, weight loss, and dyspnea. Later signs include pleuritic pain (due to pleural effusions), wheezing, and persistent infection. Other syndromes associated with lung cancer are listed in the accompanying box.

DIAGNOSIS

The history and a mass on chest x-ray suggest the diagnosis. The location of the tumor provides information regarding its histology. Squamous cell and small cell carcinomas typically arise near the hilar region, while adenocarcinomas arise peripherally. Other x-ray findings associated with lung cancer include bronchial narrowing and atelectasis. Bronchoscopy may be used for visualization and biopsy (Figure 3-3).

TREATMENT

Prognosis is generally poor, and few treatments are available. Circumscribed lesions may be surgically excised in a lobectomy, while radiation may be useful for controlling pain or compression of nerves. Five-year survival rates are less than 10%.

Lung Cancer Syndromes

Several syndromes are associated with lung cancer. The following is a brief list of those seen most commonly in a clinical setting. Paraneoplastic disorders, associated with small cell carcinoma, are described in Chapter 4.

Horner's syndrome results from the invasion of cervical sympathetic ganglia by an apical lung tumor (also known as a Pancoast's tumor). This condition results in the classic triad of miosis (pupillary constriction), ptosis (eyelid droop), and anhidrosis (lack of sweating) on the affected side.

Pancoast's syndrome is Horner's syndrome combined with pain in the arm and shoulder because of invasion of the brachial plexus.

Superior vena cava (SVC) syndrome involves obstruction of the venous drainage of the head and neck, resulting in swelling and CNS symptoms. SVC syndrome is associated more with small cell cancer than with other lung cancers but is seen in other diseases, such as TB and other neoplasms.

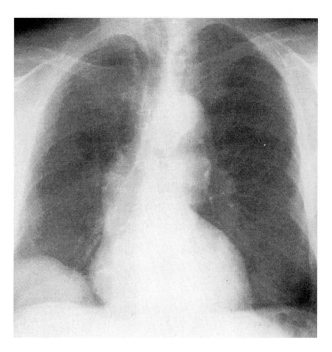

Fig. 3-3. Lung cancer. Right lower lobe mass, typical of large cell bronchogenic carcinoma. (Reprinted with permission from Khan M and Lynch J (eds.): *Pulmonary Disease, Diagnosis, and Therapy: A Practical Approach,* 1st ed. Philadelphia, Lippincott Williams & Wilkins, 1997, p 72.)

Allergy

Asthma

Asthma is a chronic disorder characterized by reversible airway obstruction, brought on by airway inflammation and increased airway sensitivity. Exacerbating factors include pollen, dust, smoke, and fumes; exercise and viral infections; and, occasionally, aspirin and sulfites (found in red wine and beer). People with asthma often have a family history of asthma, allergies, or atopic dermatitis.

Occupational asthma may result from exposure to specific particles or vapors. Symptoms in this setting may not be apparent until after work hours and will often resolve on weekends.

Up to 10% of the population may be affected by asthma, with an incidence that seems to be increasing. The disorder is typically most severe in childhood and improves in early adulthood.

SIGNS & SYMPTOMS

Recurrent episodes of wheezing, coughing, shortness of breath, and chest tightness are common. In severe attacks, patients may be cyanotic or unable to speak more than a few words. The scant sputum produced is white or yellow and has a rubbery quality. Physical examination reveals diffuse wheezing and poor air movement in the lungs. In severe cases, absence of wheezing suggests impending respiratory failure.

DIAGNOSIS

The clinical presentation is usually diagnostic. PFTs may be helpful and usually show decreased FEV_1 because of the constriction of the airways. The FEV_1 improves with a bronchodilator challenge.

Early in an asthma attack, arterial blood gases reveal a respiratory alkalosis and low CO_2 because the patient is hyperventilating. If the CO_2 rises to normal values, respiratory failure is imminent.

RESPIRATORY

Beta-adrenergic inhalers are the first-line agents for acute attacks. Common side effects are tremor and tachycardia. Corticosteroids, leukotriene modifiers, theophylline, cromolyn sodium, and anticholinergics, such as ipratropium bromide, may also be useful. Severe attacks may require oxygen and mechanical ventilation. Occupational asthma may require skin testing to diagnose the offending substance.

Long-term treatment involves prophylactic anti-inflammatory medication and episodic treatment with bronchodilators, in addition to avoidance of allergens.

Efforts should be aimed at preventing acute attacks by avoiding triggers and by using inhaled corticosteroids or leukotriene modifiers to decrease airway inflammation. Patients should monitor themselves with peak flow meters for early signs of exacerbation. Physicians and patients should have a treatment plan worked out so that patients can increase the intensity of their therapy at home at the first sign of an exacerbation.

Allergic Rhinitis

Hay fever is a seasonal form of allergic rhinitis that is usually precipitated by airborne pollens, which vary by location and season. Dust, animal dander, mold, and spores are some of the most common allergens.

Itching, tearing eyes, and clear nasal discharge are common. Coughing and wheezing may develop in severe cases. On examination, nasal membranes are erythematous and swollen, and conjunctiva are injected.

The history is generally adequate. The presence of eosinophils in nasal secretions also support the diagnosis.

A variety of nonprescription and prescription medications may be helpful. Antihistamines, decongestants, nasal glucocorticoid sprays, and cromolyn sodium may be helpful in controlling and preventing symptoms. Long-term desensitization therapy is also recommended in some cases.

Accidents

Epistaxis

Epistaxis (nosebleed) is a common condition seen in people of all ages. Simple, unilateral epistaxis arises from the anterior nasal areas, is most often due to local trauma, and can usually be controlled by pinching the nostrils shut. More severe nosebleeds can arise in elderly patients, especially those on antihypertensive or anticoagulation medications. These nosebleeds usually arise from the posterior nasal areas and may cause blood to enter the mouth and throat by leakage down the posterior pharynx. IV fluids and nasal packs are necessary for management.

Hemoptysis

Hemoptysis is the coughing up of blood or blood-tinged sputum. It can occur with bronchitis, TB, pulmonary embolism, or carcinoma. *Massive hemoptysis* refers to hemoptysis of more than 600 ml of blood within 24 hours. Conditions in which massive hemoptysis might occur include trauma, TB, pulmonary embolism, aortic aneurysm, and heart failure. Hemoptysis must be differentiated from hematemesis (vomiting blood).

Symptoms can range from the occasional expectoration of pink, frothy sputum to the ongoing expectoration of frank blood.

X-ray, CT, and bronchoscopy may be helpful in localizing the source of bleeding. Clotting studies should be performed in cases of massive hemoptysis.

If severe, the patient must be stabilized with IV fluids and blood products. Treatment depends on the diagnosis. Rarely, surgical ligation or lobectomy is necessary to stop the bleeding.

Hemothorax

Hemothorax describes the collection of blood in the pleural space, generally as a result of trauma, malignancy, TB, or pulmonary infarction. Thrombi that form may not be readily reabsorbed, and fibrosis or compromised respiratory function may result.

Signs and symptoms are similar to those of pleural effusion but include those of the underlying disorder.

Chest x-ray shows pleural effusion. Thoracentesis reveals blood.

Closed tube drainage removes blood from the pleural space. Other treatment and supportive care will depend on the underlying cause.

Pneumothorax

Pneumothorax, a collection of air in the pleural space, originates from rupture of part of the respiratory system, esophagus, or chest wall. Spontaneous pneumothorax most often occurs in 15- to 35-year-old males or in patients with severe COPD. If the chest wall is intact, it is a *closed pneumothorax;* an *open pneumothorax* involves air passage through the chest wall, usually as a result of trauma. In a *tension pneumothorax,* pressure in the pleural space can displace the heart and diaphragm. The resulting respiratory compromise and compression of the vena cava constitute a surgical emergency. Iatrogenic causes of pneumothorax include thoracentesis, subclavian or internal jugular catheter placement, lung or pleural biopsy, and other invasive procedures. Assisted ventilation may also create pneumothorax.

Patients report dyspnea and chest pain that may be referred to the ipsilateral arm and shoulder. Decreased chest wall movement, decreased breath sounds, and increased resonance may be noted on the affected side. Tension pneumothorax may be accompanied by a mediastinal shift, neck vein distension, and cyanosis.

Chest x-ray shows space between the lung and the parietal pleura and may show a mediastinal shift away from the affected side if the pneumothorax is large (Figure 3-4).

In a small, stable pneumothorax, air is reabsorbed over time and only symptomatic treatment is necessary. Otherwise, closed chest tube drainage removes the air and allows the lung to re-expand. Risk of recurrent pneumothorax is high. Chemical pleurodesis, in which irritants infused into the pleural space cause the pleura to fuse, has been recommended for recurrent disease. Thoracotomy is needed only when air leaks persist or recur frequently.

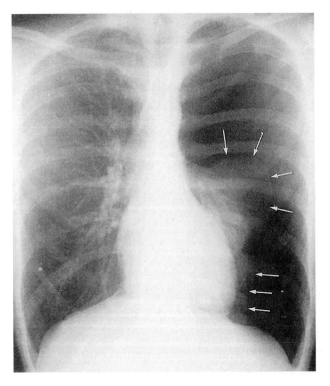

Fig. 3-4. Left pneumothorax. *Arrows* indicate the collapsed left lung tissue. (Reprinted with permission from Khan M and Lynch J (eds.): *Pulmonary Disease, Diagnosis, and Therapy: A Practical Approach,* 1st ed. Philadelphia, Lippincott Williams & Wilkins, 1997, p 55.)

Interstitial Lung Disease

Sarcoidosis

A noncaseating granulomatous disease of unknown etiology, sarcoidosis may involve the lungs, liver, spleen, joints, skin, and bones. Many patients have spontaneous resolution of their symptoms; however, one-third develop chronic disease. Sarcoidosis is much more common in blacks than in other races, with age of onset ranging from approximately 20 to 40 years.

Nonspecific symptoms of pulmonary infection are most common, as are erythema nodosum (tender, red nodules on the tibia and arms), weight loss, fatigue, malaise, and enlarged lymph nodes. Occasionally, the symptoms include dyspnea, dry cough, and fever. Extrapulmonary manifestations include arthritis, cranial nerve palsies, and visual loss.

Laboratory examination reveals increased calcium in the blood and urine. Elevated erythrocyte sedimentation rate and increased total protein (due to excess immunoglobulin production) are also seen.

The preceding symptoms with associated x-ray findings suggest the diagnosis. On chest x-ray, the presence of bilateral hilar and paratracheal adenopathy is pathognomonic. Pulmonary infiltration, with a diffuse, "ground glass" or a more nodular appearance, may also be present. Biopsy of affected sites confirms a noncaseating granuloma.

Spontaneous improvement is common. Steroids are often given, although the benefit is unproved except in cases with ophthalmologic disease or severe systemic compromise.

Asbestosis

Asbestosis, caused by chronic inhalation of asbestos fibers, is associated with increased risks of both lung cancer and malignant mesothelioma (carcinoma of the mesothelial cells of the pleura and peritoneum). Smoking greatly increases these risks. Occupations associated with asbestos use include construction workers, shipyard workers, and automobile mechanics.

Gradual onset of dyspnea and reduced exercise tolerance are typical. Productive cough and wheezing are usually not associated with asbestosis. Inspiratory crackles are noted on examination.

History of exposure and characteristic chest x-ray are diagnostic. Chest x-ray typically reveals diffuse linear opacities in the lower lungs and thickened pleura. Pleural biopsy is diagnostic.

No effective therapy is available. Preventive measures to reduce asbestos exposure, such as masks, are useful. Smoking cessation is also associated with decreased severity of disease.

Silicosis

The oldest of occupational lung diseases, silicosis follows long-term silicon dioxide inhalation. Associated industries include metal mining, pottery making, soap production, and granite cutting. Required exposure times are generally 20 to 30 years, although high exposures can precipitate disease within 10 years. These patients have an increased risk of developing TB.

Many patients are asymptomatic; others report chronic cough and dyspnea. Later stages may show signs of pulmonary hypertension and right-sided congestive heart disease.

History of exposure and characteristic chest x-ray findings, which include multiple small nodules and calcification of the hilar lymph nodes, are diagnostic. Pulmonary function abnormalities include decreased lung volumes and diffusing capacity.

No treatment is available. Effective dust control and protective measures, such as facial hoods, may prevent the development of silicosis.

Other Lung Disorders

Pulmonary Hypertension

Increased hydrostatic pressure in the pulmonary system may result from a variety of underlying diseases. Primary pulmonary hypertension is an uncommon diagnosis of exclusion that usually occurs in young women and is often fatal within a few years of diagnosis. Some causes of secondary pulmonary hypertension include pulmonary embolism, valvular heart disease, left-to-right shunts, and chronic hypoxemia, as in COPD.

Dyspnea, fatigue, retrosternal pain, cough, and syncope are common. Physical examination may show cyanosis, clubbing of the fingers, and an accentuated S_2 on cardiac examination because of pulmonic valve closure. A left parasternal heave may be evident, indicating right ventricular dilatation. Signs of right ventricular failure may be present, including jugular venous distension, hepatomegaly, and ascites.

Laboratory evaluation may show polycythemia, and ECG shows right ventricular hypertrophy. Chest x-ray reveals enlargement of the pulmonary artery and dilation of the right ventricle. Echocardiography, ventilation-perfusion (V̇/Q̇) scanning, and pulmonary angiography may assist in the diagnosis.

In secondary pulmonary hypertension, treatment of the underlying disease is most important. For primary pulmonary hypertension, supplemental oxygen, vasodilator treatment, anticoagulants, and lung transplantation are treatment options.

Pulmonary Embolism

Pulmonary embolism (PE), blockage of a branch of the pulmonary artery, usually arises from a thrombus that has been dislodged from a large vein. The resulting increase in pulmonary artery pressure increases the work of the right ventricle. This condition is particularly dangerous in a patient with pre-existing heart disease.

Most PEs arise from deep venous thromboses (DVTs) in the iliac and femoral veins. Virchow's triad of factors increasing the risk of venous thrombosis includes injury to the vascular endothelium, stasis, and increased coagulability of the blood. Therefore, risk factors for pulmonary thromboembolism include immobilization, carcinoma, recent surgery, venous disease in the lower extremities, pregnancy, oral contraceptive use, and hypercoagulable states (protein C and S deficiency, antithrombin III deficiency, factor V Leiden).

Dyspnea, tachypnea, and tachycardia are the most common symptoms. "Classic" signs are less common and include hemoptysis, pleural friction rub, gallop rhythm, cyanosis, chest pain, and chest splinting. Physical examination is often normal.

Arterial blood gases show increased alveolar-arterial oxygen gradient and hypoxia (see accompanying box). ECG may show sinus tachycardia with right heart strain or, occasionally, atrial fibrillation. The classic ECG finding is a large S wave in I, a large Q wave in III, and an inverted T wave in III (mnemonic: S1Q3⊥3). Chest x-ray can be normal but may reveal atelectasis and small effusions; wedge-shaped peripheral infiltrates may be seen on later films.

V̇/Q̇ lung scans show areas that are ventilated but not perfused. A negative V̇/Q̇ scan essentially rules out the diagnosis, whereas a positive V̇/Q̇ scan is sufficient grounds for diagnosis; both must correlate with clinical suspicion or else further testing is warranted. Identifying a DVT by ultrasound supports the diagnosis. An equivocal V̇/Q̇ scan may require pulmonary angiography, the "gold standard" of diagnosis.

Heparin may be started if there is a high clinical suspicion and continued if needed after diagnostic testing. Supportive care and anticoagulation are the mainstays of treatment. IV heparin is given until the partial thromboplastin time (PTT) is approximately 1.5 to 2.5 times the normal value. Alternatively, low-molecular-weight heparin may be given subcutaneously and PTT does not need to be monitored. Warfarin is started simultaneously and is adjusted to maintain the INR in the 2 to 3 range for at least 3 months. Thrombolysis and pulmonary embolectomy are only rarely necessary in cases of massive embolisms.

Alveolar-arterial Gradient

The **alveolar-arterial (A-a) gradient** provides a measure that compares the oxygenation status of the blood with that of the alveolar environment. The formula for its calculation is:

$$A\text{-a gradient} = PAO_2 - PaO_2$$

$$A\text{-a gradient} = \left[(713 \text{ mm Hg}) (FiO_2) - \frac{(PaCO_2)}{0.8} - PaO_2\right]$$

PAO_2 is a measure of the alveolar oxygen content. FiO_2 refers to the fraction of oxygen in the inspired air. Room air has a value of 0.21; however, patients on oxygen supplementation may have values as high as 1.0 (100% oxygen). $PaCO_2$ and PaO_2 refer to the arterial carbon dioxide and oxygen, which are obtained from the blood gas values.

The normal A-a gradient is approximately 5 to 15 mm Hg. Increased values are seen in pulmonary embolism, diffusion defects (as in pulmonary edema), and right-to-left cardiac shunts.

Pleural Effusion

Fluid collection within the pleural space may be serous, bloody, or lymphatic. **Transudative effusions** result from changes in normal hydrostatic or oncotic pressure, as seen in congestive heart failure and hepatic cirrhosis. **Exudative effusions** are protein-rich effusions that generally arise from inflammation, such as infections or neoplasms (Table 3-1). An effusion of blood (hemothorax) can occur after trauma. Lymphatic fluid may accumulate in the pleural space when the thoracic duct is ruptured or when drainage is blocked, as in mediastinal carcinomatosis. One-fourth of all effusions are associated with malignancies, and the level of suspicion for a malignancy should be high in a patient with bilateral effusions but with a normal-sized heart. *Meigs' syndrome* (pleural effusion accompanied by ascites) is associated with ovarian fibromas and other pelvic tumors.

SIGNS & SYMPTOMS

Patients may report chest tightness, shortness of breath, fever, and weakness. On examination, diminished tactile fremitus, dullness to percussion, and decreased breath sounds are evident over the area of the effusion. Egophony may be noted with larger effusions, such that the patient's voice has

Table 3-1. Differentiation of transudative and exudative pleural effusions

Effusion type	Laboratory analysis	Common causes
Transudates	Pleural to serum protein ratio <0.5	Congestive heart failure
	Pleural to serum LDH ratio <0.6	Nephrotic syndrome
	Total protein <3 g/dL	Cirrhosis
Exudates	Pleural to serum protein ratio >0.5	Neoplasms
	Pleural to serum LDH ratio >0.6	Infections
	Total protein >3 g/dL	Collagen vascular disease

LDH, lactate dehydrogenase.

a higher pitched, bleating quality when auscultated through the chest wall. Classically, the letter "E" sounds like "A" on auscultation over the effusion.

Chest x-ray confirms the diagnosis, showing the effusion as a dulling of the costodiaphragmatic angles with fluid (Figure 3-5). Thoracentesis (aspiration of pleural fluid through the chest wall) provides a fluid sample for analysis, permitting transudates to be differentiated from exudates by comparing pleural protein and lactic dehydrogenase levels with serum levels (see Table 3-1). Frank pus indicates empyema. High triglyceride levels reflect chylous effusions. Further evaluation may include cytology to look for malignant cells, pH, stains and cultures, and amylase levels (to assess pancreatitis or esophageal rupture). Pleural biopsy may be helpful to diagnose TB.

DIAGNOSIS

Thoracentesis or chest tube drainage allows for re-expansion of the lung but can be complicated by pneumothorax, infection, or fluid loculation. In addition, the underlying cause of the effusion must be treated.

TREATMENT

Pulmonary Edema

Pulmonary edema results from increased pulmonary venous pressure, causing congestion of the lung tissue. Common causes include left ventricular failure, myocardial infarction, valvular heart disease, arrhythmias, and hypertensive crises. Acute pulmonary edema may be seen in adult respiratory distress syndrome (ARDS), discussed in the next section.

Dyspnea and tachypnea are common manifestations. Orthopnea (difficulty breathing while supine), paroxysmal nocturnal dyspnea (sudden onset of breathing difficulty during sleep that requires the patient to sit upright), and pink, frothy sputum are also common. Physical examination findings include wheezing, rhonchi, gurgles, moist rales, and dullness to percussion.

SIGNS & SYMPTOMS

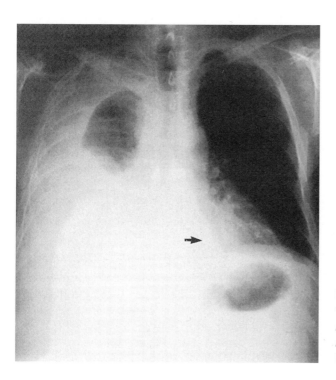

Fig. 3-5. Right-sided pleural effusion. (Reprinted with permission from Khan M and Lynch J (eds.): *Pulmonary Disease, Diagnosis, and Therapy: A Practical Approach,* 1st ed. Philadelphia, Lippincott Williams & Wilkins, 1997, p 37.)

Chest x-ray reveals the diffuse presence of fluid throughout the lung, resulting in indistinct lines and shadows. Prominent pulmonary vessels in the lung apices and Kerley's B lines (Figure 3-6), seen when the outer interlobular septa become waterlogged and fibrotic over time, are also noted. The cardiac silhouette may be enlarged if the edema is cardiac in origin.

Treatment is targeted at the underlying condition. Diuretics and salt restriction are useful for relief of symptoms. Acute pulmonary edema must be aggressively treated with oxygen, morphine, vasodilators, and rapid-acting diuretics, such as furosemide.

Adult Respiratory Distress Syndrome

ARDS describes acute lung injury that results in noncardiogenic pulmonary edema. Sepsis, major trauma, aspiration of gastric contents, near-drowning, and drug overdose are common causes. Mortality is high, particularly when ARDS is associated with sepsis. The mechanism by which ARDS occurs is still unclear, but it may be related to vascular injury and release of cytokines, causing increased vascular permeability.

Dyspnea is accompanied by rapid, shallow breathing within the first 24 to 48 hours after the causative illness or injury. Mottled or cyanotic skin and retractions may also be present. Physical examination may be normal or may reveal wheezing, rhonchi, or rales throughout the lung.

In the appropriate clinical picture, diagnosis is confirmed with arterial blood gases and a chest x-ray. Blood gases typically reveal an acute respiratory alkalosis, with low O_2 and low CO_2 (due to hyperventilation). Chest x-ray findings are typical of pulmonary edema but show diffuse infiltrates with a normal cardiac silhouette because the edema is not cardiac in origin.

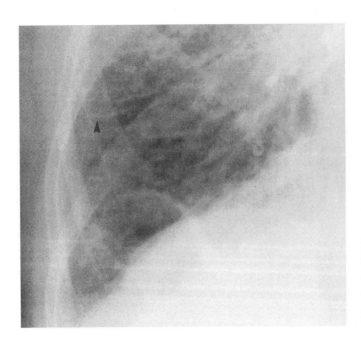

Fig. 3-6. Pulmonary edema, with Kerley's B lines. (Reprinted with permission from Khan M and Lynch J (eds.): *Pulmonary Disease, Diagnosis, and Therapy: A Practical Approach,* 1st ed. Philadelphia, Lippincott Williams & Wilkins, 1997, p 66.)

Maintenance of adequate oxygenation is crucial, and mechanical ventilation with positive end-expiratory pressure is generally used to accomplish this aim. Intravascular volume should be maintained as low as possible to decrease edema. Antibiotics are given when indicated.

Respiratory Failure

Respiratory failure refers to respiratory dysfunction that results in abnormalities of oxygenation or CO_2 elimination. It may follow a failure of ventilation, a failure of oxygenation, or a combination of the two.

Dyspnea, headache, cyanosis, and tachypnea are common, often accompanied by delirium, restlessness, and anxiety.

Arterial blood gases usually show a P_{O_2} of 50 to 60 mm Hg and a P_{CO_2} of more than 45 mm Hg.

Treatment depends on the underlying disorder causing the respiratory failure. For patients who retain CO_2 (Table 3-2), high levels of oxygen may suppress the respiratory drive and can be dangerous. COPD patients should receive low-flow oxygen, and oxygen saturation need not be raised above 90% in these patients. Non-CO_2 retainers can be given high-flow oxygen to raise P_{O_2}. Mechanical ventilation may be needed if hypoxia or hypercarbia persists.

Issues in Hospitalized Patients

Postoperative Pulmonary Complications

Respiratory complications are the single largest cause of postoperative morbidity. The five most common respiratory complications include atelectasis, pneumonia, aspiration, pneu-

Table 3-2. Conditions associated with CO$_2$ retention

CO$_2$ retainers	Non-CO$_2$ retainers
COPD	ARDS
Cystic fibrosis	Pneumonia
Asthma	Aspiration
Chest wall trauma	Pulmonary edema
Neuromuscular diseases (e.g., Guillain-Barré syndrome)	
CNS depression or drug overdose	

ARDS, adult respiratory distress syndrome; COPD, chronic obstructive pulmonary disease.

mothorax, and pulmonary embolism. Atelectasis (see next section) occurs in more than 25% of patients undergoing abdominal surgery and is responsible for more than 90% of postoperative fevers. If atelectasis persists more than 72 hours, pneumonia is likely to develop and is associated with mortality rates of more than 20%. Aspiration of gastric contents may occur as a result of CNS depression during anesthesia, especially if the patient has eaten in the 12 hours before surgery; gastric fluid aspiration may also lead to pneumonia. Pneumothorax can occur as a result of positive-pressure ventilation or central venous catheter insertion. Pulmonary embolism is especially common after abdominal, pelvic, or orthopaedic surgery and may be prevented with preoperative administration of small amounts of heparin to prevent DVT formation. Postoperative patients should be mobilized early or given elastic stockings to promote blood flow.

Atelectasis

Atelectasis refers to localized collapse of the alveoli. Postoperative atelectasis is common, especially after abdominal surgery, due to pain, anesthetic drugs, and the accumulation of secretions in the bronchioles. Newborns may experience atelectasis as part of respiratory distress syndrome because of a lack of pulmonary surfactant to help keep the alveoli open. Asthmatics may also experience patchy atelectasis. In a form of chronic atelectasis known as *middle lobe syndrome,* the right middle lobe collapses as a result of bronchial compression by surrounding lymph nodes. Poor drainage may result in infection and chronic pneumonitis. Finally, atelectasis commonly occurs after foreign body aspiration in children as a result of airway blockage.

SIGNS & SYMPTOMS

Symptoms will depend on the speed at which the atelectasis occurs. Patients may be asymptomatic or may experience pain, dyspnea, and fever. Breath sounds are decreased over the affected lobes, which are also dull to percussion.

DIAGNOSIS

Diagnosis is based on the clinical findings as well as on the chest x-ray. X-ray typically shows an airless lung area. The hemidiaphragm of the affected side may be raised.

TREATMENT

Severe atelectasis requires prompt intervention, including suctioning and chest percussion. Other measures include ambulation and encouragement of deep breathing with inspiratory spirometers. Newborns with atelectasis may be given artificial surfactant. Postoperative atelectasis should resolve within a few days.

Intubation and Tracheostomy

Intubation, insertion of a tube into the trachea, is usually done to maintain a patent airway and ventilate the lungs. The tube may be placed nasally or orally, but the oral method is preferred if the patient is unconscious. Careful visualization of the vocal cords is required to avoid damage. Once the tube is below the cords in the trachea, a balloon is inflated to

RESPIRATORY

create an airtight seal, and the patient can be ventilated. Intubation is associated with increased rates of infection and tracheal mucosal damage. If intubation is anticipated to exceed 3 weeks, a tracheostomy should be performed, as chronic ventilation through a hole in the trachea is associated with fewer complications.

Assisted Ventilation

Ventilatory support is frequently required in the intensive care unit and in the perioperative period. Assisted ventilation is indicated when there is a need for intubation (to protect the airway), or a need for respiratory assistance (for adequate gas exchange or excessive work of breathing). A variety of modes can be used, depending on the situation and condition of the patient. The two main indications for mechanical ventilation are oxygenation failure (e.g., ARDS) and ventilatory failure (e.g., decreased respiratory drive because of narcotics or respiratory muscle exhaustion). Expiration is passive and occurs through the elastic recoil of the lung. If sufficient time is not given for expiration (e.g., if the respiratory rate is too fast or if the lung's elasticity is poor, as in COPD), the ventilator will deliver the next breath while part of the last breath is in the lung. This breath "stacking" results in pressure buildup and can cause the lung to "pop" (barotrauma), resulting in pneumothorax.

When mechanical ventilation is used, adjustable parameters include tidal volume, percentage oxygen of inspired air (FIO_2), respiratory rate, and inspiratory pressure. Positive end-expiratory pressure (PEEP) is used to maintain increased lung volume by preventive collapse of marginal alveoli with expiration. It also helps to redistribute edema fluid out of the alveoli and into the interstitial space.

There are several modes of mechanical ventilation:

Controlled mechanical ventilation (CMV). In this mode, the patient makes no respiratory efforts. The machine delivers a preset volume of gas at a preset rate. This is often used during general anesthesia or in cases of drug overdose.

Assist-control ventilation. This mode is used if the patient is somewhat awake. The machine senses the patient's attempt to breathe as a negative airway pressure and "rewards" the patient by delivering a preset tidal volume. If there are no spontaneous respiratory efforts, the machine delivers breaths according to a preset backup rate.

Intermittent mandatory ventilation (IMV). In this mode, the machine delivers a preset volume of gas at a preset rate, but unlike CMV, the patient can initiate spontaneous breaths between mechanical breaths. The machine does not help the patient with the "extra" breaths.

Synchronized intermittent mandatory ventilation (SIMV). In SIMV, the ventilator is more sensitive to the patient's own efforts and tries to synchronize with them, to deliver a mechanical breath when the patient has initiated a spontaneous breath. The patient can also initiate spontaneous, unsupported breaths between mechanical breaths. If there is no spontaneous respiratory drive, a backup rate is delivered. This is used more often than IMV because it is more comfortable for the patient.

Continuous positive airway pressure (CPAP). CPAP can be delivered by mask and does not require intubation. It supplies an adequate level of pressure to allow the airways to stay open.

Extubation is attempted when it is thought that the patient will be able to breathe independently. The typical prerequisites are that the primary cause of the respiratory failure has resolved, that the patient can generate regular, spontaneous breaths, and that the patient has good nutritional status (enough to sustain the effort of breathing without tiring). Weaning is often accomplished gradually to ensure that the patient can maintain both respiration and oxygenation.

RESPIRATORY

4

Endocrine Disorders

Thyroid Disorders

Thyroid Tests

Both **thyroid hormones,** T_4 and the more active T_3, are found in free and bound states in the serum. Only the free forms are biologically active. Variations in the quantity of thyroid-binding proteins can alter the total serum T_4 without changing the amount of free T_4 available. (This also applies to T_3, but free T_3 is not routinely measured.) For example, conditions that raise levels of thyroid-binding proteins, such as pregnancy, exogenous estrogen intake, chronic heroin use, and hepatitis, will cause the total T_4 to be elevated, although the free T_4 level remains normal. Thus, hypothyroidism, which results from excessively low levels of active T_3 and T_4, can be missed in these conditions by placing too much stock in "normal" total T_4 levels. Free T_4 measurement and, where available, free T_3 measurement are therefore preferred.

Thyroid-stimulating hormone (TSH) from the pituitary induces the thyroid gland to produce T_3 and T_4. Because pituitary control over the thyroid gland is governed by a negative feedback loop (Figure 4-1), levels of TSH are low when the thyroid is hyperactive and high when the thyroid is hypoactive when the pituitary is functioning properly.

A **thyroid scan** uses a small dose of radioactive iodine or technetium, which is taken up by the thyroid gland. This procedure makes it possible to assess the size and function of the gland and is useful in determining whether a nodule is "hot" (overactive) or "cold" (underactive).

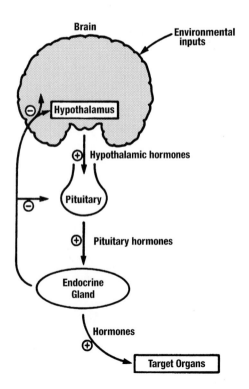

Fig. 4–1. Endocrine feedback loop.

Goiter

Any enlargement of the thyroid gland that is not the result of a neoplasm is termed a goiter. Goiters can be associated with hyperthyroidism (Graves' disease, toxic nodular goiter), euthyroidism (iodine deficiency), or hypothyroidism (Hashimoto's thyroiditis). Thyroid enlargement may result from overstimulation with TSH or a TSH-like substance or may be due to inflammation. Endemic goiter is present when a large proportion of a population has a goiter. This is usually due to iodine deficiency.

Acquired Hypothyroidism

When thyroid hormone is deficient, hypothyroidism develops. The most common cause of acquired hypothyroidism is **Hashimoto's thyroiditis,** an autoimmune disorder typically affecting middle-aged women. Note that Hashimoto's thyroiditis may begin with symptoms of hyperthyroidism. Hypothyroidism can also be iatrogenic, caused by thyroid surgery, neck irradiation, chronic lithium therapy, and some types of iodine administration. Patients who are treated with ^{131}I for hyperthyroidism can develop hypothyroidism after many years. These patients' T_4 and TSH levels should be regularly monitored. Large doses of iodine in radiographic studies can actually inhibit the release of thyroid hormone, a phenomenon called the *Wolff-Chaikoff effect.* Hypothyroidism can develop in patients undergoing these tests.

Common symptoms of hypothyroidism are lethargy, cold intolerance, constipation, weight gain despite reduced appetite, and irregular menses. Hair is coarse. Skin is dry and may show nonpitting edema in severe cases (myxedema). The relaxation phase of deep tendon reflexes may be slowed, and bradycardia may be present. In Hashimoto's thyroiditis, the thyroid is enlarged, nodular, and nontender early in the disease, but it eventually becomes small and fibrotic.

Serum free T_4 is decreased. TSH is high in primary hypothyroidism but low in secondary hypothyroidism (hypothyroidism with pituitary or hypothalamic causes). In Hashimoto's disease, high titers of antithyroperoxidase and antithyroglobulin antibodies are often found in the serum, and lymphocytic infiltrates and fibrosis are evident on needle biopsy of the thyroid.

Daily levothyroxine. Verify dose by monitoring free T_4 and TSH. Reduce dose if angina occurs or worsens.

Hyperthyroidism (Thyrotoxicosis)

Hyperthyroidism (thyrotoxicosis) is an excess of thyroid hormone. Specific etiologies are discussed in the diagnosis and treatment section.

Symptoms reflect an overactive metabolism and include nervousness, sweating, hypersensitivity to heat, palpitations, weight loss despite increased appetite, insomnia, and frequent bowel movements. Signs include tachycardia, widened pulse pressure, tremor, warm skin, and occasionally atrial fibrillation. Eye signs are found in Graves' disease only.

If the hypothalamic-pituitary axis is intact, as it is in most cases, TSH levels will be low. Usually, both free T_4 and T_3 levels are elevated. Rarely, the T_3 will be elevated with a normal T_4 (called T_3 *toxicosis*). This presentation is generally an early manifestation of thyrotoxicosis, and T_4 will rise later in the disease.

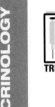

Diagnosis and treatment are based on the etiology of the symptoms.

1. **Graves' disease,** an autoimmune disorder, is the most common type of hyperthyroidism. Antibodies called thyroid-stimulating immunoglobulin (TSI) bind to the TSH receptors in the thyroid, stimulating thyroid hormone synthesis and thyroid enlargement. In addition to symptoms of hyperthyroidism, exophthalmos is typical. Pretibial myxedema is also characteristic but less common. Radioactive iodine uptake is high and TSI is present. Treatment includes symptomatic relief with propranolol as well as antithyroid medications [propylthiouracil (PTU) or methimazole], radioactive iodine (contraindicated in pregnancy), or surgery (subtotal thyroidectomy).

2. **Subacute thyroiditis,** also known as de Quervain's thyroiditis, is probably viral in origin and is characterized by a tender, enlarged thyroid gland. Symptoms of mild hyperthyroidism, neck pain, and fever are common, although a period of hypothyroidism may follow the acute phase of the illness. Radioactive iodine uptake is decreased. Sedimentation rate is elevated. Treatment involves aspirin or other NSAIDs and beta-blockers for symptom control. Thyroid replacement may be needed while the thyroid recovers.

3. **Silent lymphocytic thyroiditis** is a transient thyroiditis that is often found postpartum. Unlike subacute thyroiditis, no pain or fever is present in silent lymphocytic thyroiditis. In contrast with Graves' disease, radioactive iodine uptake is low. Biopsy shows lymphocytic inflammation, similar to Hashimoto's thyroiditis. Treatment is symptomatic (beta-blockade), and the disease is self-limited. Recurrences are common.

4. **Toxic adenoma** or **toxic multinodular goiter** occurs when one or more thyroid nodules begin to function autonomously. Also known as *Plummer's disease,* the condition is most common in older patients. The excess T_3 and T_4 depress pituitary TSH production, thereby causing hypofunction in the rest of the gland. Thyroid scan shows one or more "hot spots" with a hypoactive background. Treatment is with surgery or radioiodine.

5. **Thyrotoxicosis factitia** occurs when exogenous thyroid hormone ingestion results in symptoms of hyperthyroidism without goiter. Treatment is obvious: Stop ingestion.

Thyroid Storm

Thyroid storm is a medical emergency characterized by the extreme effects of thyrotoxicosis. It may be triggered by surgery, illness, or other stress in a patient who is already thyrotoxic.

Diaphoresis, delirium, vomiting, tachycardia, and fever are classic symptoms. Tachycardia may lead to congestive heart failure. Older patients may have myocardial infarctions.

Elevated T_4 and T_3 concentrations and the presence of the classic signs and symptoms of extreme thyrotoxicosis are diagnostic. TSH is low.

Treatment involves beta-blockers, PTU or methimazole, and IV sodium iodide to block hormone release via the Wolff-Chaikoff effect. Glucocorticoids inhibit the conversion of T_4 to T_3, the more active form of the hormone. Definitive treatment with surgery or radioactive iodide is deferred until the patient is stable.

Thyroiditis

A variety of thyroid diseases cause thyroiditis, characterized by swelling of the thyroid gland and often associated with a sensation of neck pressure and mild, often positional dyspnea. Depending on the etiology, thyroid function can be elevated or depressed. Common causes include Hashimoto's thyroiditis, the most common cause of acquired hypothyroidism; subacute thyroiditis, a common cause of hyperthyroidism; and suppurative thyroiditis. Hashimoto's thyroiditis and subacute thyroiditis have been described previously. Suppurative thyroiditis presents with thyroid tenderness, enlargement, erythema, and fluctuance, often developing during a systemic bacterial infection. Treatment involves antibiotics and surgical drainage when necessary.

Euthyroid Sick Syndrome

Euthyroid sick syndrome is a laboratory phenomenon found in acutely ill patients. Serum T_4 and T_3 levels are low because of changes in thyroid hormone metabolism, but TSH is not increased, indicating that true primary hypothyroidism is not present. Signs typically found in hypothyroidism (hypothermia, mental sluggishness) are frequently present in an acutely ill patient, but the diagnosis of primary hypothyroidism should not be made without an elevated TSH. Treatment for thyroid dysfunction is not necessary.

Thyroid Nodule

The majority of thyroid nodules are benign, although malignancy must always be considered in the workup. Both benign and malignant nodules may produce appropriate amounts of thyroid hormone, but rarely do malignancies produce excessive amounts of thyroid hormone. In contrast, those nodules that do not produce hormone, and are therefore "cold" on thyroid scan, are likely to be malignant. Risk of malignancy is increased by any of the following:

- Male gender
- Age younger than 20 or older than 70 years
- Previous head or neck irradiation
- Vocal hoarseness or dysphagia
- "Cold" nodule on radioactivity uptake scan
- Solid (not cystic) nodule on ultrasound

In the evaluation of a thyroid nodule, thyroid function tests (TSH and free T_4) and serology for antithyroperoxidase and antithyroglobulin antibodies should be performed. Fine-needle aspiration and cytology, under ultrasound guidance if necessary, makes the diagnosis. Benign nodules require treatment (surgery or ^{131}I) if symptoms of hyperthyroidism are present. Treatment for malignant nodules is discussed in the following section.

Thyroid Carcinoma

There are four main types of malignancy found in the thyroid gland:

- **Papillary carcinoma** is the most common and has the best prognosis. This slow-growing tumor usually presents as an isolated nodule but often spreads throughout the thyroid and metastasizes to local cervical nodes (check for nodal enlargement).
- **Follicular carcinoma** is more common in older patients. Prognosis of this tumor is not as good. Spread is via blood to bone, lung, brain, and liver.
- **Medullary carcinoma** is a malignancy of the parafollicular C cells, which produce calcitonin; thus, an elevated serum calcitonin is characteristic. However, elevated serum calcitonin can also be seen in thyroiditis and a number of nonthyroid malignancies. Metastases are often present at diagnosis, and prognosis is poor. This tumor often occurs as a component of familial multiple endocrine neoplasia (MEN) type 2.
- **Anaplastic carcinoma** is the least common but is the most aggressive thyroid carcinoma. Prognosis is poor. Local invasion often causes hoarseness and dysphagia.

SIGNS & SYMPTOMS

The most common presentation is an asymptomatic, nontender nodule noted by the patient or physician. Cervical lymph node enlargement, hoarseness, and dysphagia may be present.

DIAGNOSIS

If an isolated thyroid nodule is present, the workup is that of a thyroid nodule. Once fine-needle aspiration (FNA) or biopsy of the thyroid (and local lymph nodes, if enlarged) demonstrates cancer, ultrasound and other imaging modalities can assess local extension and metastasis. FNA may not be able to differentiate follicular carcinoma from a benign follicular adenoma except by demonstration of capsular or vascular invasion. Thyroid scan can be used as an indicator of whether ^{131}I will be useful in treatment, as completely cold nodules, which do not concentrate iodine, will not concentrate ^{131}I and will not respond. Medullary and anaplastic carcinomas are less likely to concentrate iodine.

TREATMENT

Surgery, with subsequent ablation of remaining thyroid tissue using radioactive iodine, is the usual treatment. Thyroid hormone replacement therapy is necessary after surgery.

Disorders of Glucose Metabolism

Diabetes Mellitus (Type 1)

Type 1 diabetes mellitus is also called *juvenile-onset diabetes* or *insulin-dependent diabetes.* Patients lose their ability to produce endogenous insulin. The mechanism is unknown, but it is thought to be autoimmune because most patients have anti–islet cell and anti-insulin antibodies at onset. (Recall, insulin is produced in the beta islet cells of the pancreas.) Type 1 diabetes is associated with HLA-DR3, HLA-DR4, and HLA-DQ, and it may run in families. The average age of onset is 11 to 13 years.

SIGNS & SYMPTOMS

The classic triad of symptoms is polyuria (caused by osmotic diuresis from glucose dumping in the urine), polydipsia (to replenish water loss), and polyphagia (in a futile effort to increase available energy). Weight loss occurs because glucose cannot get into and cannot get used by the tissues. In the absence of insulin, accelerated fat breakdown leads to ketoacidosis, and patients may present with nausea and vomiting, air hunger, or coma (see Ketoacidosis). In general, the onset of symptoms is rapid.

LABS

The presence of urine glucose and urine or serum ketones is common in such presentations. Elevated hemoglobin A_{1c} (HbA$_{1c}$) reflects hyperglycemia over the preceding 2–3 months.

DIAGNOSIS

One of the following:

1. Random plasma glucose ≥200 mg/dL and classic symptoms of diabetes
2. Fasting plasma glucose greater than 126 mg/dL on 2 separate days
3. Positive oral glucose tolerance test (plasma glucose greater than 200 mg/dL 2 hours after a 75-g oral glucose load)

TREATMENT

Insulin injections are required. Insulin doses and combinations must be titrated to maintain optimal blood glucose levels (Table 4-1 and Figure 4-2). Patients must be taught how to monitor their glucose level at home (finger-stick monitoring) and how to adjust diet and insulin accordingly. Note that type 1 diabetics often have a "honeymoon" period shortly after their diabetes is diagnosed, during which endogenous insulin levels rise. Therapy may not be needed for several months, but symptoms and insulin requirements inevitably return. The Diabetes Control and Complications Trial (DCCT) demonstrated that tight glucose control in type 1 diabetes mellitus reduces the risk of diabetic retinopathy, neuropathy, and nephropathy. However, hypoglycemia, the major detrimental effect of tight control, should be avoided.

Diabetes Mellitus (Type 2)

Type 2 diabetes mellitus is also called *adult-onset diabetes* or *non–insulin-dependent* diabetes. This type of diabetes arises when the tissues become increasingly resistant to insulin. Initially, the pancreas responds by increasing insulin production; however, the beta islet

Table 4-1. Effects of various types of insulin

Type	Peak effect (h)	Duration of action (h)
Lispro	1	3–4
Regular	2.5–5.0	8
NPH	4–12	24
Lente	7–15	24
Ultralente	10–30	36

NPH, neutral protamine Hagedorn.

ENDOCRINOLOGY

ENDOCRINOLOGY

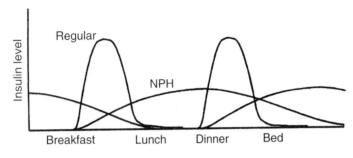

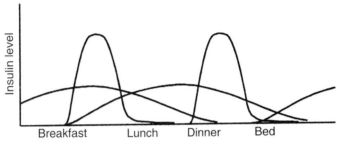

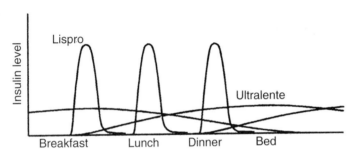

Fig. 4–2. Three examples of insulin regimens. The *top panel* shows a popular insulin regimen, consisting of regular (R) insulin and neutral protamine Hagedorn (NPH) given together before breakfast and before dinner. Two thirds of the regimen is given pre-breakfast and one third is given before dinner. The ratio of NPH:R varies but is often approximately 1:2. The *middle panel* shows a regimen useful for patients who develop nocturnal hypoglycemia and morning hyperglycemia. The pre-dinner NPH is deferred until bedtime, at which time it is often administered as a reduced dose. An alternative strategy is to divide the pre-dinner NPH dose into a pre-dinner dose as well as a pre-bedtime dose. The *bottom panel* shows a regimen designed to achieve tight control. This regimen is useful in the setting of recurrent postprandial hyperglycemia. A basal insulin is achieved with ultralente administered twice a day, and postprandial hyperglycemia is averted with the rapid-acting agent lispro given before meals.

cells' capacity to produce insulin diminishes later in the course of the disease. Thus, depending on the stage of disease at the time of diagnosis, insulin levels may be high, normal, or low. Although patients often need insulin therapy (*insulin-requiring non–insulin-dependent diabetes*), endogenous insulin production is usually sufficient to protect against diabetic ketoacidosis. Obesity and a family history of diabetes are common, but there is no association with any HLA type. Onset typically occurs after age 40 years.

SIGNS & SYMPTOMS

Although the classic symptoms are the same as in type 1, onset is more insidious. Patients may report episodic blurry vision because of osmotic changes in the lens. Ketoacidosis usually does not occur, but patients may develop hyperosmolar nonketotic coma (see Hyperosmolar Coma).

DIAGNOSIS

See diagnosis for type 1 diabetes.

TREATMENT

- Diet should be low in concentrated sugar to minimize serum glucose fluctuations. The patient should be taught to monitor serum glucose with finger-sticks.
- Weight loss and exercise generally increase insulin sensitivity in the tissues.
- Sulfonylureas (tolbutamide, tolazamide, glipizide, glyburide) stimulate insulin secretion.
- Metformin and thiazolidinediones (such as rosightazone) increase glucose uptake in peripheral tissues and reduce hepatic gluconeogenesis.

- Acarbose slows carbohydrate absorption from the GI tract.
- Insulin therapy is required in type 2 patients who do not respond to more conservative measures. Both insulin and sulfonylureas can cause hypoglycemia.

Acute Complications of Diabetes

Ketoacidosis

Insulin normally inhibits peripheral lipolysis. When the insulin level is extremely low, triglycerides are degraded into free fatty acids, which are then converted to ketoacids by the liver. Diabetic ketoacidosis (DKA) occurs in type 1 diabetics who do not take their insulin. It also occurs when infection or MI has increased the body's insulin requirements. Type 2 diabetic patients usually produce enough insulin to protect against DKA.

The prodrome involves 12 to 24 hours of weakness, polyuria, polydipsia, and hyperventilation (in an attempt to compensate for the metabolic acidosis). A fruity, acetone odor may be smelled on the breath. Abdominal pain and vomiting are also common, but care must be taken to determine if GI symptoms are due to ketoacidosis or to a precipitating infection. As dehydration worsens, mental status changes can occur.

Serum glucose is 300 to 800 mg/100 mL (compare with hyperosmolar coma; see following section).

IV fluids and insulin. Potassium must also be given and monitored carefully. Insulin will cause potassium to enter cells, and if extracellular potassium is not replaced, hypokalemia can cause fatal cardiac arrhythmias.

Hyperosmolar Coma

Hyperosmolar coma, a complication of type 2 diabetes, usually occurs after many days of infection or other illness.

The symptoms of polyuria, polydipsia, and dehydration are similar to those of ketoacidosis; however, because some insulin is present, lipolysis and ketoacidosis do not occur. Therefore, there is no hyperventilation or acetone smell to the breath, but dehydration is profound and causes significant mental status changes. Dehydration may not be immediately apparent because urine output remains normal due to osmotic diuresis. Hemoconcentration may lead to reversible gastroparesis, seizures, stroke, and thromboemboli.

Serum glucose is 600 to 2,000 mg/100 mL. Hypernatremia should be corrected for elevated glucose.

Similar to that of ketoacidosis. Adequate hydration is critical. Electrolytes should be repleted. Underlying infections should be treated.

Chronic Complications of Diabetes

Chronic complications of diabetes are due to microvascular or macrovascular disease. While patients with type 1 diabetes mellitus are more likely to develop end-stage renal disease (ESRD) and die from its complications, patients with type 2 diabetes mellitus often die from MI, strokes, and macrovascular complications. Development of complications is more severe in patients with poorly controlled diabetes and seems to correlate with the duration of diabetes after puberty. Elevated HbA_{1c}, which reflects hyperglycemia over the preceding 2 to 3 months, has prognostic value during treatment. For every 1% decrease in HbA_{1c}, there is an estimated 35% reduction in the risk of microvascular complications.

- **Retinopathy.** As many as one fifth of patients with type 2 diabetes mellitus have evidence of retinopathy at the time of diagnosis. In contrast, retinopathy often develops later after diagnosis in type 1 diabetes mellitus. The effects of **nonproliferative** or **background retinopathy** include microaneurysms, blot hemorrhages, infarcts, hard exudates, and macular edema. These changes are seen early and do not usually cause visual loss until macular edema develops. In **proliferative retinopathy,** however, new vessels grow on the retinal surface (neovascularization). These vessels are fragile and prone to hemorrhage. Fibrosis occurs during healing and may put traction on the retina, leading to retinal detachment and visual loss. Laser therapy can slow the progression of proliferative retinopathy. Other ocular complications of diabetes mellitus include premature cataracts and glaucoma.
- **Renal disease.** After 20 years of diagnosed diabetes mellitus, patients with type 1 have approximately a 35% chance of developing nephropathy, compared with a 15% chance for patients with type 2. The first sign of renal disease is proteinuria, with a subsequent decrease in creatinine clearance after 1 to 3 years. End-stage renal disease, requiring dialysis or transplant, typically occurs 3 years after that. Diabetic patients who develop renal disease may find that their insulin requirements decrease because of reduced insulin clearance by the kidneys. Preventive measures include keeping strict control of plasma glucose, eating a low-protein diet, controlling hypertension (especially with angiotensin-converting enzyme inhibitors), avoiding contrast dye, and aggressively treating urinary tract infections.
- **Atherosclerosis.** Atherosclerosis and the coronary artery disease, stroke, and peripheral vascular disease that it causes are more common in diabetic patients. Peripheral vascular disease usually presents as intermittent claudication (leg pain with exercise as a result of ischemia) and predisposes to nonhealing foot ulcers and gangrene.
- **Neuropathy. Bilateral symmetric sensory impairment** usually begins in the feet and progresses proximally in a stocking-glove distribution. Patients may report pain, paresthesias, or numbness. Foot ulcers may develop and become infected without the patient becoming aware of them, so diabetic patients should be trained to examine their feet regularly for ulcerations and implement prophylactic foot care. Repetitive trauma can also lead to multiple unidentified fractures and foot deformity (Charcot's joint). **Mononeuropathy** is caused by infarction of a single motor or sensory nerve, frequently a cranial nerve. Presentation is typically an acute onset isolated motor or sensory deficit in the distribution of a single peripheral nerve, such as foot drop or even a blown pupil. The deficit resolves spontaneously within several months. **Autonomic dysfunction** can include impotence, orthostatic hypotension, gastroparesis, constipation or diarrhea, fecal incontinence, and urinary retention. Diabetic patients are also at risk for unnoticed "silent" MI.

Hypoglycemia and Hyperinsulinism

There are several clinical entities that can cause hypoglycemia. **Reactive hypoglycemia** is lowered blood glucose that occurs 2 to 4 hours after eating. A pancreatic islet cell tumor, or **insulinoma**, can produce excess insulin, causing hypoglycemia. **Iatrogenic hypoglycemia** can result from administration of too much insulin or, less frequently, from excessive oral hypoglycemics (sulfonylureas). Other causes of hypoglycemia include alcoholism, hepatic or renal dysfunction, hypothyroidism, and sepsis.

The symptoms of hypoglycemia fall into two categories. Faintness, weakness, tremulousness, palpitations, sweating, and hunger are the epinephrine-like symptoms. Presentation of these symptoms shows that endogenous, epinephrine-induced glycogen mobilization has begun. The other symptoms are CNS-related and include headache, confusion, and personality changes. The symptoms of hypoglycemia can be masked in patients on beta-blockers.

Reactive hypoglycemia is diagnosed if hypoglycemia coincides with the occurrence of typical symptoms, which are then relieved by carbohydrate ingestion. Elevated insulin in the presence of hypoglycemia indicates insulinoma or an exogenous insulin source. If the insulin is endogenous, C-peptide will also be elevated.

Frequent small meals improve reactive hypoglycemia. Surgery is required to treat insulinoma. For iatrogenic hypoglycemia, increased care should be used in monitoring glucose and administering insulin and sulfonylureas.

Parathyroid Disorders

Parathyroid hormone (PTH) is responsible for elevating serum calcium (Figure 4-3). It mobilizes calcium stores from bone, increases reabsorption of calcium in the kidney, and increases the production of 1,25-dihydroxycholecalciferol, the vitamin D–based product that increases calcium absorption from the GI tract. Phosphate is released from bone with calcium, but PTH also decreases phosphate reabsorption in the renal tubules, resulting in a net lowering of serum phosphate.

Primary Hyperparathyroidism

Primary hyperparathyroidism occurs when excess PTH is secreted by the parathyroid gland. A single, benign adenoma is responsible in 80% of cases. Hyperplasia of all four glands accounts for most of the remaining cases. Parathyroid cancer is rare, comprising less than 2% of cases of primary hyperparathyroidism. Patients with primary hyperparathyroidism are usually older women.

The disorder is often asymptomatic, but evidence of hypercalcemia (GI disturbances, muscle weakness, emotional lability), osteoporosis (bone pain if fracture has occurred), or renal stones may be present. Recall the mnemonic: "bones, stones, abdominal groans, and psychic moans."

ENDOCRINOLOGY

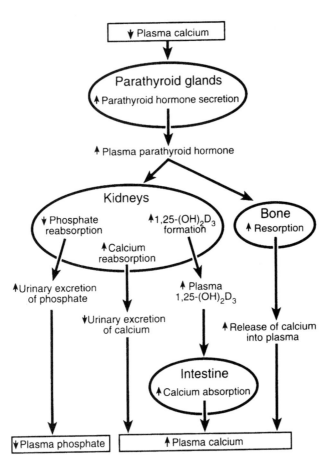

Fig. 4-3. Mechanism by which parathyroid hormone increases plasma calcium. Bone resorption increases serum phosphate as well, but this is outweighed by an increase in urinary phosphate excretion. (Reprinted with permission from Rhoades RA, Tanner GA: *Medical Physiology.* Boston, Little, Brown, 1995.)

Laboratory tests reveal high PTH, with the resulting high total and ionized serum calcium and low serum phosphate. Many malignant tumors can masquerade as hyperparathyroidism. In malignancy, however, plasma PTH is low, unless the tumor is secreting a "parathyroid-like" hormone. The hypercalcemia seen in malignancy can often exceed levels seen in hyperparathyroidism.

Treatment is surgical. Beware of postoperative hypocalcemia, as "hungry bones," freed from the power of PTH, take up the available calcium.

Secondary Hyperparathyroidism

Secondary hyperparathyroidism is parathyroid hypertrophy that develops in response to low serum calcium. Common causes of low serum calcium are vitamin D deficiency or malabsorption, renal tubular problems causing calcium loss (renal tubular acidosis, Fanconi's syndrome), and certain antiseizure medications that interfere with vitamin D metabolism (phenytoin, phenobarbital). Serum phosphate is low, unless there is renal insufficiency (see Chapter 5). Treatment addresses the underlying disorder.

Hypoparathyroidism

Hypoparathyroidism most often follows accidental removal of the parathyroid glands during thyroid surgery but also occurs when the parathyroid glands fail to develop (DiGeorge's syndrome), when they are destroyed by iron overload, or when target tissues lack responsiveness to PTH (pseudohypoparathyroidism).

The ensuing hypocalcemia causes tingling of the lips and fingers and can lead to tetany. A positive Chvostek's sign occurs when a tap on the cheek causes facial muscle spasms. Trousseau's sign is present when a blood pressure cuff inflated on the arm for 3 minutes induces carpal spasm.

Low levels of PTH, causing low ionized and total serum calcium and high serum phosphate.

Calcium and vitamin D supplementation. Note that magnesium deficiency, common in alcoholics, causes hypocalcemia and exacerbates pre-existing hypocalcemia by decreasing PTH secretion and its effect on target organs. In this case, magnesium supplementation must be added to calcium and vitamin D.

Pituitary and Hypothalamic Disorders

Diabetes Insipidus

In diabetes insipidus (DI), dysfunction of the antidiuretic hormone (ADH) pathway causes excretion of large amounts of dilute urine. Diabetes insipidus can occur through lack of ADH secretion from the posterior pituitary (central diabetes insipidus) or ADH insensitivity of the kidneys (nephrogenic diabetes insipidus). The etiology of central diabetes insipidus is most commonly head trauma, pituitary surgery, or an intracranial neoplasm. Acquired nephrogenic DI can occur with myeloma, pyelonephritis, chronic hypercalcemia, and a number of drugs, including lithium and demeclocycline. In central DI, a vasopressin challenge will reduce urine output and thirst. In nephrogenic DI, vasopressin levels are high during fluid restriction. As long as the patient can drink enough fluid to replace losses (up to 15 L per day!), dehydration, hypernatremia, and hyperosmolality will not occur. An X-linked form of nephrogenic DI usually presents neonatally and affects males more often than females. Permanent brain damage will occur, however, if hydration is not maintained. Treatment of central DI is with vasopressin or its analogs. Nephrogenic DI often responds to hydrochlorothiazide and indomethacin.

Syndrome of Inappropriate Antidiuretic Hormone Secretion

The syndrome of inappropriate ADH (SIADH) secretion occurs when excess ADH is secreted, causing free water to be absorbed in the kidneys. This results in hypotonic hyponatremia and overly concentrated urine. The etiology can be a cranial lesion (trauma, tumor, infection), pulmonary disease (tuberculosis, pneumonia, positive pressure ventilation), ectopic ADH production (usually from a lung tumor), and certain drugs. Despite their low serum osmolarity and hyponatremia, patients are euvolemic. Fluid restriction will correct serum osmolality and serum sodium. If sodium is below 120 mEq/L, normal saline with furosemide is useful. Sodium should be corrected slowly to avoid central pontine myelinolysis.

Panhypopituitarism

Panhypopituitarism is a deficiency of all anterior pituitary hormones (Figure 4-4). A variety of pituitary or hypothalamic lesions, including hypophysectomy from trauma, can cause this syndrome. Some hormones are stored in large quantities and other target glands maintain some autonomous function, so symptoms of deficiencies appear at varying times. Follicle-stimulating hormone and luteinizing hormone levels are usually the first to decrease, with resulting menstrual irregularities and sexual organ atrophy. Adrenocorticotropic hormone (ACTH) and TSH decreases follow, leading to hypoadrenalism and hypothyroidism. Patients often seem depressed and apathetic. Treatment is with replacement hormones.

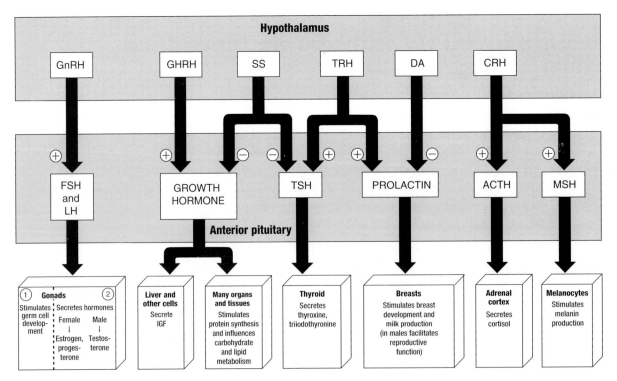

Fig. 4-4. Hormones of the hypothalamic-pituitary axis and their target tissues. ACTH, adrenocorticotropic hormone; CRH, corticotropin-releasing hormone; DA, dopamine; FSH, follicle-stimulating hormone; GHRH, growth hormone–releasing hormone; GnRH, gonadotropin-releasing hormone; IGF, insulin-like growth factor; LH, luteinizing hormone; MSH, melanocyte-stimulating hormone; SS, somatostatin; TRH, thyroid-releasing hormone; TSH, thyroid-stimulating hormone.

Acromegaly

Acromegaly is a condition in which continued bone growth in adults results in a characteristic enlargement of the jaw, forehead, hands, and feet. It is caused by the excessive production of growth hormone by a pituitary adenoma. Soft tissues (tongue, heart, liver, kidneys) also enlarge. Osteoarthritis is common, as is diabetes mellitus, a result of glucose intolerance caused by growth hormone. The offending pituitary tumor can cause visual disturbances and headaches if it becomes large enough. Treatment is via transsphenoidal surgery, or local radiation therapy if surgery fails.

Adrenal Disorders

Primary Corticoadrenal Insufficiency (Addison's Disease)

Destruction of both adrenal cortices results in a deficiency of mineralocorticoids (most important, aldosterone) and glucocorticoids (most important, cortisol) (Figure 4-5). Etiology is usually autoimmune, infectious (tuberculosis, fungal, late human immunodeficiency virus), or hemorrhagic (usually due to anticoagulant therapy).

SIGNS & SYMPTOMS

Symptoms are nonspecific, including fatigue, weakness, anorexia, weight loss, nausea, and vomiting. A notable feature is hyperpigmentation of the skin, which develops because ACTH and melanocyte-stimulating hormone (MSH) are made from the same precursor (see Figure 4–4). When ACTH production is increased in an attempt to stimulate cortisol production, MSH increases as well, causing darkening, especially of the folds of the skin. Some degree of hypotension is common.

LABS

Loss of aldosterone causes hyponatremia (with associated dehydration and orthostatic hypotension) and hyperkalemia. Eosinophilia is also characteristic.

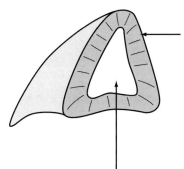

Adrenal cortex
- Mineralocorticoids
  (aldosterone)
- Corticosteroids
  (cortisol)
- Androgens
  (androstenedione)

Adrenal medulla
- Catecholamines
  (epinephrine)

Fig. 4-5. Hormones of the adrenal gland.

Diagnosis is made by using the Cortrosyn stimulation test, in which serum cortisol is assessed before and after Cortrosyn (synthetic $ACTH_{1-24}$) is given. If serum cortisol does not increase when ACTH is given, the diagnosis is established.

Glucocorticoid and mineralocorticoid replacement. Glucocorticoid doses should be increased in times of stress and illness. (John F. Kennedy had Addison's disease, and he was healthy enough to become president only after cortisol was developed.)

Secondary Corticoadrenal Insufficiency

Secondary corticoadrenal insufficiency is due to a lack of ACTH. It most commonly occurs in patients who have received corticosteroids for more than 4 weeks. Exogenous steroids suppress ACTH, thus allowing the adrenal glands to atrophy. If steroid use is abruptly discontinued, the adrenals are not able to produce a sufficient supply of endogenous steroid. Because of this phenomenon, patients should be tapered off their steroid medication. Symptoms are similar to those of primary disease, but without hyperpigmentation or hyponatremia. A corticosteroid taper is sufficient treatment.

Acute Corticoadrenal Insufficiency Crisis (Addisonian Crisis)

Because patients with corticoadrenal insufficiency cannot make cortisol—the "stress" hormone—even a minor illness can cause profound weakness, shock, fever, and even coma. Treatment is with IV glucose, saline, and hydrocortisone.

Cushing's Syndrome

The excess of glucocorticoids causing Cushing's syndrome has several possible etiologies, including pituitary adenoma, paraneoplastic ACTH production, adrenal cortical tumor, and chronic glucocorticoid therapy.

The characteristic body habitus is central obesity with a "buffalo hump" (think "cushion"), moon facies, and peripheral muscle wasting. Obesity in Cushing's syndrome is caused by cortisol, the "stress" hormone, mobilizing energy stores from the periphery to the body's core. Other symptoms include vertebral fractures from osteoporosis, atrophic skin with purple striae, easy bruising, hypertension, and psychiatric changes (depression or euphoria). In women, high adrenal androgens may cause hirsutism, acne, and menstrual irregularities. In men, cortisol may inhibit gonadotropin secretion by the pituitary, causing impotence and a loss of libido.

Hyperglycemia with positive urine glucose and leukocytosis are common.

Dexamethasone suppression test diagnoses Cushing's syndrome. Dexamethasone is a potent glucocorticoid. In people who do not have Cushing's syndrome, low dose (1 to 2 mg) dexamethasone, given at night, feeds back to inhibit ACTH release from the pituitary and results in lower serum cortisol levels the next morning. This serum cortisol suppression does not occur in people with Cushing's syndrome. In addition, 24-hour urine free cortisol is elevated in Cushing's syndrome. The combination of low- and high-dose dexamethasone suppression tests can often differentiate between pituitary and ectopic causes of Cushing's syndrome (see below). Serum ACTH is low in adrenal cortical adenomas secreting cortisol and high in pituitary and ectopic adenomas secreting ACTH.

Treatment is based on the etiology of the symptoms.
- **Cushing's disease,** caused by a pituitary adenoma, is the most common cause of Cushing's syndrome. The adenoma produces ACTH, which causes adrenal hyperplasia. ACTH levels may be normal or elevated. (Either is inappropriate, given the high levels of cortisol in blood.) A high-dose dexamethasone suppression test (8 mg/day for 2 days) will suppress cortisol levels somewhat because the pituitary still has some feedback regulation intact. Treatment is transsphenoidal removal of the pituitary tumor.
- **Ectopic ACTH production** is usually associated with a lung tumor. This ACTH is not suppressible, even with a high-dose dexamethasone suppression test. If the tumor is not resectable for cure, treatment is symptomatic and palliative.
- An **adrenal cortical tumor** may produce high levels of cortisol. ACTH levels are suppressed, and dexamethasone suppression tests do not affect cortisol levels. Treatment is with surgical resection of the tumor. Glucocorticoids must be given postsurgically while the atrophied contralateral adrenal gland recovers.
- In **chronic glucocorticoid therapy,** there are no symptoms of increased androgens. Other signs of steroid use (cataracts, glaucoma, hypertension) may be present. Elevated cortisol levels are not suppressible by dexamethasone. Exogenous steroids should be tapered if possible.

Adrenogenital Syndrome

Adrenogenital syndrome includes any condition in which high levels of adrenal androgens cause virilization (see Hirsutism and Virilization in Chapter 6). Effects are more obvious in women and can include hirsutism, male-pattern baldness, acne, voice changes, amenorrhea, and clitoral hypertrophy. The condition can be congenital, in which an enzyme defect causes precursors of cortisol and aldosterone synthesis to be shunted to androgen synthesis. Later in life, adrenal hyperplasia, adenoma, or adenocarcinoma can increase androgen production and cause symptoms.

Hyperaldosteronism

Aldosterone is a mineralocorticoid secreted by the adrenal cortex. It acts on the distal renal tubules to increase sodium retention and potassium loss. Its release is stimulated by low sodium or low blood pressure (via the juxtaglomerular cell-renin-angiotensin system) and by hyperkalemia.

ENDOCRINOLOGY

Primary hyperaldosteronism is caused by unilateral adrenal adenoma (Conn's syndrome) or bilateral adrenal hyperplasia. Patients have muscular weakness, hypertension, polyuria, and hypokalemia. Diagnostic findings include low plasma renin and high 24-hour urine aldosterone. Treatment is with the aldosterone antagonist spironolactone. Adenomas are surgically resected.

Secondary hyperaldosteronism is generally caused by increased activity of the renin-angiotensin system. The most common cause is a decrease in the blood pressure perceived by the juxtaglomerular cells, as in congestive heart failure, cirrhosis, nephrotic syndrome, and chronic diuretic therapy. Other causes include renal vascular disease, oral contraceptives, and black licorice. The underlying disorder is treated.

Pheochromocytoma

Pheochromocytoma is a condition in which a tumor of the adrenal medulla or sympathetic ganglion secretes bursts of catecholamines, usually norepinephrine. The increased sympathetic activity causes headaches, palpitations, anxiety, and hypertension (episodic or sustained). Diagnosis is confirmed with a 24-hour urine collection showing elevated levels of catecholamines and their metabolites, metanephrines and vanillylmandelic acid (VMA). Treatment is surgical, although symptoms may be temporarily controlled with alpha- and beta-blockers.

Disorders of Mineral Metabolism

Hypercalcemia

Hyperparathyroidism and malignancy are the most common causes of hypercalcemia. Bony metastases and osteolytic tumors (multiple myeloma, lymphoma, leukemia) may raise calcium levels by increasing bone resorption. Bronchogenic tumors may produce a substance similar to PTH, PTH-related protein (PTHrP), that acts on the PTH receptors to increase serum calcium. Prolonged bed rest may aggravate hypercalcemia in cancer patients. Other causes include increased intestinal absorption (sarcoidosis, hypervitaminosis A or D), increased renal reabsorption (thiazide diuretics, Addison's disease), and ingestion of large amounts of calcium carbonate and milk (milk-alkali syndrome).

SIGNS & SYMPTOMS

"Bones (bony pain), stones (renal stones), abdominal groans (constipation, nausea, vomiting), and psychic moans (emotional lability, fatigue)." Renal stones may result in acute urinary tract obstruction. Polyuria occurs because the excess calcium blocks ADH receptor sites in the distal convoluted tubules. A small subset of patients develops pancreatitis.

DIAGNOSIS

A large proportion of calcium is bound to albumin in the serum. Patients with low albumin levels have low total calcium levels, although their free calcium levels may be normal. To adjust for the effect of low albumin, the lower limit of normal for calcium (usually 8.4 mg/dL) should be shifted down by 0.8 mg/dL for every 1.0 g/dL of albumin below normal (4.0 g). For example, if the patient's albumin level is 3.0 (1.0 g below normal), a total calcium level of 7.6 mg/dL (0.8 mg/dL below normal) would still be considered normal.

The diagnosis is made by demonstrating high levels of calcium, after adjusting for albumin level. Extreme hypercalcemia is more likely to be malignancy than hyperparathyroidism. PTH is high in hyperparathyroidism and low in malignancies that produce PTHrP.

Aggressive, continuous hydration, followed by furosemide (not thiazide diuretics!) to promote calciuria after the patient is well hydrated. Bisphosphonates such as pamidronate, calcitonin, and gallium nitrate help by inhibiting bone resorption.

Hypocalcemia

Etiologies of hypocalcemia include hypoparathyroidism, vitamin D abnormalities (deficiency, malabsorption, or impaired metabolism, for example in renal failure), renal tubular defects, alcoholism, diuretic therapy, and acute pancreatitis.

Tetany and seizures occur in severe cases. Chvostek's sign (tapping the facial nerve in front of the ear elicits facial contraction) and Trousseau's sign (inflating a blood pressure cuff for 3 minutes causes carpal spasm) may be present. QT prolongation can predispose to ventricular arrhythmias.

Both total serum calcium corrected for albumin and ionized serum calcium are low. Serum phosphate is high in hypoparathyroidism and renal failure but not in vitamin D deficiency. If serum magnesium is low, it can exacerbate hypocalcemia by decreasing PTH secretion and tissue responsiveness to PTH.

IV or oral calcium, depending on the urgency of the presentation. Vitamin D. Magnesium if necessary.

Hemochromatosis

Hemochromatosis is a common autosomal-recessive disease in which there is increased GI absorption of iron. Iron accumulation over time causes multiple organ damage. Clinical disease is much more common in men because women lose some of the excess iron during menses. As many as 15% to 20% of patients with cirrhosis develop hepatocellular carcinoma.

Hepatomegaly with eventual cirrhosis; diabetes mellitus; and bronze pigmentation of the skin. The last two characteristics give rise to the commonly used name "bronze diabetes." Testicular atrophy, cardiomyopathy (cardiomegaly, heart failure, and arrhythmias), and hypopituitarism also occur.

Serum ferritin (reflecting the body's iron stores) and transferrin saturation (the ratio of serum iron to total iron-binding capacity) are increased.

Liver biopsy shows increased iron content.

Regular phlebotomy (removal of blood) is used to decrease iron stores. Deferoxamine, an iron-chelating agent, may also be given. Screening of family members may be helpful in early diagnosis.

Wilson's Disease

Wilson's disease is a rare autosomal-recessive disease that involves impaired copper excretion into the bile, thereby resulting in copper retention. It is most commonly diagnosed in patients 10 to 40 years of age.

Copper accumulation in the liver causes chronic hepatitis and cirrhosis. Copper in the CNS causes tremor, ataxia, psychoses, and dementia. All patients with neuropsychiatric signs have the pathognomonic Kayser-Fleischer rings, which are golden-brown or gray-green rings of pigment at the edge of the cornea that are often grossly visible but can otherwise be visualized by slit-lamp examination.

Low serum ceruloplasmin, the copper-binding protein, increased copper stores on liver biopsy, and increased urinary copper. LFTs may be normal.

Penicillamine chelates copper and reverses most of the disease process. Family members should be screened for the disease as well.

Heat-related Illness

Heat Stroke

Both the autonomic nervous system and the endocrine system contribute to temperature regulation. Heat stroke occurs when inadequate heat loss leads to hyperpyrexia, with core body temperatures exceeding 40°C. It is fundamentally different from **heat exhaustion**, in which excessive fluid loss precipitates hypovolemic shock. Although the prognosis of heat exhaustion is often good (in the absence of extended circulatory collapse), heat stroke has a mortality rate approaching 50%. Rhabdomyolysis, consumption coagulopathy, and brain, myocardial, hepatic, and renal dysfunction can occur. Heat stroke can be exertional or nonexertional in origin. Impaired awareness (e.g., intoxication or dementia) or inability to escape the heat often contributes to nonexertional heat stroke. Accordingly, risk factors for heat stroke include many medications, drug use, and extremes of age.

SIGNS & SYMPTOMS

Weakness, dizziness, confusion, nausea, and vomiting may precede acute loss of consciousness. The skin is hot and red, often with minimal signs of sweating. Body temperature is high, often exceeding 40°C, and pulse rate is rapid.

DIAGNOSIS

The preceding presentation suggests heat stroke. Creatine kinase, LFTs, coagulation tests, BUN, creatinine, urinalysis, and ECG should be checked to assess complications.

TREATMENT

Immediate emergency cooling is essential because heat stroke can lead to permanent brain damage and death. Rehydration may also be necessary. Complications should be treated. Predisposing conditions should be identified and corrected.

Neoplasms

Multiple Endocrine Neoplasia Syndromes

Multiple endocrine neoplasia (MEN) syndromes are a group of autosomal-dominant syndromes involving hyperplasia or neoplasms in more than one endocrine gland (Table 4-2). All patients who have hyperplasia or neoplasms in one endocrine gland should be evaluated for these syndromes, and the family history should be thoroughly reviewed. **MEN type 1** (Wermer's syndrome) includes parathyroid hyperplasia or neoplasm (90% of those with the disorder); pituitary adenomas (65%); and pancreatic islet tumors (75%), which may secrete insulin, gastrin, somatostatin, ACTH, vasoactive intestinal polypeptide (VIP), serotonin, or prostaglandin. One third of patients also have adrenal cortical adenomas or hyperplasia, usually without functional consequences. **MEN type 2a** (Sipple's syndrome) includes parathyroid hyperplasia or neoplasm (20%), medullary thyroid carcinoma (90%), and pheochromocytoma (20%). **MEN type 2b** includes the same tumors as type 2a, with medullary thyroid carcinoma (80%) and pheochromocytoma (60%), but parathyroid tumors are much less common. In addition, most patients with type 2b have a marfanoid habitus and neuromas of the eyes, mouth, GI tract, and upper respiratory tract. Treatment of all the syndromes depends on the presentation and is frequently surgical. Mutation of the *Ret* proto-oncogene causes the vast majority of MEN 2a and much of MEN 2b. Screening of family members is advisable for all MEN syndromes.

Table 4-2. Common tumors of MEN syndromes

MEN 1	MEN 2a	MEN 2b
Parathyroid	Parathyroid	Neuromas
Pituitary	Medullary thyroid CA	Medullary thyroid CA
Pancreatic	Pheochromocytoma	Pheochromocytoma
		Marfanoid habitus

CA, carcinoma; MEN, multiple endocrine neoplasia.

ENDOCRINOLOGY

Hormone-susceptible Neoplasms

Cancers that develop in cells along the hypothalamic–pituitary–end-organ axis are often responsive to hormones that function in that axis. Hormone susceptibility is common in breast cancer, endometrial cancer, prostate cancer, leukemia, and lymphoma. Although hormones promote growth of some cancers, they suppress growth of others. Endocrine chemotherapy attempts to suppress tumor growth through the use of either hormone receptor agonists or antagonists. It is often combined with cytotoxic chemotherapy or surgery.

Paraneoplastic Disorders

Paraneoplastic disorders are syndromes caused by the indirect effects of tumors at sites removed from the tumor site. Most paraneoplastic disorders result from secretion of ectopic hormones from tumor cells. Destruction of bone with resulting hypercalcemia is another mechanism. Ectopic hormone secretion occurs in approximately 10% of patients with advanced malignancies, most often involving small cell and squamous cell lung cancers, breast cancer, and thyroid cancer. Commonly secreted hormones include insulin, VIP, norepinephrine, ACTH, ADH, calcitonin, and PTH.

SIGNS & SYMPTOMS

The effects are determined by the specific hormone secreted. For example, insulinomas cause hypoglycemia, whereas pheochromocytomas, which secrete epinephrine and norepinephrine, lead to palpitations and hypertension. Other possible clinical manifestations include Cushing's syndrome that is due to ectopic ACTH secretion, hyperthyroidism that is due to ectopic TSH secretion, and hypercalcemia that is due to ectopic PTH secretion.

DIAGNOSIS

The constellation of symptoms should suggest the diagnosis in a patient with a known malignancy. Otherwise, the malignancy must be sought.

TREATMENT

Treat the underlying malignancy as much as possible. Control of symptoms may be achieved with medications specific to the hormonal effects.

5

Genitourinary Disorders

Disorders of the Bladder and Ureters

GENITOURINARY

Definitions

Dysuria

Painful urination is a symptom commonly associated with bacterial infections of the lower and upper urinary tract. If bacteria are not present and symptoms are persistent, other sources of inflammation, including neoplasms, must be ruled out.

Hematuria

Blood in the urine can be macroscopic or microscopic. If pain is also present, blood is often due to infection or a stone passing in the ureter. If no pain is present, blood may be due to a kidney or bladder tumor, renal cysts, or prostatic disease. Glomerulonephritis is indicated by the presence of RBC casts in the urine.

Pyuria

White blood cells in the urine are prominent in urinary tract infections (UTIs) but may also be a nonspecific sign of inflammation. In particular, WBC casts in the urine indicate nephritis, which may or may not be infectious.

Obstruction

Obstruction of urine flow can occur at the kidney, ureter, bladder, or urethra. Possible causes include stones, tumors, fibrosis at sites of injury, and, in men, an enlarged prostate gland. The complications of obstruction include hydronephrosis and urinary stasis, leading to stone formation, infection, and loss of kidney function.

Oliguria and Anuria

Oliguria is the reduction of urine output to less than 500 ml/day, whereas anuria is the absence or severe reduction of urine output, generally less than 100 ml/day. These conditions may occur as a result of prerenal factors (dehydration, bilateral renal artery occlusion), renal factors (acute renal failure), or postrenal factors (bladder outlet obstruction).

Azotemia

Azotemia is the accumulation of excess nitrogenous wastes in the blood in the form of urea, creatinine, ammonia, or uric acid. It is often a sign of kidney failure but may also be the result of increased protein digestion (e.g., during a gastrointestinal bleed) or increased protein catabolism (e.g., severe burns). Uremia is often used as a synonym for azotemia, but uremic syndrome is a separate clinical entity.

Cystitis

Bladder infections, or cystitis, are common in sexually active women. They are more rare in children, especially boys, and should prompt a search for congenital abnormalities or vesicoureteral reflux (see Chapter 8), which can lead to renal scarring and insufficiency. Infections in the elderly have an equal gender distribution. *Escherichia coli* is the most common causative organism. Hospitalized patients with indwelling Foley catheters may be infected with *Pseudomonas*.

The classic symptoms are urinary frequency, urgency, dysuria, nocturia, and suprapubic pain. Gross hematuria may be present.

A urine specimen is obtained using a "clean catch" (midstream urine), urethral catheterization, or suprapubic bladder aspiration. WBCs and more than 100,000 bacteria/mL indicate infection.

Trimethoprim-sulfamethoxazole, fluoroquinolones, or other appropriate antibiotics are started empirically and may be adjusted based on culture results.

Urolithiasis

Most stones of the urinary tract contain calcium, and hypercalciuria predisposes to the formation of calcium stones. Patients with hypercalciuria should be worked up, as they may have a treatable disorder (e.g., primary hyperparathyroidism). However, more than half of the cases of hypercalciuria are due to a hereditary condition called **idiopathic hypercalcinuria.** Individuals with this condition can take preventive measures (outlined in Prevention) to avoid developing urinary stones. Struvite stones compose 10% to 15% of urinary tract stones and develop when a UTI with a urea-splitting bacteria (e.g., *Proteus, Klebsiella,* or *Pseudomonas*) makes the urine basic enough to precipitate struvite (magnesium ammonium phosphate). Stones may also form from uric acid or, rarely, cystine.

Sudden and severe pain, known as *renal colic,* results from the backup of urine that occurs when a stone blocks the urinary collecting system. The pain may be in the flank, abdomen, or groin, and, depending on the location of the blockage, may be referred to the inner thigh or either the labia majora or the testicle. The pain typically lasts 20 to 60 minutes. Dysuria, frequency, and nausea and vomiting may also be present. Hematuria occurs in most cases. Patients are typically uncomfortable lying still but unable to find a comfortable position.

Urinalysis shows hematuria. Abdominal x-rays reveal 85% of stones. IV urogram shows filling defects at the site of obstruction. CT scan and ultrasonography may also show stones or hydronephrosis.

Aggressive hydration may help flush the stone out. Narcotics are often necessary to relieve pain. Lithotripsy (ultrasound) can shatter small stones and allow them to be passed through the system. If lithotripsy is not possible and pain continues, surgery is indicated.

Drinking plenty of water and avoiding calcium reduce the risk of forming calcium stones. Thiazide diuretics lower urinary calcium in patients with idiopathic hypercalcinuria. Acidification of the urine and aggressive treatment of UTIs may help prevent struvite stone formation.

Neurogenic Bladder

Bladder control requires intact sensation (to feel when the bladder is full), motor function (to initiate emptying the bladder), and cerebral control (to inhibit sympathetic-mediated sphincter tone and allow voiding). Damage at any level of this complex loop results in neurogenic bladder.

An atonic, distended bladder with overflow dribbling occurs in acute spinal cord injury ("shock bladder") or when the sensory component of control is impaired, as occurs in diabetic patients. If the motor component is damaged, as in polio, trauma, and some cases of tumor invasion, the patient can sense a full bladder but cannot initiate voiding. An autonomous bladder develops in spinal cord–injured patients after their acute recovery. The bladder fills and empties by reflex, and there is no cerebral control.

Evaluation includes urodynamic studies to assess bladder sensation, capacity, postvoid residual volume, and sphincter control. Voiding cystourethrogram is used to rule out obstruction and reflux.

Medications can improve sphincter control, decrease detrusor spasticity, or increase autonomic stimulation. Regular catheterization can be done by the patient or an assistant. Surgical redirection of the urinary tract is also possible.

Bladder Carcinoma

Transitional cell carcinoma is the most common type of bladder cancer. Risk factors include smoking, schistosomiasis infection, and aniline dyes. Men are affected three times more often than women. Squamous cell cancer and adenocarcinoma are less common.

Painless hematuria is the most common finding. Frequency or dysuria may occur as the tumor grows and occupies the bladder space or invades the bladder wall. A suprapubic mass may be palpable.

GENITOURINARY

Urine cytology shows malignant cells, and IV urogram may reveal the presence of a mass. Cystoscopy and biopsy provide definitive diagnosis.

Surgical resection, radiation, and chemotherapy are used, depending on the stage of the tumor. Bladder tumors tend to recur, so patients should be carefully monitored.

Avoid chemical exposures, particularly cigarette smoke.

Disorders of the Kidneys

Hydronephrosis

Dilation of the renal pelvis because of increased pressure in the urinary system can occur with or without accompanying dilation of the ureter, depending on the site of obstruction. If not corrected, this condition eventually leads to progressive damage of the renal parenchyma and loss of renal function. Obstruction is most commonly due to calculi, neoplasms, or prostatic enlargement.

If chronic, hydronephrosis may be asymptomatic or associated with dull flank pain. Colicky pain is typical in acute cases. UTIs are common, and GI symptoms are particularly frequent in children with congenital ureteropelvic obstruction.

Ultrasound or IV urogram.

Temporary drainage via a nephrostomy tube will relieve acute symptoms. The underlying obstruction must be addressed, usually with lithotripsy or surgery.

Pyelonephritis and Pyelitis

Pyelonephritis (infection of the renal parenchyma) and pyelitis (infection of the renal pelvis) are clinically indistinguishable and are usually due to *E. coli,* which ascends from the lower urinary tract. Obstruction, urinary stasis, foreign bodies, and immune compromise predispose to infection.

Fever, chills, flank pain, nausea, and vomiting are the classic symptoms. There may be associated symptoms of a lower UTI (e.g., frequency, dysuria). On examination, there is costovertebral angle tenderness on the affected side. Septic shock occurs in severe cases.

Pyelonephritis can be distinguished from cystitis by the presence of systemic symptoms and WBC casts in the urine.

Many patients require hospitalization and IV treatment with a fluoroquinolone (e.g., ciprofloxacin) or cephalosporin for 1 to 2 days. After stabilization or in moderately ill patients, oral treatment with a fluoroquinolone for 2 weeks is standard.

Hypertensive Renal Disease

Hypertension is a frequent complication of renal disease and is usually due to salt and water retention. Hypertension can, in turn, worsen renal failure, so careful control of blood pressure is required to break this vicious cycle. Salt and water restriction and antihypertensive medications are appropriate. Angiotensin-converting enzyme (ACE) inhibitors should be used with caution, depending on the patient's renal function. Although ACE inhibitors have been shown to slow progression of renal disease in diabetic patients and reduce renal damage from high blood pressure on the kidney, in some patients they reduce renal perfusion enough to result in renal insufficiency.

Renovascular Hypertension

Stenosis or occlusion of the renal artery causes hypertension via the renin-angiotensin system. The affected kidney receives less blood flow than normal and is fooled into "thinking" that there is systemic hypotension. It releases renin to increase blood pressure. This is the most frequent cause of curable hypertension, although it accounts for only 5%–10% of all cases of hypertension. In the elderly, the most common cause of renovascular hypertension is atherosclerotic disease, whereas in young women, renal artery stenosis is due to fibromuscular hyperplasia of the artery wall.

Persistent hypertension is noted. A renal artery bruit is heard in the upper quadrants of the abdomen in half of patients.

Decreased renal blood flow is seen by Doppler or radioisotope studies after a dose of ACE inhibitors. Arteriography is the gold standard to visualize the lesion.

Angioplasty, renal artery bypass surgery, and vascular stents are common treatment options.

Renal Cell Carcinoma

Renal cell carcinoma, an adenocarcinoma, is the most common renal tumor in adults and is more common in men than in women. Like bladder cancer, it is associated with tobacco use.

The classic triad is hematuria, flank pain, and an abdominal mass. Other symptoms include hypertension, fever, and weight loss.

Polycythemia because of erythropoietin activity is occasionally seen. Urinalysis may show hematuria.

IV urogram, ultrasound, and magnetic resonance imaging can help identify the extent of the tumor.

Surgery of localized disease is the only curative option.

Trauma

Injury to the bladder from external trauma is uncommon, resulting only when serious other injury, including pelvic fracture, occurs. Retrograde cystogram is diagnostic, although treatment of other injuries usually takes precedence.

Most injuries to the kidney result from blunt, rather than penetrating, trauma. Hematuria is present, and intravenous urography or CT scan is diagnostic. Minor injuries may be managed expectantly; others require surgical repair.

Nephritic and Nephrotic Syndromes

Glomerulonephritis

Glomerular injury can arise in a variety of clinical situations.

- **Poststreptococcal glomerulonephritis** is an immune complex–mediated disease that presents as *acute glomerulonephritis*. Group A beta-hemolytic streptococcal antigen-antibody complexes lodge in the glomerular capillary walls and trigger an immune response. This condition is usually preceded by several weeks with an upper respiratory tract infection and is most common in children older than age 3 years.

- **Goodpasture's syndrome** classically presents as a *rapidly progressive glomerulonephritis*. It is an antibody-mediated disease that, although rare, is most common in young men. Immunoglobulin G is deposited in the kidney and the lung, and the associated hemoptysis may be severe.
- **Diabetic glomerulosclerosis** is a *chronic glomerulonephritis* in which proteinuria gradually progresses to renal failure and uremia. Lupus is another common cause of chronic glomerulonephritis, discussed below.

There are several patterns by which glomerulonephritis can present. In acute glomerulonephritis, oliguria, periorbital edema, and hypertension are present in addition to the typical laboratory findings. In rapidly progressive glomerulonephritis, uremia develops within 3 to 9 months. In chronic glomerulonephritis, renal function is preserved for many years, but eventually hypertension and uremia develop.

The classic laboratory findings are hematuria, RBC casts, and proteinuria. Oliguria and hypertension may be present.

In poststreptococcal glomerulonephritis, antibiotics are only useful if the underlying infection has not resolved. Otherwise, supportive care is indicated, and resolution occurs within 2–3 months. Goodpasture's syndrome is treated with high-dose corticosteroids, cyclophosphamide, and plasmapheresis to reduce the level of circulating antibodies. ACE inhibitors may forestall the development of diabetic glomerulosclerosis.

Lupus Nephritis

Renal disease is a frequent complication of systemic lupus erythematosus (SLE) and accounts for half of SLE fatalities. There are several types of disease, including mesangial, membranous, focal proliferative, and diffuse proliferative nephritis.

Patients may be asymptomatic or have signs and symptoms of nephritic or nephrotic syndrome.

Proteinuria with WBC and RBC casts on urine microscopy. Renal biopsy confirms diagnosis.

Corticosteroids or cyclophosphamide, an immunosuppressant, can improve survival of the kidney.

GENITOURINARY

Nephrotic Syndrome

Nephrotic syndrome exists when there is proteinuria in excess of 3 g per day. It can be caused by any glomerular disease, but **minimal change disease** is the most common cause in children and **diabetes mellitus** is the most common cause in adults. Albuminuria leads to hypoalbuminemia, which stimulates the liver to produce more proteins. In addition to albumin synthesis, lipoprotein synthesis also increases, leading to hyperlipidemia.

Generalized edema, pulmonary edema or pleural effusion, ascites, pericardial effusion, and hypertension occur because of hypoalbuminemia.

Hypoalbuminemia and hyperlipidemia, which cause the serum to appear milky. Prothrombin time (PT) and partial thromboplastin time (PTT) may be decreased because of the urinary loss of protein C, which normally inhibits clotting. Urine appears foamy, and urinalysis confirms proteinuria.

Proteinuria greater than 3 g per day with edema, hypoproteinemia, and hyperlipidemia is the classic tetrad. Kidney biopsy can identify the pathologic process.

A low-salt diet, corticosteroids, and diuretics can be used. Prognosis is excellent for minimal change disease, although recurrences are common. End-stage renal disease develops in slightly less than half of adults with idiopathic glomerulonephritis. Any underlying disease should be addressed.

Interstitial Nephropathy

Because of its rich blood supply, the kidney is susceptible to damage by substances that do not reach toxic concentrations in other areas of the body. Most often, these substances damage the renal tubules, causing acute tubular necrosis, but the interstitial cells of the kidney can also be damaged, causing tubulointerstitial nephritis. The list of potential toxins is enormous; it includes antibiotics (especially aminoglycosides, amphotericin B, and sulfa drugs), analgesics [both acetaminophen and all nonsteroidal anti-inflammatory drugs (NSAIDs)], heavy metals, iodine-containing contrast dye, pesticides, and mushrooms. Interstitial nephropathy can also be due to infectious or autoimmune processes. Renal insufficiency occurs with sudden onset. It may take good detective work to find the source of nephropathy in an individual patient. The offending agent should be removed and any available antidote given. Supportive care for acute renal failure is indicated.

Renal Failure

Acute Renal Failure

Acute tubular necrosis is the most common cause of acute renal failure not related to pre- or postrenal etiologies. It can be due to toxins (see preceding section) or ischemic injury to the kidney (e.g., from shock, surgery, or rhabdomyolysis after a crush injury). Other causes of acute renal failure include prerenal disease, interstitial nephritis, glomerulonephritis, vascular disease, and obstruction.

The history may provide clues to the etiology of the renal failure (e.g., drug exposure, signs of sepsis, hemorrhage, hypotension). Oliguria or anuria may be present and have an associated increased mortality rate. Uremic symptoms may be present; however, peripheral neuropathy and renal osteodystrophy are only associated with chronic failure (see Uremic Syndrome).

Elevated BUN and creatinine and fractional excretion of sodium indicate a decreased glomerular filtration rate. Urinalysis and urinary sediment may help establish the etiology.

Whether or not the patient is oliguric, fluid intake and output must be carefully balanced to prevent fluid overload. Electrolytes should be monitored. Protein intake must be kept at a minimum to minimize azotemia. Dialysis may be necessary if conservative measures fail. Recovery usually takes several weeks, although irreversible damage can occur.

Potentially nephrotoxic medications (e.g., radiocontrast, NSAIDs, aminoglycosides) should be avoided or accompanied by adequate hydration and renal function monitoring.

Chronic Renal Insufficiency and Failure

The kidney has a great deal of reserve, and chronic renal insufficiency does not manifest symptoms until 90% of the nephrons have been destroyed. Thus, failure can develop over the course of many years. The most common causes of chronic renal failure by far are hypertension and diabetes mellitus, accounting for more than 60% of cases. The problems of renal failure are related to decreased glomerular filtration rate and loss of tubular function.

Symptoms of uremia develop gradually (see Uremic Syndrome). Most patients have hypertension, either primary (leading to renal disease) or secondary (resulting from renal insufficiency).

Serum potassium is high and serum sodium may be low. The kidney is unable to metabolize vitamin D and unable to absorb calcium and excrete phosphate, resulting in hyperphosphatemia and hypocalcemia. This leads to the development of renal osteodystrophy as the bones are broken down to maintain calcium levels. Anemia results from decreased erythropoietin secretion. A metabolic acidosis develops and the urine osmolarity is fixed at approximately 300 mOsm/L.

Azotemia (increased BUN) on a routine laboratory examination is usually the first finding. Abdominal ultrasound typically shows hydronephrosis or small kidneys, except in polycystic kidney disease, amyloidosis, and diabetic nephrosclerosis.

Salt and protein intake should be restricted and metabolic disturbances corrected as much as possible. Dialysis and renal transplantation are indicated if symptoms are uncontrollable with conservative management.

Uremic Syndrome

Symptomatic renal failure is termed uremic syndrome and usually does not develop until the glomerular filtration rate has fallen below 20 ml/min. The wide variety of symptoms develops as a result of fluid and electrolyte imbalances, buildup of toxins, and depletion of necessary substances.

Neurologic symptoms begin to develop first and can include drowsiness, impaired mentation, asterixis (flapping tremor), encephalopathy, coma, and seizures. Hypertension as a result of hypervolemia is common, and congestive heart failure may occur. GI manifestations are also quite common and include anorexia, nausea and vomiting, GI bleeding, and an unpleasant taste in the mouth. The skin develops a yellow-brown color, and in extreme cases, urea from sweat may crystallize on the skin (known as *uremic frost*). Peripheral neuropathy occurs only in chronic uremic syndrome.

A normochromic normocytic anemia results from decreased renal erythropoietin. A moderate metabolic acidosis is present because of impaired hydrogen ion excretion. Serum phosphorus is high and calcium is low, which may lead to renal osteodystrophy (see following section).

Elevated BUN and creatinine in the presence of symptoms is usually diagnostic. Urine volume does not respond to changes in fluid intake, and urine osmolality is close to plasma osmolality because of the kidneys' inability to change the concentration of the urine.

Progression of renal disease can be slowed but generally not halted. Dialysis or transplant may ultimately be necessary.

Renal Osteodystrophy

Renal osteodystrophy develops in chronic renal failure and leads to bony disorders, such as osteitis fibrosa cystica, osteomalacia, osteoporosis, and osteosclerosis. Because of poor renal function, phosphorus builds up in the serum and calcium is spilled in the urine. Vitamin D metabolism in the kidney is also impaired, leading to decreased absorption of calcium in the GI tract. These factors lead to secondary hyperparathyroidism, and parathyroid hormone (PTH) draws calcium out of the bone to restore serum calcium levels to normal. If left untreated, bone pain and fractures occur. Dietary phosphorus restriction and calcium supplementation can halt the course of this disease by raising serum calcium and eliminating the need for PTH to release calcium from the bone.

GENITOURINARY

Dialysis and Transplantation

The ultimate treatments for renal failure are dialysis or transplantation. **Hemodialysis** involves using a machine to filter the blood and redeliver it to the patient. **Peritoneal dialysis** involves infusing dialysis fluid into the peritoneal cavity via a permanent catheter. The peritoneum acts as the dialysis membrane, and substances in the blood diffuse into the dialysis fluid. This fluid is removed after 4 to 6 hours, and new fluid is infused. This procedure can be performed at home, which is often preferred by the patient. Infection is a danger with both methods, but peritonitis is a particular risk of peritoneal dialysis.

Kidney transplantation can be performed using a kidney from a living, related donor or from a cadaver. Donors are HLA-matched before transplantation, but graft rejection is still the biggest concern (see Chapter 9). Cyclosporine and prednisone help suppress rejection. Despite the cost of surgery and immunosuppressive drugs, transplantation is still more cost-effective than long-term dialysis.

Inherited Disorders of the Kidney

Polycystic Kidney Disease

Polycystic kidney disease is an autosomal-dominant disorder with 100% penetrance. Multiple, bilateral renal cysts result in large but poorly functioning kidneys. Some patients have associated intracranial aneurysms.

The disease is usually asymptomatic until adulthood, when it gradually progresses to end-stage renal disease. Hypertension and flank pain are common presenting symptoms. Chronic UTIs, episodic gross hematuria (due to ruptured cysts or dislodged stones), and, ultimately, uremic symptoms are characteristic. Fifteen percent of polycystic kidney disease patients will have subarachnoid hemorrhages, and intracerebral bleeds due to hypertension are equally common. In advanced stages, the kidneys may be palpable.

SIGNS & SYMPTOMS

Proteinuria, hematuria, and pyuria are common. BUN and creatinine are elevated, and anemia may be present.

LABS

Ultrasound or IV urogram shows large kidneys with multiple cysts.

DIAGNOSIS

Aggressive management of UTIs and hypertension extend kidney function. Dialysis or transplantation is required to treat kidney failure; however, familial donation of kidneys may be difficult because half of family members will also have the disease. Genetic counseling should be provided.

TREATMENT

Hereditary Nephritis (Alport's Syndrome)

Hereditary nephritis (Alport's syndrome) is an X-linked disorder of type IV collagen that affects the glomerular basement membrane. Affected males develop renal insufficiency in early adulthood.

Sensorineural deafness and symptoms of renal insufficiency.

The signs and symptoms are usually diagnostic. Tissue analysis confirms the diagnosis.

Dialysis and transplantation are used when uremia occurs. Genetic counseling is advised.

Electrolyte Metabolism

Hypernatremia

Blood sodium concentrations of more than 155 mEq/L most commonly result from dehydration from decreased fluid intake or from increased loss of fluid from skin (burns, sweating) or the intestinal tract (diarrhea and vomiting). Diabetes insipidus, in which a deficiency of antidiuretic hormone (ADH) causes the body to spill dilute urine even in the presence of severe dehydration, is another cause.

Clinical features include decreased urine output (except in the case of diabetes insipidus) and CNS depression from neuronal shrinkage, leading to seizures, coma, and death.

Treatment involves gradual hydration. Patients with diabetes insipidus require ADH analogues such as desmopressin.

Hyponatremia

Hyponatremia refers to blood sodium concentrations of less than 135 mEq/L and is most commonly due to renal retention of excess water. This type of hyponatremia occurs in diseases associated with edema (e.g., congestive heart failure, cirrhosis, and nephrotic syndrome), in the syndrome of inappropriate antidiuretic hormone (SIADH), and in patients taking thiazide diuretics (salt wasting causes hypovolemia, which stimulates ADH secretion). An iatrogenic cause is excessive absorption of irrigant during some endoscopic procedures. Osmotic hyponatremia can occur in patients with hyperglycemia. The excess glucose draws water into the extracellular volume, thereby diluting the sodium concentration. Because this will correct rapidly when the hyperglycemia is treated, the measured sodium level can be adjusted up by 1.6 mEq for every 100 mg/dL of glucose above normal levels.

True hyponatremia should be differentiated from **pseudohyponatremia,** which may be seen in the context of hyperlipidemia. In hyperlipidemia, a large proportion of the plasma volume is taken up by nonpolar lipids, and sodium is excluded from this volume because it is a polar molecule. When plasma electrolytes are measured, it is assumed that sodium is equally distributed throughout the volume, when, in fact, the lipid-containing fraction contains little sodium. This faulty assumption leads to the diagnosis of hyponatremia, although the sodium concentration in the fraction of plasma that contains sodium may be normal.

Sodium levels below 125 mEq/L may lead to irreversible CNS damage as a result of edema of the brain cells. If untreated, this condition eventually results in seizures, coma, and death.

Treatment includes fluid restriction, salt-sparing diuretics, such as spironolactone, and hypertonic saline infusions. **Central pontine myelinolysis** is the destruction of CNS cells when hyponatremia is corrected too rapidly. It occurs most commonly in alcoholics, diuretic users, and patients with malnutrition. Symptoms include progressive weakness of the face and extremities, resulting in a "locked-in" state, in which the patient can only communicate via eye movements. Prognosis is poor.

Hyperkalemia

Hyperkalemia is defined as serum potassium levels of more than 5.5 mEq/L. It is often seen in metabolic acidosis, when hydrogen ions are buffered inside cells, causing potassium to exit from the cells. The kidney is responsible for eliminating excess potassium from the body, so oliguria, potassium-sparing diuretics, and aldosterone deficiency can all result in hyperkalemia. Massive cell damage (e.g., crush injury, hemolysis, and burns) may release enough potassium to cause hyperkalemia as well.

Pseudohyperkalemia is due to hemolysis or release of potassium from blood cells and platelets, after blood is drawn. To avoid this faulty measure, plasma potassium level should be measured immediately, and serum should be inspected for pinkish discoloration that signifies hemolysis.

Clinical features include neuromuscular weakness and cardiac arrhythmias, which can be fatal. The initial ECG finding is peaked T waves.

Treatment involves calcium (to antagonize cardiac effects) and sodium bicarbonate, glucose, and insulin (to stimulate potassium uptake by cells). Potassium binders, such as sodium polystyrene sulfonate (known commercially as Kayexalate), increase potassium loss from the GI tract. Acute treatment may also include dialysis.

Hypokalemia

Serum potassium levels of less than 3.5 mEq/L usually occur with GI or renal loss, although poor dietary intake can be a cause as well. GI loss occurs with vomiting, diarrhea, or chronic laxative use. Renal causes include adrenal steroid excess, potassium-wasting diuretics, osmotic diuresis, and renal tubular disease. Anise, found in some licorice, can mimic aldosterone and cause hypokalemia. In addition, insulin administration can cause acute hypokalemia because potassium accompanies glucose entering the cells.

SIGNS & SYMPTOMS

The most significant symptoms are those of muscle weakness, which may lead to respiratory failure, and cardiac arrhythmias.

TREATMENT

Treatment involves oral or IV potassium administration, usually in the form of potassium chloride.

Acid-base Disorders

Acid-base Survival

We all agree that acid-base disorders are confusing. Just when you think you've got it, a new complicating factor pops up. If you're completely overwhelmed, remember that most questions on the Step 2 exam deal with simple (not mixed) acid-base disorders. To answer these questions correctly, you should be able to carry out steps 1, 2, and 3 in the section on Approach to Acid-base Analysis. A flowchart of these steps is pictured in Figure 5-1. Other details can wait until internship! If you're OK with the basics, adding the compensation and mixed disorders may give you an extra little boost on the exam. Good luck!

Acid-base Physiology

The pH of the blood is normally kept constant by a series of buffers and by the body's ability to excrete excess acid through the lungs and kidneys. The main buffering system is the bicarbonate-carbonic acid buffer, which is described by the following reaction:

$$CO_2 + H_2O \rightleftharpoons H_2CO_3 \rightleftharpoons HCO_3^- + H^+$$

Normal values for the pH, P_{CO_2}, and HCO_3^- are as follows:

pH = 7.40	(7.38 to 7.42)
P_{CO_2} = 40 mm Hg	(35 to 45 mm Hg)
HCO_3^- = 24 mEq/L	(22 to 26 mEq/L)

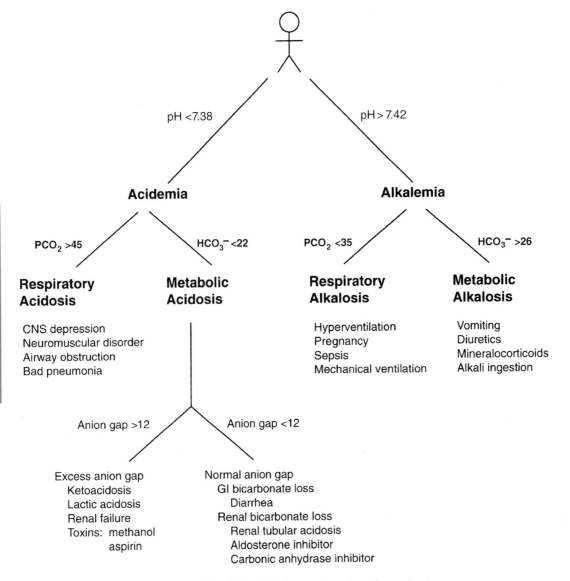

Fig. 5-1. Acid-base disorders flow chart.

In an arterial blood gas measurement, the pH and the P_{CO_2} are directly measured; HCO_3^- is calculated using the Henderson-Hasselbalch equation. However, the HCO_3^- value in a chemistry panel is directly measured, so the directly measured value should be used whenever possible.

When the pH of the blood is >7.42, the blood is **alkalemic;** when the pH is <7.38, the blood is **acidemic.** Note that these terms are different from alkalosis and acidosis, which are based on the physiologic causes of the abnormality. For example, a patient with a blood pH of 7.3 has an acidemia, but physiologically, the patient may have both a metabolic acidosis and a simultaneous respiratory alkalosis.

Disorders of acid-base balance occur when there is a buildup or depletion of CO_2, HCO_3^-, or H^+ driving the equilibrium of the bicarbonate-carbonic acid buffer more in one direction or the other. There are four basic disorders, each caused by a variety of pathologic processes (see Figure 5-1).

- In conditions causing **respiratory acidosis,** such as hypoventilation, CO_2 accumulates in the blood. This forces the bicarbonate-carbonic acid equation to the right, resulting in an increased concentration of H^+ ions (a pH drop).
- The opposite occurs in hyperventilation, in which rapid breathing causes the concentration of CO_2 to fall, the bicarbonate-carbonic acid equation is pulled to the left, and the concentration of H^+ ions drops (pH rises). This condition is called **respiratory alkalosis.**
- **Metabolic acidosis** can occur in two different ways. First, loss of bicarbonate (by the GI tract or kidneys) can pull the reaction to the right, increasing the concentration of H^+. Second, there can be a direct increase in H^+ from another source (e.g., acid ingestion or excess production). Either way, the H^+ concentration rises and pH falls.
- **Metabolic alkalosis** is caused by increased loss of H^+ from the kidneys or GI tract. The drop in H^+ correlates to a rise in pH.

As mentioned, patients can have more than one acid-base abnormality at the same time. This is known as a **mixed acid-base disorder** and can be identified by calculating the corrected serum bicarbonate and by checking that compensatory responses are occurring to the degree expected (Table 5-1). Note that the formulas involve a factor of 0.08 for acute compensation and a factor of 0.03 for chronic compensation.

GENITOURINARY

Table 5-1. Compensation formulas

Metabolic acidosis with respiratory compensation:

Expected $Pco_2 = 1.5 \times (HCO_3^-) + (8 \pm 2)$

- If $Pco_2 <$ expected, a respiratory alkalosis is present.
- If $Pco_2 >$ expected, a respiratory acidosis is present.

Metabolic alkalosis with respiratory compensation:

In metabolic alkalosis, respiratory compensation will not bring the Pco_2 above 50. If $Pco_2 > 50$, a primary respiratory acidosis is present. Conversely, if $Pco_2 < 40$, a primary respiratory alkalosis is present.

Respiratory acidosis, acute (limited renal compensation):

Expected decrease in pH $= \dfrac{0.08 \times (Pco_2 - 40)}{10}$

Respiratory acidosis, chronic (full renal compensation over several days):

Expected decrease in pH $= \dfrac{0.03 \times (Pco_2 - 40)}{10}$

Respiratory alkalosis, acute (limited renal compensation):

Expected increase in pH $= \dfrac{0.08 \times (Pco_2 - 40)}{10}$

Respiratory alkalosis, chronic (full renal compensation over several days):

Expected increase in pH $= \dfrac{0.03 \times (Pco_2 - 40)}{10}$

Anion Gap

The serum anion gap is the difference between the concentration of sodium (the main positive ion in the extracellular space) and the concentrations of chloride and bicarbonate (the main negative ions in the extracellular space). The overall ion balance in the extracellular space is neutral, but there are negative ions (anions) that are not commonly measured. The anion gap quantifies the concentration of these unmeasured ions:

$$\text{Anion gap} = (Na^+) - [(Cl^-) + (HCO_3^-)] \text{ (Normal = 8 to 12)}$$

Typical contributors to a normal anion gap include negatively charged proteins, phosphates, and organic acids.

In metabolic acidosis, the anion gap can be normal or elevated. In normal anion gap acidosis, the acidosis is caused by a loss of HCO_3^- and is offset by a gain in chloride, thus maintaining the anion gap. In anion gap acidosis, the acidosis is caused by the addition of an acid to the system. For example, in lactic acidosis, there is an accumulation of lactic acid. The H^+ is buffered by HCO_3^-, and lactate remains as an unmeasured anion. This leads to a reduction of HCO_3^- and an increase in the anion gap.

The causes of anion gap acidosis can be memorized using the mnemonic **MUDPILES:**

*M*ethanol ingestion
*U*remia (renal failure)
*D*iabetic, alcoholic, or starvation ketoacidosis
*P*araldehyde ingestion
*I*schemia, isoniazid, iron
*L*actic acidosis (hypoxemia, shock)
*E*thanol or ethylene glycol
*S*alicylates (aspirin overdose)

Beyond the Scope

Although it is beyond the scope of the Step 2 exam, it is important to remember in clinical settings that a "normal" anion gap of 8 to 12 is based on patients with a normal albumin level (albumin is one of the most important unmeasured anions). Therefore, if a patient's albumin level is low, as is the case in patients with cirrhosis or nephrotic syndrome, the normal anion gap range should be adjusted down by 2 mEq for every 1 g/dL decrease in the serum albumin level. For example, a patient with an albumin level of 2 g/dL should have an anion gap in the 4 to 8 range.

Also beyond the scope of the Step 2 is the occurrence of an anion gap in alkalosis. If the blood pH is >7.5, additional negative charges on albumin molecules are exposed, increasing the concentration of unmeasured anions and thus the anion gap.

Corrected Serum Bicarbonate

As discussed in the previous section, a higher-than-normal anion gap develops when an acid is added to the system and bicarbonate is used up to buffer the excess hydrogen ions. The corrected serum bicarbonate level is calculated to make sure that the serum bicarbonate would otherwise be normal if bicarbonate had not been used for this purpose. The calculation is as follows:

Excess anion gap = Measured anion gap − Normal anion gap (usually 12)

Corrected bicarbonate = Excess anion gap + Measured HCO_3^-

- If the corrected bicarbonate is in the normal range (22 to 26), then any decrease in measured bicarbonate is due solely to the anion gap acidosis.
- If the corrected bicarbonate is high (>26), then there is an underlying metabolic alkalosis in addition to the anion gap metabolic acidosis.
- If the corrected bicarbonate is low (<22), then there is an underlying nonanion gap metabolic acidosis in addition to the anion gap metabolic acidosis.

Compensation

Whenever there is a primary disturbance in acid-base equilibrium, the lungs and kidney attempt to compensate for the disturbance and return the pH back to normal. If the initial disturbance is respiratory, the compensatory response will be metabolic and vice versa. The amount of compensation for a particular abnormality is fairly predictable but is usually not adequate to completely correct the pH abnormality (see Table 5-1). Renal compensation mechanisms include suppression of acid secretion and extra production or excretion of bicarbonate, but these adjustments take several days to occur. Respiratory compensations, on the other hand, occur rapidly. If the compensation does not correlate with the predictions, a mixed disorder must be sought.

Approach to Acid-base Analysis

On the exam, you will be given arterial blood gas values and serum chemistry levels, and you will be asked to determine which acid-base abnormalities are present. The following provides one stepwise method that can be used for this determination (see Figure 5-1):

Step 1: Is the primary disturbance **acidemia** or **alkalemia**? Remember, acidemia is pH <7.38 and alkalemia is pH >7.42.
Step 2: Is the primary disturbance **respiratory** or **metabolic**?
    In acidemia:
        Respiratory acidosis if PCO_2 >45
        Metabolic acidosis if HCO_3^- <22

In alkalemia:

Respiratory alkalosis if $P_{CO_2} < 35$

Metabolic alkalosis if $HCO_3^- > 26$

Step 3: What is the **anion gap**?

$$\text{Anion gap} = (Na^+) - [(Cl^-) + (HCO_3^-)]$$

Normal anion gap is 8 to 12. If there is a metabolic acidosis and the anion gap is >12, it is an anion gap acidosis. If the anion gap is >20, there is an underlying anion gap acidosis regardless of which other primary disorders are present.

Step 4: If there is a high anion gap, what is the **corrected serum bicarbonate**?

$$\text{Corrected bicarbonate} = \text{Excess anion gap} + \text{measured } HCO_3^-$$

If the corrected bicarbonate is high, there is an underlying metabolic alkalosis. If the corrected bicarbonate is low, there is an underlying nongap acidosis.

Step 5: In metabolic disorders, is the degree of **compensation** appropriate? In respiratory disorders, is the disorder **acute** or **chronic**?

Now you are ready for a few practice problems!

Practice Problems

As with everything in medicine, the more times you practice, the easier it gets. Figure out the acid-base disorders in each of the following:

1. $pH = 7.50$, $P_{CO_2} = 25$, $HCO_3^- = 22.5$, $Na^+ = 138$, $K^+ = 3.2$, $Cl^- = 105$

2. $pH = 7.26$, $P_{CO_2} = 15$, $HCO_3^- = 5$, $Na^+ = 133$, $K^+ = 2.8$, $Cl^- = 118$

3. $pH = 7.50$, $P_{CO_2} = 47$, $HCO_3^- = 36$, $Na^+ = 138$, $K^+ = 3.8$, $Cl^- = 92$

4. $pH = 7.11$, $P_{CO_2} = 16$, $HCO_3^- = 5$, $Na^+ = 140$, $K^+ = 5.3$, $Cl^- = 110$

5. $pH = 6.86$, $P_{CO_2} = 81$, $HCO_3^- = 16$, $Na^+ = 139$, $K^+ = 6.5$, $Cl^- = 84$

Answers:

1. The patient is alkalemic. The P_{CO_2} is low, indicating a respiratory alkalosis. The anion gap of 11 is normal range. The compensation formula for acute respiratory alkalosis more accurately predicts the actual pH [$0.08 \times (40 - 25)/10 = 0.12$ and $7.5 - 0.12 = 7.38$, a pH in the normal range]. Thus, this patient has an acute respiratory alkalosis. Excessive mechanical ventilation can cause this disorder.

2. The patient is acidemic. The bicarbonate is low, indicating a metabolic acidosis. The anion gap is normal at 10. The expected P_{CO_2} matches the actual P_{CO_2} ($1.5 \times 5 + 8 = 15.5$). This patient has a nonanion gap metabolic acidosis with respiratory compensation. Severe diarrhea could account for this picture.

3. The patient is alkalemic. The bicarbonate is high, indicating a metabolic alkalosis. The anion gap is normal at 10. The P_{CO_2} of 47 is consistent with appropriate respiratory compensation. This patient has metabolic alkalosis with respiratory compensation. This could be caused by intractable vomiting.

4. The patient is acidemic. The bicarbonate is abnormally low, indicating a metabolic acidosis. The anion gap is increased at 25, indicating an anion gap metabolic acidosis. The excess anion gap is $25 - 12 = 13$, so the corrected serum bicarbonate is $13 + 5 = 18$, which is below the normal bicarbonate range and indicates that a nongap metabolic acidosis is present as well. The expected P_{CO_2} is $1.5 \times 5 + 8 = 15.5$, so there is adequate respiratory compensation for the acidosis. This patient has both a gap and nongap metabolic acidosis with respiratory compensation. A clinical situation with this set of disorders is diabetic ketoacidosis with early renal failure causing renal bicarbonate loss.

5. The patient is acidemic. Both the bicarbonate and the carbon dioxide levels are abnormal in the direction of the pH, indicating that both a respiratory acidosis and a metabolic acidosis are present. The anion gap is 39, indicating that there is an anion gap acidosis. The corrected serum bicarbonate is $39 - 12 + 16 = 43$, which is above normal bicarbonate levels. This indicates that there is a hidden metabolic alkalosis present as well. This patient has a "triple disorder"—a respiratory acidosis, an anion gap metabolic acidosis, and a metabolic alkalosis. Alcohol ingestion to the point of ketoacidosis, vomiting, and obtundation could cause this picture.

Disorders of the Male Reproductive System

Urethritis

Urethritis in males is most commonly caused by *Neisseria gonorrhoeae* or *Chlamydia trachomatis* and is classified as "gonococcal" urethritis and "nongonococcal" (chlamydial) urethritis.

SIGNS & SYMPTOMS

Purulent urethral discharge is seen in gonorrhea, and thin, white, mucoid discharge is seen in chlamydia. Dysuria, frequency, and urgency may also occur.

DIAGNOSIS

Gonorrhea is diagnosed by finding gram-negative diplococci within WBCs on Gram's stain or by a positive Thayer-Martin culture. Chlamydia is presumed if the Gram's stain is negative. DNA probes are also diagnostic.

TREATMENT

Ceftriaxone (for gonorrhea) and doxycycline or azithromycin (for chlamydia) are used together because of the high incidence of co-infection. If left untreated, urinary strictures can develop. Sexual partners should be treated.

GENITOURINARY

Urethral Stricture

Congenital strictures are rare and usually result from a thin diaphragm across the urethra. Acquired strictures may result from trauma, instrumentation, or infection (especially gonorrhea). Symptoms include dysuria, weak or spraying urine stream, urinary retention, or UTIs. Retrograde urethrogram demonstrates the location of the stricture. Treatment is by surgical incision.

Epididymitis

Epididymitis is inflammation of the epididymis, which is the coiled tube continuous with the vas deferens that lies posterior to the testis. It often coexists with orchitis (inflammation of the testicles). Epididymitis and orchitis can be caused by urinary reflux, prostatitis, urethral instrumentation, and sexually transmitted diseases.

SIGNS & SYMPTOMS

Induration and intense tenderness of the spermatic cord. Supporting the testis relieves pain somewhat. As the inflammation progresses, the epididymis and testicle become one large inflamed mass.

DIAGNOSIS

Urinalysis reveals bacteria and WBCs. Culture for gonorrhea and chlamydia should be performed.

TREATMENT

Tetracycline, or other broad-spectrum antibiotic. If gonorrhea or chlamydia is suspected, they should be treated appropriately as above.

Torsion of the Testis

Torsion of the testis is caused by the twisting of the spermatic cord, cutting off blood supply to the testis. This condition occurs most commonly in adolescent boys.

SIGNS & SYMPTOMS

Exquisitely tender, swollen, and superiorly displaced testis. Supporting the testis does not relieve pain (compare with epididymitis). Sometimes, a knot can be felt in the spermatic cord above the testis. Nausea, vomiting, and fever may also be present.

DIAGNOSIS

If the diagnosis is in doubt, a testicular perfusion or color flow Doppler ultrasonography scan may be used.

Emergency surgery to restore blood supply to the testis and prevent gangrene is required within 4–7 hours (this is no time for long emergency room waits!). Orchiopexy (attachment of the testes to the scrotum) is then performed bilaterally to prevent recurrence.

Hydrocele

If a painless scrotal lump can be transilluminated (i.e., light passes through it when it is lit from behind), it is most likely an accumulation of sterile fluid called a hydrocele. No treatment is necessary unless the cystic mass becomes larger and painful. A congenital hydrocele results when the processus vaginalis remains in open communication with the abdominal cavity. This condition may resolve spontaneously, but if it does not, the child is at risk for developing indirect inguinal hernias.

Varicocele

A varicocele is a collection of veins that occurs most often in the left scrotum. A "bag of worms" can be palpated when the patient is standing, but it is absent when the patient lies down. The etiology is unclear but may be due to compression of venous flow. When occurring in children, a search for intra-abdominal or retroperitoneal pathology is indicated. Varicocele is associated with infertility, presumably because of increased temperature in the testes, inhibiting sperm production. Surgical treatment may be helpful if infertility or pain is a problem.

Testicular Neoplasms

Of the several types of testicular neoplasms, seminomas are the most common and have the best prognosis. This is the most common neoplasm in males 15 to 35 years old. Men who have a history of undescended testes are at increased risk.

Patients present with a painless testicular mass that does not transilluminate. Symptoms of metastasis, such as cough or lymphadenopathy, may be present.

Transillumination and ultrasound localize the tumor to the testis. Biopsy is diagnostic.

Chemotherapy and irradiation are used to treat some seminomas. Orchiectomy is necessary for other types of tumor. Five-year survival rates of patients with seminomas are higher than 80%, and cure is possible even if disease is metastatic.

GENITOURINARY

GENITOURINARY

Prostatitis

Bacterial infection of the prostate can be acute or chronic. Gram-negative GI organisms are most commonly involved. Nonbacterial prostatitis is more common than bacterial but the etiology is unknown.

Low back and perineal pain are accompanied by urinary frequency, urgency, and pain on urination. Acute prostatitis may cause chills and fever. The hallmark of chronic prostatitis is recurrent UTIs. Rectal examination usually reveals a tender, warm, boggy prostate.

Bacterial counts from prostatic specimens are high. Prostatic secretions from nonbacterial prostatitis have WBCs but no bacteria. Hematuria may result from UTIs.

Trimethoprim-sulfamethoxazole or ciprofloxacin are used because of their ability to achieve high concentrations in prostatic secretions. Treat for gonorrhea and chlamydia in men younger than 35 years of age. Antibiotic use is controversial for non-bacterial prostatitis.

Benign Prostatic Hyperplasia

Benign adenomatous hyperplasia of the prostate gland is common in older men. Because the hyperplasia is usually periurethral, varying degrees of bladder outlet obstruction occur. Bladder distention, UTIs, hydronephrosis, and altered renal function may develop.

Symptoms of urinary obstruction include hesitancy, straining, decreased stream, dribbling, sense of incomplete emptying, and urinary retention. Irritative symptoms, including frequency, urgency, nocturia, and urge incontinence, may be the result of incomplete bladder emptying or UTIs.

Digital rectal examination may reveal a large, fleshy prostate, but transrectal ultrasound is a more accurate test. Measurement of urinary flow rate can document urinary obstruction. Prostate-specific antigen (PSA) may be mildly elevated.

Alpha-blockers (prazosin, terazosin) inhibit contractions of the urinary bladder sphincter. If symptoms cannot be controlled medically, surgical treatment is indicated. The most common intervention is transurethral prostatectomy.

Prostate Carcinoma

Adenocarcinoma of the prostate is the most common cancer found in men other than skin cancer. Its incidence increases with age. In contrast to benign prostatic hyperplasia, prostate cancer usually develops in the peripheral regions of the prostate. Prognosis is good with early recognition and treatment.

Patients are often asymptomatic. On examination, the prostate is firm, nodular, or irregular. Symptoms occur late in disease and include bladder outlet obstruction, hematuria, and pyuria. Many patients present with back pain from bony metastases.

Serum alkaline phosphatase and PSA are elevated.

Ultrasound is used to direct biopsies. Bone scan will show bony metastases.

Radical prostatectomy and radiation are both used; however, impotence and incontinence are common side effects of these treatments. In late-stage disease, hormone therapy may prolong life for several years. Older men with well-differentiated tumors may choose to delay treatment ("watchful waiting") because tumors tend to progress quite slowly.

After age 50, PSA is recommended as a screening test for prostate cancer; however, false-positives are common because patients with benign prostatic hyperplasia may also have elevated PSA levels. A free PSA can be measured, and lower free PSA values correlate with a higher risk of a cancer diagnosis.

Impotence

Impotence, or erectile dysfunction, is a consistent inability to obtain and maintain an erection. Penile erection and ejaculation require intact penile innervation, intact penile circulation, and a normally functioning hypothalamic-pituitary-gonadal axis. Impotence may be psychogenic or organic; however, patients with organic causes of impotence often develop components of psychogenic impotence as well as a result of "performance anxiety." The most common cause of organic impotence is vascular insufficiency. Diabetic patients are especially prone to impotence, with both vascular insufficiency and diabetic neuropathy as the primary causes. Impotence is also a side effect of many drugs, such as antihypertensives (e.g., beta-blockers and vasodilators), antidepressants, and tranquilizers. Chronic abuse of alcohol or street drugs may cause impotence as a result of testicular atrophy or neuropathy.

Patients may need to be specifically questioned about sexual dysfunction because many are reluctant to address the topic independently. Testes may be atrophied, indicating testosterone deficiency. Distal pulses may be diminished or absent, and patients may report claudication, indicating peripheral vascular disease. Absence of anal wink on stimulation indicates possible neuropathy.

LABS

Serum testosterone, luteinizing hormone, and prolactin levels may identify an endocrinologic abnormality. Glucose level and thyroid function tests may be performed.

DIAGNOSIS

History and physical examination. Nocturnal penile tumescence measurement helps differentiate between psychogenic and organic impotence because nocturnal erections continue in psychogenic impotence.

TREATMENT

Addressing the primary cause (e.g., testosterone injections in cases of deficiency, changing medications) is often helpful. Other treatments include vacuum devices, penile prostheses, papaverine injections, and the oral medication sildenafil (Viagra).

GENITOURINARY

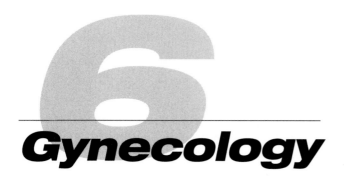

Gynecology

Normal Physiology

The normal ovulatory cycle consists of a **follicular phase** and a **luteal phase** (Figure 6-1). The follicular phase begins on the first day of menses and is characterized by the development of the ovarian follicle. Follicle-stimulating hormone (FSH) secretion from the pituitary gland increases, stimulating growth of the ovarian follicle, which then secretes estradiol. Estradiol (in the absence of progesterone) drives the proliferation of the endometrium. Thus, the fol-

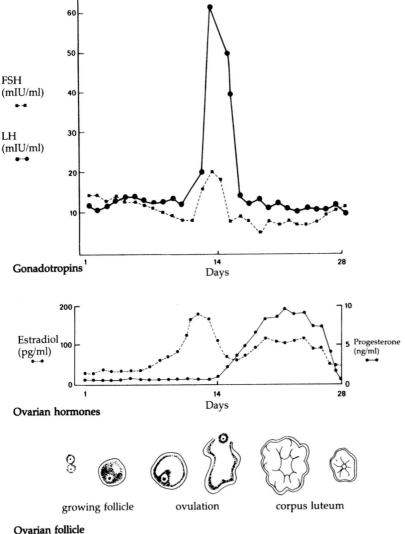

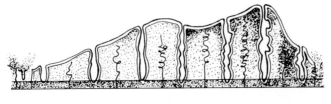

Fi. 6-1. Physiology of the normal ovulatory menstrual cycle. FSH, follicle-stimulating hormone; LH, luteinizing hormone. (Reprinted with permission from Emans S, Goldstein D: *Pediatric and Adolescent Gynecology,* 3rd ed. Boston, Little, Brown, 1990.)

licular phase of the ovary corresponds to the **proliferative phase** of the uterus. Luteinizing hormone (LH) secretion from the pituitary begins to increase after a lag of several days. As ovarian estradiol levels rise, a positive feedback loop develops, with the increasing estradiol enhancing LH and FSH levels. This process culminates in the midcycle LH and FSH surge that precipitates ovulation.

The luteal phase begins with the LH surge and its accompanying ovulation and ends with the onset of menses. After ovulation, the follicle is called the **corpus luteum.** The corpus luteum continues to secrete estradiol and begins to secrete progesterone. After the LH surge, a negative feedback loop is re-established such that the elevated estradiol and progesterone levels now suppress LH and FSH secretion. The elevated progesterone levels also cause the endometrial lining to develop secretory ducts. Thus, the luteal phase of the ovary corresponds to the **secretory phase** of the uterus, during which the endometrium prepares to accept a fertilized egg. If no egg is fertilized, the decreased LH level allows the corpus luteum to regress, leading to a decline in progesterone and estradiol levels. This decline results in ischemia and sloughing of the endometrial lining (menstruation). The decrease in estradiol and progesterone allows FSH to increase, driving follicular growth in the next cycle.

If fertilized, the egg will implant in the endometrium. The early placental tissue secretes human chorionic gonadotropin (hCG), which acts like LH to maintain the corpus luteum. The corpus luteum continues to secrete progesterone to maintain the uterine lining until approximately week 6 of pregnancy, when the placenta begins to produce its own progesterone for this purpose.

The production of mature sperm occurs continuously throughout a man's life. Sperm generation occurs in the seminiferous tubules of the testis. The sperm then travel to the epididymis, gaining motility and nutrients to prepare for the further journey. The development process takes approximately 70 days.

In contrast to spermatogenesis, the number of diploid precursors of ova in girls is fixed before birth. Each month, FSH causes a group of follicles to begin maturation. One follicle will dominate and be expelled from the ovary (ovulation). Unlike spermatogenesis, in which each precursor develops into four equal sperm cells, each ovum precursor develops into one ovum and three smaller polar bodies.

Contraception

Behavioral Methods

- **Abstinence** means never having intercourse. Effective, but dull.
- The **rhythm method** involves monitoring monthly cycles, basal body temperature, and cervical mucus to estimate the date of ovulation each month. Sexual intercourse is avoided for several days surrounding this date. This method is safe, free, and acceptable to most religions. However, effectiveness rates vary widely, and this method is ineffective if cycles are irregular.
- **Coitus interruptus** (withdrawal of the penis from the vagina just before ejaculation) is only approximately 75% effective, in part because sperm-containing fluid may leak from the penis before ejaculation occurs. It is also associated with decreased pleasure and is ineffective if withdrawal is not timed properly.

Barrier Methods

- **Diaphragms** and **cervical caps,** used with **spermicide,** provide barriers that block sperm from entering the cervix. These barriers must be inserted before intercourse and must remain in the vagina for 6 to 8 hours after intercourse. If used correctly, effectiveness is more than 98%; however, in practice, effectiveness rates are closer to 80% because of inconvenience and accompanying lack of compliance.
- **Condoms** are sheaths that cover the penis during intercourse, preventing sperm from entering the vagina. Made of either latex or lambskin, they are often used in conjunction with spermicidal cream or foam. Under perfect conditions, condoms are 95% effective in preventing pregnancy; however, in practice, effectiveness rates are less than 85% because of breakage and improper use. Condoms made of latex are the most effective method of protection against STDs, including HIV.
- **Intrauterine devices** (IUDs) are placed into the uterus, where they inhibit sperm passage and embryonic implantation. These are inserted by clinicians and can remain in the uterine cavity for 1 to 10 years. Some IUDs contain progesterone for further inhibition of implantation. IUDs are associated with spontaneous abortion, uterine perforation, and ectopic pregnancy. In women at risk for sexually transmitted disease, IUDs may increase rates of PID.

Hormonal Methods

- **Birth control pills** (BCPs), consisting of low doses of estrogen and progesterone, work by preventing ovulation and by changing the quality of the endometrial lining to interfere with implantation. BCPs are available by prescription only and must be taken daily to be effective. Theoretically, effectiveness rates approach 100%; however, in practice, rates range from 90% to 95%. Side effects include nausea, headache, hypertension, and weight gain. The risk of thromboembolic disease is slightly increased, and smokers older than age 35 years should not be given BCPs because of a higher rate of clots. Progestin-only pills ("mini-pills") are associated with fewer side effects but are slightly less effective than estrogen-containing pills.
- **Medroxyprogesterone acetate suspension** (Depo-Provera) is a progestin analogue that prevents pregnancy by suppressing endometrial development. It is administered via injection every 3 months. Side effects are similar to those of BCPs and include weight gain, headache, nausea, and irregular spotting.
- **Levonorgestrel implants** (Norplant) are a set of progestin capsules placed subcutaneously that provide long-term pregnancy prevention. Typically, six capsules are implanted, and protection lasts for 5 years. Side effects are similar to those of medroxyprogesterone acetate suspension and include weight gain and menstrual irregularities. Patients who wish to become pregnant may have the capsules removed and are usually able to ovulate within 3 months.
- **Emergency contraception,** also called postcoital or "morning after" pills, is used after unprotected intercourse and is frequently recommended after sexual assault. There are several possible regimens. The most common involves two doses of two norgestrel and ethinyl estradiol (Ovral) tablets (a widely available BCP) taken 12 hours apart. This regimen is 97% effective in preventing pregnancy but is associated with high rates of nau-

sea and vomiting. Using levonorgestrel alone (marketed as Plan B) causes fewer side effects and has a 99% efficacy.

Sterilization

Permanent sterilization in men can be achieved with a **vasectomy,** in which the vas deferens is cut and sealed. Follow-up semen analysis verifies results. This surgery is simple and effective, and the success of reversal, if desired, is approximately 60%.

Tubal ligation in women can be done at the time of cesarean section, immediately postpartum, or with laparoscopy at any other time. Efficacy is generally excellent, but ectopic pregnancy must be excluded in a woman with a prior tubal ligation if she presents with pregnancy. Reversal is often effective but places the woman at a particularly high risk for ectopic pregnancies.

Sexually Transmitted Diseases

Gonorrhea

Neisseria gonorrhoeae can cause acute infection of the cervix, urethra, rectum, and pharynx, depending primarily on sexual practices. Disseminated gonococcal infection is the most common cause of septic arthritis among young people. Untreated disease may cause pelvic inflammatory disease in women and urethral strictures in men. Even asymptomatic infections in women can lead to infertility and an increased risk of ectopic pregnancy.

Symptoms depend on the location of the infection and typically begin 1 to 3 weeks after inoculation. Cervicitis may be asymptomatic or may be associated with a purulent discharge. Urethritis is also associated with a purulent discharge and dysuria. Whereas rectal infection is frequently asymptomatic in heterosexual women (who may or may not have engaged in anal intercourse), it is associated with a bloody discharge and pain in homosexual men. Pharyngeal infection is frequently asymptomatic.

Gram's stain shows gram-negative intracellular diplococci. Culture or DNA probes are usually diagnostic.

Ceftriaxone or cefixime. Doxycycline is also given for presumptive co-infection with chlamydia. Sexual partners should be treated.

Chlamydia

Chlamydia trachomatis is an obligate intracellular organism that invades only columnar epithelium. Like gonorrhea, untreated chlamydia in women may result in pelvic inflammatory disease, infertility, and increased risk of ectopic pregnancy. Chlamydia may account for half of the cases of nongonococcal urethritis in men. Anal sex with an infected partner may cause

GYNECOLOGY

chlamydial proctitis. Half of all patients with gonorrhea have co-infection with chlamydia. Infants born of infected mothers are at risk for chlamydial conjunctivitis and pneumonia.

Most women are asymptomatic, but some have urethritis or cervicitis with a mucopurulent discharge. Pain with intercourse, abnormal bleeding, and low-grade fever may be present. Men have a thin, mucopurulent urethral discharge.

DNA probes and immunofluorescence studies of the discharge are diagnostic. Gram's stain is not useful because chlamydia is an intracellular organism.

Doxycycline or azithromycin are effective treatments. Azithromycin or erythromycin can be used during pregnancy and lactation. Sexual partners should be treated.

Pelvic Inflammatory Disease

Pelvic inflammatory disease (PID) can include endometritis, salpingitis, tuboovarian abscess, and peritonitis. It is a polymicrobial infection that is primarily associated with *N. gonorrhoeae* or *Chlamydia,* but *Bacteroides, Escherichia coli,* and streptococci are also frequently involved. Risk factors include multiple sex partners, young age, prior episode of PID, current or past IUD use, vaginal douching, and cervical instrumentation. Long-term complications of PID include adhesions, ectopic pregnancy, infertility, and chronic pelvic pain.

Low abdominal pain is the primary symptom. It often starts within a few days of menses, during which flow may be heavier than normal. Nausea, vomiting, fever, and chills may be severe, and there may be purulent discharge from the cervix. If the urethra is involved, the patient will have dysuria, frequency, and urgency. Abdominal examination reveals uni- or bilateral lower quadrant tenderness; guarding and rebound tenderness are present if the peritoneum is inflamed. Bimanual examination reveals characteristic *cervical motion tenderness* as well as adnexal tenderness.

Leukocytosis with neutrophilia and an elevated erythrocyte sedimentation rate are characteristic.

Diagnosis is frequently based on presentation, but a culdocentesis yielding pus is confirmatory. Gram's stain of cervical discharge may reveal gram-negative intracellular diplococci.

Broad-spectrum antibiotic combinations are started immediately. Patients should be hospitalized if they have fever higher than 38°C, are pregnant, are teenagers, or are not able to tolerate oral intake. Sexual partners should be tested and treated appropriately.

Trichomonas **Vaginitis**

Trichomonas vaginitis is caused by the protozoan *Trichomonas vaginalis* and is generally transmitted by sexual intercourse.

Vaginal discharge is yellow-green, thin, copious, frothy, and malodorous. Pruritus and burning may be mild or severe. A few patients have the classic vaginal or cervical petechiae or "strawberry patches."

Saline wet mount shows the pear-shaped, flagellated, motile organism, often with many WBCs.

Metronidazole for the patient and for her partner.

Syphilis

Syphilis is caused by the spirochete *Treponema pallidum.* It enters the body through tiny abrasions in the skin, multiplies locally, and then spreads systemically.

Approximately 3 weeks after exposure, a *chancre* develops. A chancre is a firm papule that later becomes a painless ulcer with rolled edges and a punched-out base. There may be associated rubbery adenopathy. The chancre heals spontaneously in 6 to 9 weeks if left untreated. **Secondary syphilis** develops as the chancre heals. It involves *condyloma lata* (flat, coalescing papules containing spirochetes) on moist areas of the skin, generalized rubbery lymphadenopathy, a maculopapular rash on the palms and soles, and constitutional symptoms (malaise, headache, anorexia). These symptoms resolve in 3 to 12 weeks and are followed by latent syphilis, an asymptomatic phase. If left untreated for many years, 20% to 30% of patients will develop **tertiary syphilis.** Manifestations can include gummatous syphilis (granulomatous reactions in any tissue of the body) or cardiovascular syphilis (endarteritis of the vasa vasorum leading to injury of the large arteries and occasionally resulting in dilation of the aortic root with aortic insufficiency). **Neurosyphilis** (meningitis; cerebral atrophy caused by spirochetes in the parenchyma; and tabes dorsalis, which involves damage to the posterior columns causing multiple impairments and general paresis) can develop at any stage.

Serologic tests, such as rapid plasma reagin (RPR) and the VDRL test, are positive in 80% to 90% of cases. Diagnosis is confirmed with the fluorescent treponemal antibody absorption (FTA-ABS) test or microhemagglutination assay for antibodies to the treponemes (MHA-TP). *T. pallidum* can be isolated from a primary chancre or lymph node and viewed with dark-field microscopy.

Penicillin G in one intramuscular dose treats all but late latent or tertiary syphilis, which requires repeated doses. Doxycycline or tetracycline are options for penicillin-allergic patients. Pregnant patients or those with advanced disease who are allergic to penicillin require in-hospital penicillin desensitization.

GYNECOLOGY

Chancroid

Caused by the gram-negative rod *Haemophilus ducreyi,* chancroid is a highly contagious venereal disease seen primarily in tropical and subtropical climates.

Within 1 to 14 days of inoculation, a small papule develops on the vulva or penis. The papule then ulcerates, forming a painful ulcer (in contrast to the painless ulcer of syphilis) with a gray base and undermined borders. Inguinal lymphadenopathy occurs in half of cases and can be severe.

Gram's stain of material from the ulcer edge may show the gram-negative rods. Gram's stain and culture of inguinal node aspirates may also be diagnostic.

Ceftriaxone, erythromycin, or azithromycin.

Herpes Genitalis

Herpes simplex virus (HSV) is the most common cause of genital ulcers. It is transmitted in oral or genital secretions. Herpes genitalis infection is most frequently caused by HSV type 2. After the primary infection, HSV DNA remains in the sensory ganglia and may reactivate at any time. During recurrences, new virus particles travel down the nerve to the skin and produce active lesions. Patients should avoid sexual contact while lesions are present because of the high risk of transmission, although they may also shed virus when they are not symptomatic.

Symptoms of initial infection usually appear 3 to 5 days after exposure. Patients with primary infections often have generalized malaise, inguinal lymphadenopathy, and a low-grade fever. Clear vesicles appear, rupture, and form painful ulcers. Lesions later recur in half of infected individuals and are usually preceded by 24 hours of itching, tingling, or burning in the region. Secondary lesions are less severe, smaller, and of shorter duration than primary lesions.

The clinical presentation is usually diagnostic, but a Tzanck smear or a culture of vesicular fluid will reveal multinucleated giant cells with intranuclear inclusion bodies.

Acyclovir, famciclovir, or valacyclovir are not curative but may shorten the duration of the episode and decrease shedding of the virus. Prophylactic antiviral treatment may be used in immunocompromised patients and in those with frequent outbreaks.

Condyloma Acuminata

Also known as *venereal warts,* lesions of condyloma acuminata are caused by human papillomavirus (HPV) 6 and 11. These subtypes are not associated with cervical or penile cancer risk.

Lesions appear on the external genitalia, perineum, anus, or cervix and may be small and discrete or large and cauliflower-like.

Inspection is usually sufficient for diagnosis.

Trichloroacetic acid, cryosurgery, or laser ablation are used for treatment.

Molluscum Contagiosum

Probably caused by a mildly contagious virus, molluscum contagiosum is a benign syndrome that is spread only by direct contact.

Pink, umbilicated nodules ranging up to 1 cm in diameter are visible on the genitalia.

Inspection is sufficient for diagnosis.

Treatment options include liquid nitrogen or removal of the papules with a curette, with subsequent cauterization of the base of the lesions. If untreated, the infection generally resolves within 6 months.

Other Infections

Candida Vulvovaginitis

Most "yeast" infections are due to *Candida albicans,* although other *Candida* species may be involved. Predisposing risk factors include oral contraceptive use, antibiotic use, pregnancy, diabetes mellitus, and HIV infection.

GYNECOLOGY

Intense pruritus and a "cottage cheese" discharge are the primary symptoms. The vulva is tender, red, and swollen. The pH of the discharge is low (4 to 5).

A KOH wet mount shows pseudohyphae and spores. An acidic pH of 4–5 also suggests *Candida*.

Vaginal antifungal medication (miconazole, clotrimazole) or a single dose of oral fluconazole is usually curative. Consider screening for diabetes or HIV if infections are recurrent. Treatment of partners is not necessary.

Bacterial Vaginosis

Bacterial vaginosis is a polymicrobial infection caused by overgrowth of normal vaginal flora. Lactobacilli are replaced with predominantly anaerobic bacteria, generally including *Gardnerella vaginalis*.

An unpleasant vaginal odor occurs, usually with a white discharge. Vaginal or vulvar irritation may be present.

On a saline wet mount, characteristic *clue cells* (epithelial cells with intracytoplasmic coccobacilli) are observed. A fishy odor is released when 10% KOH is added to the discharge (the "whiff test").

Metronidazole. Treatment of partners is not recommended.

Urinary Tract Infections

The majority of urinary tract infections (UTIs) are due to *E. coli*. The remainder are generally caused by other gram-negative organisms. *Chlamydia* may cause urethritis.

Dysuria, frequency, urgency, and suprapubic pain are the typical symptoms. Fever, chills, and costovertebral angle tenderness indicate that the infection has ascended to the kidneys.

Urinalysis showing positive leukocyte esterase, centrifuged urine with WBCs and bacteria, and urine culture with more than 100,000 bacteria/mL are indicative of UTI. Persistent pyuria without bacteriuria may indicate chlamydial infection.

Trimethoprim-sulfamethoxazole, fluoroquinolones, or, if *Chlamydia* is suspected, doxycycline.

Bartholin's Gland Abscess

An abscess often occurs from secondary infection of a Bartholin's cyst.

An uninfected cyst presents as a unilateral swelling in the lateral posterior introitus. It may be painful. An abscess is tender and inflamed.

Cysts do not need treatment, but they can be drained if they are troublesome to the patient. Sitz baths can be used to treat an abscess, but they generally require incision and drainage. For a recurrent abscess, marsupialization is suggested.

Toxic Shock Syndrome

The multisystem condition toxic shock syndrome is caused by the exotoxin from certain strains of *Staphylococcus aureus*. Most frequently associated with tampon use, it has also resulted from prolonged use of intravaginal contraception and from nasal packing, septic abortions, and postpartum infections.

Patients usually present with sudden high fever, a sunburn-like rash, and a constellation of systemic symptoms, including diarrhea, vomiting, sore throat, and headache. Hypotensive shock develops within several hours. Severe cases may involve adult respiratory distress syndrome and disseminated intravascular coagulation. Desquamation of the palms and soles occurs approximately 10 days into the illness.

The clinical presentation suggests the diagnosis. Culture of the vagina (or other site of infection) may reveal *S. aureus*.

Remove any foreign bodies. Aggressively treat hypotension with fluids, transfusions, and dopamine, as necessary. Penicillinase-resistant penicillins will not affect symptoms, which are caused by the exotoxin, but will reduce recurrences.

GYNECOLOGY

Disorders of Pelvic Support

Pelvic Relaxation

The pelvic organs are supported by the muscles of the pelvic floor and their ligaments. Pelvic relaxation is a weakness of these ligaments resulting in prolapse of pelvic organs. **Uterovaginal prolapse** is the descent of the uterus through the urogenital diaphragm into the vagina. **Cystocele** is the descent of the bladder into the upper anterior vaginal wall (Figure 6-2). **Urethrocele** describes the bulging of the urethra into the lower anterior vaginal wall without urethral dilation. A **rectocele** involves prolapse of the rectum into the lower posterior vaginal wall (Figure 6-3), and an **enterocele** is the prolapse of a loop of intestine into the upper posterior vaginal wall. Enteroceles are almost always due to herniation of the pouch of Douglas.

SIGNS & SYMPTOMS

Patients may report a bulge or the feeling that "something is falling out." Cystocele may be associated with urinary urgency, frequency, incontinence, and, rarely, retention. Symptoms of rectocele include difficulty emptying the rectum.

DIAGNOSIS

Vaginal examination is required for the diagnosis of pelvic relaxation. If prolapse is not apparent, having the patient strain may precipitate it.

TREATMENT

Asymptomatic pelvic relaxation does not require any intervention. For symptomatic cases, definitive treatment is surgical, although perineal exercises ("Kegel exercises") and pessaries may be helpful.

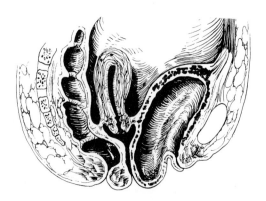

Fig. 6-2. Cystocele. (Reprinted with permission from DeCherney A, Pernoll M (eds): *Current Obstetric and Gynecologic Diagnosis and Treatment,* 8th ed. Norwalk, Appleton & Lange, 1994, p 810.)

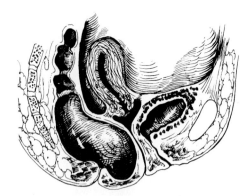

Fig. 6-3. Rectocele. (Reprinted with permission from DeCherney A, Pernoll M (eds): *Current Obstetric and Gynecologic Diagnosis and Treatment,* 8th ed. Norwalk, Appleton & Lange, 1994, p 814.)

GYNECOLOGY

Urinary Incontinence

Involuntary loss of urine is a common symptom, particularly in postmenopausal women. **Stress incontinence** occurs when sudden increases in intra-abdominal pressure (e.g., coughing, sneezing, or exercise) cause leakage of small amounts of urine because of poor bladder support. **Urge incontinence,** also called detrusor instability, generally involves the loss of large amounts of urine due to contraction of the bladder. It is generally preceded by a strong urge to void.

A detailed history about the incontinent episodes, with a voiding diary that includes precipitating factors, should be obtained. UTI and diabetes should be ruled out.

The history is generally diagnostic, but cystometry and urethral pressure studies may be useful. Physical examination may involve the "Q-tip test," which measures the angle of the urethra at rest and during a Valsalva maneuver. If the urethra moves significantly, an anatomic defect is present.

Kegel exercises may improve stress incontinence. Both behavior modification, with biofeedback and bladder retraining, and anticholinergic agents are useful in urge incontinence. Estrogen replacement therapy in postmenopausal women will improve both types of incontinence. Surgery is available for stress incontinence if an anatomic defect is present.

Gynecologic Neoplasms

Vulvar Neoplasms

Malignant tumors of the vulva usually occur after menopause. The majority are squamous cell carcinomas. Pruritus is the most common presenting symptom, although many lesions are asymptomatic until late in the disease. Biopsy confirms the diagnosis and should be followed by surgical excision with lymph node dissection. This type of neoplasm is generally fairly advanced by the time of diagnosis, however, so the prognosis is often poor.

Cervical Dysplasia

Cervical dysplasia is a preinvasive phase of cervical cancer that can be diagnosed by Pap smear. If left untreated, 10% to 15% of mild and moderate dysplasias will progress to invasive cancer, but the majority of lesions will resolve spontaneously. HPV typing is newly available to differentiate lesions that are likely to progress to cancer from those that are likely to be benign, and this typing test is changing the way cervical lesions are followed. Traditionally, however, all lesions are followed closely until they are treated or have resolved. Dysplasia and carcinoma of the cervix are due to infection with HPV types 16, 18, 31, and 33. Other risk factors for dysplasia are consistent with a sexual mode of transmission (multiple sexual partners, early age at first intercourse, and so forth).

Dysplasia is asymptomatic.

During a Pap test, both the ectocervix and the endocervical canal should be sampled. Abnormal lesions can also be visualized by colposcopy because they turn white after the application of acetic acid. Biopsy provides definitive diagnosis. According to the Bethesda system, lesions are categorized as atypical squamous cells of undetermined significance (ASCUS), low grade squamous intraepithelial lesion (LGSIL), high grade squamous intraepithelial lesion (HGSIL), carcinoma in situ (CIS), or carcinoma.

A mild lesion with a low risk HPV type may now be followed with annual Pap smears, although serial Pap tests every 3 months have been the standard of care for ASCUS or LGSIL. Persistent or high grade lesions are treated at the time of diagnosis. Superficial ablation is appropriate if the entire transformation zone (see box) is visible and invasive disease has been excluded. Techniques available include laser ablation, cryosurgery, and electrocautery. For more extensive carcinoma in situ, a cone biopsy or deep electrosurgical excision can be curative.

The **squamocolumnar junction** is the junction between the columnar epithelium of the endocervix and the squamous epithelium of the ectocervix and vagina. Throughout life, this junction moves progressively closer to the os, eventually moving into the endocervical canal. The **transformation zone,** the site most likely to show cervical dysplasia and neoplastic transformation, is the area between the new squamocolumnar junction and the original junction.

Cervical Cancer

Cervical cancer is a direct progression from cervical dysplasia, so risk factors and etiology are the same as for dysplasia. Because of widespread cervical cancer screening, which detects the disease at a more treatable stage, mortality from cervical cancer in the United States is quite low. Histologically, 85% of cervical cancer is squamous cell carcinoma, while the remainder is adenocarcinoma.

Patients with cervical cancer are most often asymptomatic, but some may present with postcoital bleeding or bloody discharge.

An abnormal Pap test suggests the diagnosis, and biopsy confirms it.

Treatment of early stages of cervical cancer is primarily surgical (hysterectomy and pelvic node dissection), and radiation is used in advanced disease (Table 6-1).

GYNECOLOGY

Table 6-1. Stages of gynecologic neoplasms

Stage	Cervical cancer	Endometrial cancer	Ovarian cancer
I	Confined to cervix	Confined to endometrium	Confined to ovary and peritoneal fluid (from ruptured capsule)
II	Extension beyond cervix but not pelvic wall or lower third of vagina	Extension to cervix	Extension into pelvic tissues or organs
III	Extension to pelvic wall or lower third of vagina	Metastasis to or invasion of adnexa, vagina, pelvic nodes, or para-aortic nodes	Extension into abdominal cavity
IV	Extension beyond true pelvis, invasion of bladder or rectum, or distant metastasis	Invasion of bowel or bladder or distant metastasis	Distant metastasis

Uterine Myoma

Uterine myoma, also called *leiomyoma* or *fibroids,* are extremely common, benign masses composed of smooth muscle tissue. They are hormonally responsive, growing only in the reproductive years and generally regressing after menopause.

Many fibroids are asymptomatic. Symptoms may include long and heavy menses, a sensation of pelvic fullness, urinary frequency or obstruction, infertility, and spontaneous abortion. Necrosis of fibroid tissue can cause bleeding and severe pain. On examination, a mass may be palpable.

Anemia, due to excessive bleeding, is common.

Examination, ultrasound, and hysterosalpingography are used to confirm the presence of a uterine mass and are generally satisfactory to establish the diagnosis.

Treatment is not necessary for asymptomatic, slow-growing masses. Myomectomy or hysterectomy are the surgical options.

Endometrial Cancer

Endometrial cancer, an adenocarcinoma, is strongly correlated with high estrogen states. Risk factors include unopposed exogenous estrogen, anovulatory cycles, obesity, early menarche, late menopause, and nulliparity.

GYNECOLOGY

Vaginal bleeding is the most common presenting symptom. Any postmenopausal woman with vaginal bleeding must be evaluated for endometrial cancer.

Endometrial biopsy.

Hysterectomy is usually curative for early stages. Radiation, hormone therapy, and chemotherapy may be used in more advanced disease (see Table 6-1).

Ovarian Neoplasms

Ovarian cancers have a large variety of histologic types and, taken together, make up almost one-fifth of all gynecologic neoplasms. They occur most often in middle-aged women. Most ovarian neoplasms are diagnosed after the disease has spread beyond the ovary, traveling initially by "seeding" into the peritoneal cavity and by lymphatics to regional lymph nodes, and eventually by hematogenous dissemination to the liver and lung. Because diagnosis is often delayed, prognosis is typically poor.

Ovarian tumors are asymptomatic until late in disease. The earliest symptoms are often related to mild gastrointestinal distress or abdominal discomfort. Later, ascites, pain, anemia, and cachexia develop. Early bimanual examination may reveal an enlarged ovary.

The CA-125 level is often elevated in ovarian cancer, although this is not a good screening test because it can be elevated by many other conditions. CA-125 is used in individual patients to follow tumor load.

Workup usually involves an ultrasound to diagnose a mass. Laparotomy, with excision and lymph node dissection, provides tissue for definitive histologic diagnosis.

In a young patient with low-grade disease, a unilateral oophorectomy may be sufficient treatment. More extensive disease requires radical surgery and chemotherapy (see Table 6-1).

Menstrual and Endocrinologic Disorders

Primary Amenorrhea

Primary amenorrhea is the absence of menarche by age 16 years in a woman with otherwise normal secondary sexual characteristic development or the absence of both menarche and secondary sexual characteristics by age 14 years. The keys to diagnosis often lie in a careful history and physical examination and in appropriate laboratory studies. Pregnancy, the most common cause of amenorrhea, should be ruled out regardless of the history.

SIGNS & SYMPTOMS

The patient should be asked about growth and development, exercise and dietary habits, and family history of genetic anomalies. Symptoms of hyperandrogenism (e.g., excess hair growth), thyroid dysfunction, and galactorrhea should be addressed. A history of medications may also be important. On examination, breast development and pubic hair growth should be evaluated (see Physical Changes of Puberty in Chapter 8). Pelvic examination is necessary to check for the presence of a normal vaginal orifice, vagina, uterus, and ovaries.

LABS

Initial appropriate studies include beta-human chorionic gonadotropin (β-hCG) to rule out pregnancy, thyroid function tests, prolactin levels to rule out prolactinoma, and FSH levels to assess the hypothalamic-pituitary axis. A progesterone challenge, with or without estrogen, evaluates for anatomic abnormalities.

DIAGNOSIS

Etiologies of primary amenorrhea include:

- **Anatomic abnormalities.** Imperforate hymen, transverse vaginal septum, vaginal agenesis, and müllerian dysgenesis (congenital absence of the uterus and the upper two-thirds of the vagina) can all cause amenorrhea. Cyclic pain and a vaginal bulge may be noted with imperforate hymen or transverse vaginal septum.
- **Ovarian failure.** These disorders are associated with low levels of estradiol. FSH and LH are elevated (hypergonadotropic hypogonadism) in enzyme defects of the estradiol synthesis pathway and in ovarian dysgenesis (which may be related to the XO karyotype of Turner's syndrome). Ovarian dysfunction, seen in polycystic ovary (PCO) syndrome (discussed later in this chapter), can cause primary or secondary amenorrhea.
- **Pituitary defects.** A prolactinoma of the pituitary may cause amenorrhea by unclear mechanisms. Galactorrhea is a common symptom. Bromocriptine inhibits prolactin secretion and is the treatment of choice. A prolactinoma may also be the cause of secondary amenorrhea.
- **Hypothalamic amenorrhea.** Low levels of FSH and LH are associated with hypogonadotropic hypogonadism, which can be caused by anorexia nervosa, excessive exercise, and emotional stress. These factors may also cause secondary amenorrhea.
- **XY karyotype.** Congenital androgen insensitivity, also called testicular feminization, causes female genitalia to develop in a genetically male fetus. There is no uterus, and the undescended testicles should be surgically removed to eliminate the risk of testicular cancer.

GYNECOLOGY

GYNECOLOGY

Secondary Amenorrhea

Secondary amenorrhea is the absence of menses for at least 6 months in a woman with previously regular menses or the absence of menses for at least 12 months in a woman with a history of oligomenorrhea. Once again, pregnancy must be ruled out.

Galactorrhea may indicate a prolactinoma, whereas hirsutism suggests PCO.

The first step in establishing a diagnosis is a progestin challenge, in which oral progestin is given to see if the patient has a functioning endometrium. If so, she should bleed within 2 weeks of the progestin challenge. If bleeding occurs and the patient is hirsute, PCO is likely. If the patient is not hirsute, mild hypothalamic dysfunction is the likely etiology. If the patient does not bleed, an FSH level should be measured. Low FSH indicates severe hypothalamic dysfunction (usually due to extreme weight loss or exercise), whereas high FSH indicates gonadal failure (as seen in menopause).

PCO and mild hypothalamic dysfunction may be treated with cyclic progestin or oral contraceptives. Ovarian failure may be treated with estrogen replacement therapy. The cause of severe hypothalamic dysfunction should be sought and treated.

Premenstrual Syndrome

Premenstrual syndrome (PMS) occurs only in ovulating women and is independent of the presence of a uterus. After hysterectomy, cyclic symptoms continue if the ovaries are preserved. Although most menstruating women experience some adverse symptoms of PMS, 5% to 10% of women experience severe symptoms that interfere with daily living. A specific etiology for PMS has not yet been identified.

Typical physical symptoms are abdominal bloating, edema and consequent weight gain, breast swelling and tenderness, headache, pelvic ache, altered bowel habits, and decreased coordination. Common psychological symptoms are irritability, depression, anxiety, fatigue, and a change in sleep, appetite, or libido.

Supportive evidence for the diagnosis of PMS includes the regular occurrence of symptoms at the same time in each cycle, onset well after menarche and worsening with age, a positive family history, a history of postpartum depression, and improvement with drugs that inhibit ovulation. When applicable, organic disease should be excluded.

The main treatment options are NSAIDs, oral contraceptives, and progestins. There is some evidence that antidepressants in the selective serotonin reuptake inhibitor family may help with PMS symptoms.

Primary Dysmenorrhea

Primary dysmenorrhea, a common syndrome of cyclic pain associated with menses, frequently begins in adolescence. Prostaglandins (PGF_{2a} and PGE_2) cause uterine contractions and decreased uterine blood flow, which leads to tissue ischemia and pain.

SIGNS & SYMPTOMS

Crampy pain is typical, usually strongest over the lower abdomen and back. The dysmenorrhea usually starts a few hours before the onset of menstruation and may last several days. Nausea, vomiting, fatigue, headache, and diarrhea may be associated.

DIAGNOSIS

The history is usually diagnostic, but further evaluation is indicated if symptoms are severe and cannot be controlled with medication.

TREATMENT

NSAIDs and oral contraceptives may be used alone or in combination.

Secondary Dysmenorrhea

Secondary dysmenorrhea is acquired dysmenorrhea because of an identifiable underlying pathology. It typically occurs in young and middle-aged women. Endometriosis is the most common etiology, but pelvic inflammatory disease, adenomyosis (presence of endometrial glands within the myometrium), uterine fibroids, ovarian cysts, uterine polyps, cervical stenosis, and pelvic congestion should be considered. Laparoscopy is required to diagnose endometriosis. Hysterosalpingogram or ultrasound may be useful to diagnose other etiologies. The underlying disorder must be addressed.

Abnormal Uterine Bleeding

Normal menstruation occurs every 21 to 35 days and generally lasts 3 to 7 days. Normal blood loss is less than 80 cc. Abnormal uterine bleeding involves a change in menstrual frequency, duration, or volume. Menorrhagia is defined as heavy menstrual flow, while metrorrhagia is defined as uterine bleeding between periods. A wide variety of gynecologic and nongynecologic diseases can lead to abnormal uterine bleeding, including uterine fibroids, cervical or endometrial polyps, cervical or endometrial carcinomas, disorders of the hypothalamic-pituitary-ovarian axis, and blood-clotting disorders. Dysfunctional uterine bleeding indicates an abnormal pattern without a clear etiology, and it is often due to anovulatory cycles. Hormonal therapy is used to regulate cycles.

GYNECOLOGY

Endometriosis

Endometriosis is the presence of endometrial tissue outside the uterine cavity. It is estimated that 25% to 50% of infertile women have endometriosis, although many fertile women are affected as well.

Cyclic symptoms are produced when the ectopic endometrial tissue undergoes the same changes during the menstrual cycle as normal endometrial tissue. Progressive dysmenorrhea, dyspareunia, and infertility are the most common symptoms. Examination is usually normal, but rarely lesions are seen on the genitalia or cervix.

Laparoscopy and biopsy are required for definitive diagnosis.

Medical treatment attempts to minimize ovarian stimulation of endometrial tissue. Continuous oral contraceptives, androgens, and gonadotropin-releasing hormone (GnRH) agonists may be used. Surgical treatment includes laparoscopic ablation of ectopic endometrial tissue, which preserves reproductive potential. Postsurgery fertility rates range from 40% to 70%, depending on the severity of initial disease. Surgery for intractable symptoms involves a hysterectomy and bilateral salpingo-oophorectomy.

Hirsutism and Virilization

Androgens are produced in the adrenal glands and in the ovaries. Hirsutism and virilization are the clinical manifestations of increased androgen effects. One cause is **congenital adrenal hyperplasia,** in which a defect of an enzyme in the steroid synthesis pathway (21-hydroxylase, 11β-hydroxylase, or 3-hydroxysteroid dehydrogenase) leads to the overproduction of androgens. Cushing's syndrome, PCO syndrome, adrenal neoplasms, and ovarian neoplasms are other possible etiologies.

Hirsutism is defined as excess body hair in a male hair pattern and is often accompanied by acne and oily skin. Virilism occurs in severe hyperandrogenism and is characterized by the development of increased body hair, muscle bulk, and a deepening voice in a female. Clitoromegaly may be present. In the most severe form of congenital adrenal hyperplasia, the deficiency leads to ambiguous genitalia in female neonates and to life-threatening salt wasting.

A pattern of serum hormone level elevation is helpful in diagnosis.

Glucocorticoid replacement treats congenital adrenal hyperplasia. Treatment of Cushing's syndrome depends on the specific etiology (see Chapter 4). Neoplasms are typically treated surgically.

Polycystic Ovary Syndrome

PCO syndrome affects 1% to 4% of women of reproductive age. It is characterized by a constellation of androgen excess, chronic anovulation, and, frequently, obesity. Hyperandrogenism is typically secondary to androgen overproduction by both the ovary and the adrenal gland. Excess androgen is peripherally converted to estrogen which, when unopposed by progesterone, can cause endometrial hyperplasia or carcinoma. Increased estrogen in turn stimulates excess ovarian androgen production. Chronic anovulation occurs because of both chronic, mild suppression of FSH release and the androgen's antagonism of the follicular response to FSH. Women with PCO syndrome are also at risk for insulin resistance and diabetes.

SIGNS & SYMPTOMS

Hirsutism and menstrual irregularity are present in 90% of patients, infertility in 75%, obesity in 50%, and virilization in 15%.

DIAGNOSIS

Serum LH is high. Multiple ovarian cysts may be seen on ultrasound. A progestin challenge test confirms normal uterine anatomy in an amenorrheic patient.

TREATMENT

Clomiphene, an orally active antiestrogen, is useful in patients who wish to conceive. It blocks estrogen's negative feedback on FSH and allows FSH levels to rise normally, thereby permitting the stimulation of follicular maturation. Otherwise, cyclic oral progestin or oral contraceptives can be used to induce periodic sloughing of the endometrium and eliminate the increased risk of endometrial cancer. Oral contraceptives are also useful in treating patients with hirsutism and acne.

Infertility

Infertility is generally defined as the failure to conceive after 1 year of regular intercourse without contraception. It affects 15% of all couples and 20% of American women older than age 35 years who are attempting to conceive. Abnormalities generally fall into the following four categories:

- **Male factor:** Semen analysis assesses sperm morphology, semen volume (>1 mL), concentration of sperm (>20 million/mL), and sperm motility (greater than 50%). A golden hamster assay is performed, in which the semen is tested for the ability to fertilize a hamster egg. Major causes for decreased semen viability are congenital, chromosomal, and hormonal (e.g., hyperprolactinemia) etiologies and varicoceles (incompetent vein valves). Abnormal tests should be repeated.
- **Cervical mucus:** Functional sperm must be able to interact properly with cervical mucus to travel to the egg. This interaction can be tested by evaluating the postcoital cervical mucus on the day before ovulation. If numerous immobile sperm are seen in the mucus, the sperm may have been destroyed by an overactive immune response. Antibody tests may be appropriate for both partners, and intrauterine insemination may help.

GYNECOLOGY

- **Pelvic factor:** Scarred fallopian tubes can often lead to infertility. A history of damage, such as with PID, STDs, previous ectopic pregnancy, or previous tubal surgery, suggests a tubal factor. Endometriosis or structural abnormalities, such as uterine myoma, can prevent successful implantation. A hysterosalpingogram can assess tubal patency. Surgery may be curative.
- **Ovulatory factor:** Most women who menstruate regularly are ovulating, but this can be evaluated by monitoring the basal body temperature (BBT), which should rise by 0.4°F at ovulation. Sufficient progesterone levels in the luteal phase also reflect ovulation. Abnormal BBT or a history of spontaneous abortion may indicate an inadequate luteal phase, even if ovulation is occurring. This can be evaluated with an endometrial biopsy, which is dated histologically and in relationship to menses. If these dates differ by more than 2 days, a luteal phase defect is present and should be treated with cyclic progesterone. Treatment with clomiphene citrate may enable certain anovulatory women to conceive.

Menopause

The average age of menopause is 51 years, although there is considerable variation. During the perimenopausal period, ovarian response to FSH and LH is reduced, resulting in decreased production of estrogen and progesterone. Without the negative feedback of estrogen, the circulating FSH and LH levels rise substantially.

Premature menopause is defined as ovarian failure before age 40 years. Smoking, chemotherapy, exposure to radiation, and surgery that limits the ovary's vascular supply are all associated with premature menopause. Artificial menopause occurs after bilateral ovary removal or pelvic irradiation.

SIGNS & SYMPTOMS

Symptoms of menopause include hot flushes and sweating, which arise from vasomotor instability; intermittent dizziness, palpitations, tachycardia, and paresthesias; insomnia, fatigue, irritability, and nervousness; nausea, flatulence, diarrhea, and constipation; and myalgias and arthralgias.

Long-term changes associated with menopause develop gradually and are related to the low-estrogen state. They include urogenital atrophy (with associated vaginal dryness, dyspareunia, and urinary frequency and urgency), osteoporosis, and cardiovascular disease.

DIAGNOSIS

The history is frequently diagnostic, but an elevated FSH is confirmatory.

TREATMENT

Estrogen replacement therapy (ERT) relieves acute symptoms and prevents the development of long-term symptoms. ERT may also reduce the risk of cardiovascular disease, osteoporosis, Alzheimer's, and colon cancer. If the patient's dietary calcium intake is insufficient, calcium supplementation is recommended. Progestin must be given with ERT to reduce the risk of endometrial cancer in all patients with a uterus.

Absolute contraindications to estrogen replacement include a history of estrogen-dependent endometrial or breast neoplasms, a history of thromboembolic disease or thrombophlebitis, and severe liver disease. A controversial slight increase in breast cancer risk discourages many women from using ERT.

Vaginal atrophy can be managed with estrogen creams or the use of lubricants during intercourse.

Postmenopausal Bleeding

Postmenopausal bleeding is always abnormal, and malignancy must be excluded. Exogenous estrogens are the cause of 30% of postmenopausal bleeding, but bleeding in this context should only occur during the progesterone withdrawal period. Atrophic endometritis or vaginitis is responsible for another 30% of postmenopausal bleeding. Fifteen percent of cases are caused by uterine polyps or endometrial hyperplasia. The remaining 15% are caused by endometrial cancer.

Disorders of the Breast

Breast Cysts

Solitary breast masses are either solid or cystic. The difference can be established by examination and ultrasound. If cystic, a fine-needle aspiration is indicated. If clear fluid is found and the cyst resolves, no further intervention is necessary, as fluid-filled cysts are generally benign. If, however, bloody fluid is found or there is residual thickening after the fluid is drawn off, excisional biopsy is indicated.

Fibrocystic Change of the Breast

Fibrocystic change of the breast is a common condition of premenopausal women. It is found postmenopausally only in women who take exogenous estrogens.

SIGNS & SYMPTOMS

Multiple, bilateral masses that are tender and fluctuate in size are typical. Minor discomfort frequently increases during the premenstrual period.

DIAGNOSIS

Although the term fibrocystic disease is often used as an umbrella term for mastalgia, breast cysts, and breast lumpiness, the diagnosis is histologic when biopsy is performed. Fibrocystic disease involves hyperplastic changes of the ductal epithelium, lobular epithelium, or breast connective tissue. Only in the 5% of cases with cellular atypia is there an increased risk of breast cancer.

TREATMENT

Women with fibrocystic change should have a baseline mammogram. Fine-needle biopsy of suspicious cystic lesions is indicated, as this disorder can be indistinguishable from carcinoma. Cysts may be present and can be aspirated. If the aspirated fluid is non-bloody and the cyst resolves completely, no further workup is required. However, with bloody aspirate, any remaining nodule, or recurrence, a biopsy is indicated. Oral contraceptives, progesterone, tamoxifen, or androgen therapy is useful in some patients. Diuretics and decreased salt intake may relieve premenstrual, edema-associated mastalgia. The role of decreased caffeine consumption is controversial, but many women report that decreasing caffeine intake relieves their symptoms.

GYNECOLOGY

Abscess of the Breast

Peripheral breast abscesses are typically due to streptococci or to *S. aureus.* Subareolar abscesses are usually due to anaerobes. More than 50% of subareolar abscesses are secondary to mammary duct ectasia, an inflammation and thickening of the large mammary ducts associated with breast-feeding. Infections are actually rare in the non-lactating breast and, if persistent despite antibiotics, may represent inflammatory cancer.

A red, swollen, painful mass in the breast.

Clinical presentation.

Incision, drainage, and appropriate antibiotics, such as dicloxacillin or clindamycin, are used for treatment. Most peripheral breast abscesses do not recur, but subareolar abscesses may reappear. Recurrent abscesses may cause fistula formation, and excision of the large duct system may be necessary for cure.

Fibroadenoma

Fibroadenomas are the most common benign breast tumors. Although they can occur in women of any age, they are most common before age 30 years. Pregnancy may stimulate their growth, and they often regress and calcify after menopause.

These tumors present as sharply circumscribed, mobile masses that are usually solitary.

Fine-needle aspiration can establish the diagnosis, but excisional biopsy is often necessary to rule out carcinoma.

Surgical excision is the treatment of choice and provides tissue for diagnosis. Fibroadenomas frequently recur.

Breast Cancer

Breast cancer accounts for approximately one-third of cancer in women. There are a number of associated risk factors (Table 6-2). The increased risk from hormone replacement

Table 6-2. Breast cancer risk factors

Category	Risk factor
Genetic	First-degree relative, particularly premenopausal and/or bilateral cancer
	History of ovarian or endometrial cancer
	Personal history of breast or ovarian cancer
Demographic	Nulliparity
	First pregnancy after age 35 years
	Early menarche
	Late menopause
	Older age
	Caucasian race
Dietary	High fat intake
	Postmenopausal obesity
Morphologic	Fibrocystic change with cellular atypia

therapy in postmenopausal women is highly controversial. Invasive ductal tumors compose approximately 90% of breast cancers, particularly, nonspecific infiltrating ductal carcinoma. The remaining 10% arise primarily in the breast lobule.

There are two types of in situ cancer, ductal and lobular. Ductal carcinoma in situ (DCIS) may present as a lump or as a mammographic abnormality. It is more aggressive than lobular carcinoma in situ (LCIS) and requires lumpectomy and sometimes radiotherapy. LCIS, in contrast, is not generally apparent on mammography or as a palpable mass. It is usually an incidental finding and is, in fact, unlikely to progress to invasive cancer. Women with LCIS, however, are at high risk of developing an invasive cancer (in either breast) and require careful monitoring.

SIGNS & SYMPTOMS

The typical early presentation is a firm, painless breast lump, most frequently in the upper outer quadrant of the breast. A bloody or serous nipple discharge may be present (although this is more commonly a sign of *benign intraductal papilloma*). The mass may be freely mobile, but with progressive growth it affixes to the deep fascia and becomes immobile. Nipple retraction secondary to ductal involvement or skin retraction and dimpling secondary to skin invasion may be present. *Peau d'orange* (obstruction of skin lymphatics causing lymphedema and skin thickening such that the skin resembles an orange peel) may also be observed. Axillary or supraclavicular lymphadenopathy suggests tumor spread.

DIAGNOSIS

Mammography and biopsy are used for diagnosis. Fine-needle aspiration (FNA) can precede open biopsy, but a negative FNA requires follow-up open biopsy because of the high rate of false-negatives with this procedure (20%). Chest x-ray may show pulmonary metastases.

TREATMENT

Modified radical mastectomy (total mastectomy plus axillary dissection) and segmental mastectomy (lumpectomy) with subsequent radiation are standard surgical options, depending on the size of the tumor. Hormonal therapy may also be used in tumors positive for estrogen and progesterone receptors. Chemotherapy appears to delay recurrence, but there is no evidence that it will cure patients who do not respond to radiotherapy or mastectomy. Better prognosis is seen in older patients and in those with estrogen receptor-positive tumors who are treated with tamoxifen, an antiestrogen. Involvement of the axillary lymph nodes is the most important negative prognostic indicator.

PREVENTION

Most early breast cancers are found by patients, so monthly self-examinations of the breast should be encouraged. All women should have a clinical breast examination once a year. Women older than age 40 years should have mammograms every year or two. Annual mammography is recommended after age 50 years. Tamoxifen prophylaxis has recently been demonstrated to prevent breast cancer in high-risk women, although it introduces a significant risk for uterine cancer.

Paget's Disease of the Breast

Paget's disease of the breast is an intraductal carcinoma that involves the main excretory ducts of the breast and accounts for only 3% of breast cancer cases. The first sign of disease is typically a crusting erosion of the nipple, with or without discharge. The tumor is apparent on palpation in only two-thirds of patients. Diagnosis is made by biopsy of the nipple, and treatment is similar to that of other breast tumors. Prognosis depends on the extent of disease at diagnosis.

GYNECOLOGY

7
Obstetrics

Physiology and Endocrinology of Normal Pregnancy

Conception and Implantation

For effective conception, an egg and a sperm cell must meet to form a zygote and then implant in the endometrium. Fertilization typically occurs in the fallopian tube within 12 hours of ovulation. Repeated cleavage of the zygote produces a solid morula and then a hollow blastocyst. The blastocyst reaches the uterine cavity approximately 3 days after ovulation. On day 6 or 7, the developing embryo implants. At this time, the trophoblastic cells, which will develop into the placenta, invade the endometrial lining and begin to produce beta-human chorionic gonadotropin (β-hCG). The syncytiotrophoblasts, the cells closest to the endometrium, form lacunae that will fill with maternal blood for exchange of oxygen and nutrients. By 17 days after fertilization (around the time of the missed menses), fetal and maternal blood vessels have a functional exchange, and a placental circulation exists.

Fetal Development

Weeks 2 through 8 after fertilization is the embryonic period. It is during this time that organogenesis of all major systems begins. It is also during this time that teratogenic agents are likely to have the greatest effect. The entire fetus forms from three layers of cells, called *germ layers:* the endoderm, mesoderm, and ectoderm. The central nervous system begins to develop from the endoderm in the third week and continues to mature throughout gestation. The heart begins to form at the end of the third week and can be seen via ultrasound in the fourth week (6 weeks after the last menstrual period begins). The gut forms during weeks 4 through 8, bile is produced at week 12, and the pancreas begins to function at week 20. The kidneys migrate from the pelvis to their adult position by week 9, and urine becomes a large component of the amniotic fluid in the second and third trimesters. Lungs are, of course, not needed by the fetus and develop rather late. Buds form at 5 weeks, but alveoli do not form and surfactant is not made until at least 24 weeks. Limbs are complete by 8 weeks, although the mother does not feel fetal movement until 17 to 20 weeks.

Prior to 6 weeks, male and female embryos are indistinguishable. If testosterone is present, the wolffian ducts develop into the epididymis, vas deferens, and seminal vesicles, and the penis and scrotum develop. Without testosterone, the müllerian ducts develop into the uterus, fallopian tubes, and vagina.

Maternal Physiology

The mother must provide oxygen, nutrients, and a safe environment for the developing fetus. These demands put a tremendous stress on the maternal system. Plasma volume increases to 50% above nonpregnant levels with resulting increased cardiac output and glomerular filtration rate by the kidneys. A systolic murmur is not uncommon in pregnant women. Despite an associated red blood cell mass increase, hematocrit falls slightly because of dilution and anemia often results. Human placental lactogen antagonizes the effects of insulin and can lead to glucose intolerance.

OBSTETRICS

The Placenta

The placenta, derived from fetal trophoblastic cells, is the site of maternal-fetal exchange. Fetal and maternal blood flow to the placenta, both at approximately 400 cc/min. Although the blood does not actually mix, these large volumes of blood allow for the necessary exchanges over thin membranes. Steroids, often synthesized by the placenta itself, are exchanged, in addition to oxygen, nutrients, and waste products. Most diffuse across the membranes, although peptides are exchanged by active transport and glucose is transferred by facilitated diffusion. Among the hormones produced by the placenta are human chorionic gonadotropin, human chorionic somatomammotropin (also called human placental lactogen), progesterone, and estrogens (primarily estriol).

Human Genetics

Every pregnancy has a 3% to 4% risk of a genetic disorder or structural congenital anomaly. Congenital and hereditary disorders include chromosomal abnormalities (e.g., Down syndrome, with trisomy 21), autosomal-dominant disorders (e.g., adult polycystic kidney disease), autosomal-recessive disorders (e.g., cystic fibrosis), X-linked disorders (e.g., hemophilia), and multifactorial disorders (e.g., spina bifida, anencephaly). Table 7-1 lists some of the most important genetic disorders. A personal or family history of any of these disorders suggests the need for counseling before pregnancy. If a patient decides to become pregnant or has her first visit while she is already pregnant, prenatal testing and pregnancy options must be discussed.

Teratology

A teratogen is any agent that causes a permanent abnormality in the fetus. Most teratogens pass from the maternal circulation through the placenta to the developing fetus. If a teratogen reaches the embryo within the first 2 weeks after conception, it will either cause embryonic demise or have no effect, in an "all or nothing" phenomenon. During organogenesis, especially in weeks 2 through 8, teratogen effects vary depending on which organ system is forming when the substance reaches the embryo. The U.S. Food and Drug Administration (FDA) has classified medications based on the associated fetal risks (Table 7-2). Because

Table 7-1. Genetic disorders

Autosomal dominant	Autosomal recessive	X-linked recessive
Achondroplasia	Cystic fibrosis	Androgen insensitivity
Ehlers-Danlos syndrome	Gaucher's disease	Duchenne's muscular dystrophy
Huntington's chorea	Phenylketonuria	Hemophilia A and B
Intestinal polyposis	Sickle cell anemia	Lesch-Nyhan syndrome
Marfan syndrome	Tay-Sachs disease	
Neurofibromatosis	Wilson's disease	
Adult polycystic kidney disease	Most enzyme diseases	
von Willebrand's disease		

Table 7-2. U.S. Food and Drug Administration classification of medications and associated fetal risk

Class	Fetal risk
A	Controlled studies in humans have demonstrated no fetal risk.
B	Animal studies indicate that there are no fetal risks, or animal studies show fetal harm but well-controlled human studies demonstrate no fetal risk.
C	No adequate studies have been done.
D	Evidence of fetal risk, but benefits may outweigh risk.
E	Proved fetal harm and contraindicated during pregnancy.

of the difficulty in using pregnant women as research subjects, most drugs are designated Class C. Most antibiotics are considered relatively safe in pregnancy, with the exception of streptomycin and tetracycline.

Maternal Mortality

Maternal mortality is defined as a woman's death from any pregnancy-related cause, irrespective of the site or duration of the pregnancy, at any time during the pregnancy or within 6 weeks of its termination. The mortality rate is generally described as the number of maternal deaths per 100,000 live births. Ninety-five percent of maternal deaths occur in developing countries. In the United States, the most frequent causes are hemorrhage and embolism, followed by cardiac and pulmonary problems, pregnancy-induced hypertension, and anesthetic complications.

Prenatal Care

Prenatal Visits

The goals of prenatal care are to prevent, detect, and manage conditions that can cause adverse outcomes in pregnancy. Prenatal visits require careful assessment for preterm labor and delivery, intrauterine growth retardation (IUGR), diabetes, hypertension, perinatal infections, and post-term pregnancy. Some important historical points include previous pregnancy outcomes, smoking and drug use, past medical history, and family history.

At an early visit, the physician should perform a Pap test; complete blood count; blood type, including Rhesus factor (Rh); syphilis test; hepatitis B screen; HIV test; and rubella antibody screen. The rubella screen provides information about the risk of congenital infection; however, nonimmune women should not be immunized until after delivery. A hepatitis B surface antigen test will determine if the mother is a chronic carrier of the hepatitis B virus. If so, the newborn must be treated with hepatitis B immune globulin and the hepatitis B vaccine to reduce the high risk of developing chronic infection. Between 24 and 28 weeks, a glucose tolerance test screens for gestational diabetes. If it is abnormal, it is followed by a 3-hour fasting glucose tolerance test.

Evaluation at every prenatal visit includes the following:

- **Maternal weight:** Desired weight gain varies depending on prepregnancy weight, but 30 pounds is average and appropriate for a nonobese woman. Even obese women should gain a small amount of weight; weight loss is not recommended. Inadequate weight gain is associated with preterm labor and IUGR, and excessive weight gain is associated with gestational diabetes and, in the third trimester, preeclampsia.
- **Urinalysis:** This simple screen can identify urinary tract infections; glucosuria, which may indicate diabetes; and proteinuria, which may indicate preeclampsia.
- **Blood pressure:** A rise may indicate preeclampsia.
- **Fundal height:** Appropriate fetal growth can be followed, and after 28 weeks, the fetal position can be assessed using Leopold's maneuvers.
- **Fetal heart tones:** The fetal heart should be auscultated at every visit to ensure fetal well-being.

Nutrition

Many nutritional requirements increase during pregnancy, and proper nutrition is necessary for the health of both mother and fetus. Patients at particularly high risk for under-nutrition include teenagers, women of low economic status, underweight women, alcoholics, and drug addicts. Weight gain should be monitored particularly closely in these women.

Ideal weight gain in pregnancy is 25 to 35 pounds, with about half of that gain occurring in the first and second trimester. (Rapid weight gain in the third trimester may be a sign of preeclampsia.) Nausea may interfere with weight gain in the first trimester. Patients should be counseled to eat frequent, small meals if this is a problem.

It is common to provide vitamin supplements to pregnant women. The most important are iron and folate. Iron demand is increased by the needs of the fetus and the expanding maternal blood supply, and anemia is common during pregnancy. Folate is required by dividing cells, and folate supplementation decreases the incidence of neural tube defects. Ideally, women should take 0.4 mg of folate each day starting prior to conception, and women at risk for neural tube defects should take 4 mg. In addition, women should be counseled to increase their calcium intake. If intake is insufficient, fetal bone formation will be maintained at the expense of maternal bone.

Prenatal Diagnosis

Many fetal abnormalities can be detected prenatally using a number of diagnostic tests. Common indications for a prenatal workup include women 35 years old or older (who have an increased risk of fetal chromosomal abnormalities), a history of several spontaneous abortions, a history of neonatal morbidity or mortality, a history of exposure to teratogens during the current pregnancy, and any maternal conditions (such as diabetes) that are associated with an increased fetal risk of congenital abnormalities. Frequently used tests include the following:

- **Ultrasonography** is used at any stage of pregnancy and can often identify fetal structural abnormalities. It presents no associated risk and is the most common diagnostic device used to assess the effects of teratogens on fetal development. Structural abnormalities that may be detected include anencephaly, spina bifida, gastrointestinal defects, renal anomalies, and congenital heart defects. Ultrasound is also used to evaluate gestational age. Accuracy is better earlier in the pregnancy.

- **Expanded maternal serum alpha-fetoprotein** (MSAFP), or a "triple marker screen," is performed between weeks 15 and 20 of gestation to evaluate risk of neural tube defects, Down syndrome (trisomy 21), and trisomy 18. From the maternal serum, levels of alpha-fetoprotein (AFP), unconjugated estradiol, and hCG are measured. Elevated MSAFP suggests neural tube defects (e.g., anencephaly or spina bifida), ventral abdominal wall defects, multiple gestation, fetal demise, or inaccurate estimated age of gestation. A pattern of markers, including low MSAFP, indicates a possibility of Down syndrome or trisomy 18. Subsequent ultrasound can detect many of these defects. If desired, amniocentesis may then be used to determine the amniotic fluid AFP level (to better rule out neural tube defects) and the fetal karyotype (to rule out Down syndrome and trisomy 18).

- **Amniocentesis** can be performed after week 16. Amniotic fluid is withdrawn through a needle placed in the abdominal wall. Amniocentesis assesses the amniotic fluid AFP content and the fetal karyotype, so it identifies both neural tube defects and chromosomal disorders with high accuracy. This test has a 1 in 200 risk of spontaneous abortion. Earlier amniocentesis, although slightly riskier, is now being performed so that pregnancy termination remains an option for some women.

- **Chorionic villus sampling** is a more invasive test performed transabdominally or transcervically between 9 and 12 weeks of gestation. It permits first-trimester identification of chromosomal abnormalities and genetic disorders that have biochemical markers (e.g., Tay-Sachs disease).

- **Percutaneous umbilical blood sampling** is typically performed between 10 and 22 weeks of gestation. This test involves withdrawing blood from the umbilical vein for a rapid karyotype or identification of some genetic disorders.

- **Doppler flow studies,** done by ultrasound, measure flow through the uterine, umbilical, and intracranial arteries. They are primarily used to evaluate the degree of compromise in growth-retarded fetuses.

- **Lung maturity studies** can be performed on amniotic fluid obtained via amniocentesis in the third trimester. A high lamellar body count, the presence of phosphatidyl glycerol, or a lecithin-sphingomyelin ratio greater than two (L/S >2) all predict fetal lung maturity. These studies are used in decisions regarding timing of delivery.

Medical Complications of Pregnancy

Hyperemesis Gravidarum

Severe nausea and vomiting occasionally arise during early pregnancy and may cause dehydration or poor weight gain. Symptoms usually peak in the first trimester and then decline, paralleling the levels of β-hCG. Hyperemesis gravidarum is more common in nulliparas, patients with recent stressful experiences, and patients with gestational trophoblastic disease who have an elevated β-hCG.

A history of intractable nausea and vomiting typically accompanies signs of weight loss and dehydration.

Diagnosis is based on the clinical presentation after other GI complications have been ruled out. The presence of ketonuria and electrolyte disturbances, including hypokalemia, hyponatremia, and hypochloremic alkalosis, must be monitored.

Patients should have frequent, light meals of solid food. Antiemetics are useful, and prevention of dehydration is critical.

Gestational Diabetes Mellitus

Gestational diabetes mellitus (GDM) refers to glucose intolerance beginning or newly recognized during pregnancy. The etiology is unknown. Insulin-antagonist hormones produced by the placenta may be responsible, or the stress of pregnancy may unmask a subclinical abnormality in insulin activity. GDM is associated with many pregnancy complications, including macrosomia and its associated risks for traumatic delivery, delayed fetal lung maturity and respiratory distress syndrome of the neonate, congenital anomalies, neonatal hypoglycemia, and intrauterine fetal death. The pregnant diabetic mother is also prone to complications, including preeclampsia, polyhydramnios, hypoglycemia, ketoacidosis, diabetic coma, and the typical end-organ involvement of diabetes. Risk factors include obesity, family history of diabetes, maternal age older than 25 years, and personal history of macrosomia, polyhydramnios, stillbirth, a congenitally deformed baby, or recurrent abortions. Although GDM generally resolves after delivery, as many as half of women with GDM will develop diabetes later in life.

GDM is usually asymptomatic. A large-for-gestational-age fetus or polyhydramnios may be warning signs.

Half of all women who develop GDM do not have an associated risk factor, so glucose screening between 24 and 28 weeks is mandatory for all patients. Earlier screening is recommended for women with risk factors. Nonfasting women ingest a glucose load, and plasma glucose is measured 1 hour later. If the value is high, a 3-hour glucose tolerance test is performed. This involves measuring a fasting glucose level, ingesting a larger glucose load, and measuring glucose levels at 1, 2, and 3 hours. Two or more abnormal values indicate GDM.

Strict glucose control during pregnancy decreases perinatal morbidity and mortality. Appropriate diet and exercise can often maintain normal glucose levels, but glucophage or insulin is sometimes necessary for adequate control. Periodic fetal monitoring, including nonstress tests and ultrasound, is

OBSTETRICS

indicated. Given the association with birth trauma, macrosomic babies are sometimes delivered by cesarean section.

Preeclampsia

Also known as *pregnancy-induced hypertension,* preeclampsia is a multisystem disease that involves the development of hypertension, proteinuria, and edema. Its cause is not known. It develops after 20 weeks of gestation and affects 5% of pregnancies. Preeclamptic patients are usually primiparous. Other risk factors include pre-existing hypertensive states, advanced maternal age, multiple gestation, and other vascular disease. Preeclampsia may result in a number of complications, including stroke, seizure, and IUGR. The HELLP syndrome is an associated condition consisting of *h*emolysis, *e*levated *l*iver enzymes, and *l*ow *p*latelets. Complications include abruptio placenta, disseminated intravascular coagulation (DIC), acute renal failure, pulmonary edema, and encephalopathy.

SIGNS & SYMPTOMS

Most signs and symptoms are due to endothelial injury and vasoconstriction. In addition to hypertension, proteinuria, and edema, patients may experience headache, blurred vision, scotomata, epigastric pain, hyperreflexia, and oliguria.

DIAGNOSIS

Hypertension and nondependent edema or 2+ proteinuria is diagnostic of preeclampsia. Hypertension during pregnancy is defined as a 30 mm Hg rise in systolic pressure or a 15 mm Hg rise in diastolic pressure during the course of the pregnancy. If baseline values are not known, an alternate definition is pressure above 140/90 mm Hg after 20 weeks of gestation. Blood pressure must remain elevated at a second measurement at least 6 hours after the initial elevated reading. Severe preeclampsia is diagnosed with blood pressure above 160/110, oliguria, 3+ proteinuria, or evidence of end organ damage including fetal compromise.

TREATMENT

Therapy attempts to minimize complications and avoid progression to full-blown eclampsia. The definitive cure is delivery, and the patient's blood pressure returns to baseline within 1 to 2 days.

For mild preeclampsia, bed rest and close monitoring are appropriate. If the fetus is term, prompt delivery is indicated. IV magnesium is used for seizure prophylaxis.

For severe preeclampsia, the mother's condition should be stabilized and the baby delivered. Magnesium is important for seizure prophylaxis. Fluid restriction may help, but enough fluid must be given to maintain urine output. Hydralazine or other antihypertensives may be used, but severe drops in blood pressure may compromise placental perfusion. Antihypertensive medications and seizure prophylaxis should continue for at least 24 hours postpartum.

Eclampsia

Eclampsia is diagnosed when seizures occur in a preeclamptic patient, and it can be fatal if left untreated. Other types of seizure disorders should be excluded for this diagnosis to apply.

Treatment of eclampsia is similar to that of severe preeclampsia. The patient must be stabilized and the baby delivered. IV diazepam helps to control the seizures. Magnesium is used to prevent additional seizures, and antihypertensives lower blood pressure. Vaginal delivery is generally preferable.

OBSTETRICS

Gestational Hypertension

Also known as *late transient hypertension,* gestational hypertension is sometimes difficult to differentiate from preeclampsia. It involves idiopathic hypertension during the second half of gestation or in the first day postpartum, without proteinuria or edema. It is a retrospective diagnosis only, made at least 1 week after delivery, when proteinuria never appears and blood pressure has returned to normal.

Chronic Hypertension

Patients with known hypertension or with high blood pressure detected before the twentieth week of pregnancy have chronic hypertension. This primarily includes long-standing, clinically recognized disease, but the physiologic stress of pregnancy is also capable of exacerbating a previously subclinical hypertensive disorder. Methyldopa, beta-blockers, and hydralazine can be used throughout the pregnancy, but diuretics and angiotensin-converting enzyme inhibitors are contraindicated. Blood pressure should be monitored closely.

Urinary Tract Infections

Urinary tract infections (UTIs) occur more frequently during pregnancy for several reasons, including obstruction of outflow by the enlarging uterus and progesterone inhibition of ureteral peristalsis. Asymptomatic bacteriuria is not more common in pregnancy per se, but it is more likely to cause pyelonephritis in pregnant women because of increased urinary stasis. Because of this, asymptomatic bacteriuria is treated in pregnancy.

SIGNS & SYMPTOMS

Symptoms of cystitis and pyelonephritis are no different from those in the nonpregnant woman and include dysuria, frequency, and urgency, as well as fever and flank pain in cases of pyelonephritis.

DIAGNOSIS

Urinalysis reveals white blood cells and bacteria. Urine culture identifies the causative organism and can be used to verify antibiotic sensitivities.

TREATMENT

Antibiotics should be targeted at the probable organisms and then readjusted, if necessary, when culture results become available. Women with pyelonephritis or recurrent infections should remain on suppressive antibiotics for the duration of their pregnancies.

Genital Herpes

Genital herpes—herpes simplex virus (HSV)—is a common, sexually transmitted infection discussed in detail in Chapter 6. Treatment of herpes infection in pregnant women revolves around minimizing the incidence of neonatal herpes infection, a devastating neurologic disease (see Chapter 8). Among women who develop their first herpes lesion around the time of labor, there is a 40% risk of infecting a vaginally born infant. In women with recurrent herpes and prodromal symptoms or active lesions at the time of vaginal birth, less than 5% of infants will become infected. Only 0.1% of vaginally born infants of asymptomatic HSV-infected mothers will become infected. Because of these probabilities, women who have active lesions or prodromal symptoms at the time of labor are typically delivered via cesarean section. Otherwise, a vaginal delivery is preferred. Acyclovir may be given near term to women with frequent infections in an attempt to avoid an outbreak.

Group B Streptococcal Infection

Group B streptococcus (GBS) is frequently found in the vaginal flora and is not normally a pathogen. During labor, however, it can be transmitted to the neonate and cause life-threatening infection (see Neonatal Sepsis in Chapter 8). The difficulty in screening for and treating infection in pregnant women is that GBS comes and goes from the vagina, with the rectum serving as a reservoir. Two strategies for preventing neonatal infection are currently in practice. One involves culturing for GBS at 36 weeks, and giving antibiotics in labor to women with positive cultures or any risk factors. The other strategy simply is to treat presumptively any women who present with certain risk factors for neonatal infection, including preterm labor, preterm premature rupture of membranes, prolonged rupture of membranes, intrapartum fever, and a previous neonate with GBS infection. Antibiotics (typically penicillin) can be stopped if culture results are negative before the infant is delivered.

Deep Venous Thrombosis

Several factors are known to increase the incidence of clotting disorders during pregnancy, including venous stasis, vascular damage, and hypercoagulability of the blood due to an increase in clotting factors II, VII, VIII, and X. An underlying blood disorder may also be unmasked during this time. The presentation, diagnosis, and treatment are virtually the same as in the nonpregnant state and are discussed in detail in Chapter 3. It is important to remember that warfarin is contraindicated during pregnancy, so treatment involves heparin only. In patients at risk for clotting (with a known clotting disorder or past history of thrombosis), prophylaxis throughout the pregnancy and postpartum period is warranted. Heparin or low molecular weight heparin may be used.

Surgical Complications of Pregnancy

Occasionally pregnancies are complicated by a condition requiring surgery. Fortunately, anesthesia is not thought to be teratogenic, although rates of spontaneous abortion and preterm labor are somewhat increased after surgery. The safest time for any procedure is the second trimester.

Acute appendicitis is the most common surgical complication during pregnancy, followed by ovarian masses and then gallstones. Ovarian masses are almost always benign and immediate surgery is not mandatory. However, torsion is a risk and all factors must be weighed. Removal of the ovary, even with the corpus luteum, is not a threat to the pregnancy once the placenta has begun secreting hCG.

Gestational Trophoblastic Disease

Molar "pregnancies" are actually neoplasms of trophoblastic cells, the cells that form the placenta. Gestational trophoblastic disease ranges in severity from the benign hydatidiform mole (the great majority of cases) to malignant and metastatic choriocarcinoma. Locally invasive disease also occurs. Because excessive placental tissue develops, levels of β-hCG increase, usually to levels higher than expected for a normal pregnancy.

Hydatidiform Moles

Hydatidiform moles are benign growths of trophoblastic tissue; however, they occasionally develop into cancer. It is critical to monitor these patients carefully to assess for development of choriocarcinoma. Complete moles have a 46,XX karyotype, whereas partial moles have a 69,XXY karyotype and are usually associated with an abnormal fetus.

SIGNS & SYMPTOMS

Hydatidiform moles usually present with heavy or irregular painless uterine bleeding during the first half of pregnancy. A uterus that is large for dates and hyperemesis gravidarum are also common first warnings. On examination, expulsion of vesicles resembling a "bunch of grapes" may be evident. There is no fetal movement or heart tones. Preeclampsia in the first half of pregnancy is pathognomonic of hydatidiform mole.

DIAGNOSIS

Higher than normal β-hCG titers are a suspicious finding. Ultrasound provides definitive diagnosis, showing a "snowstorm" pattern with no sac or fetus. A chest x-ray is important to rule out metastases to the lung.

TREATMENT

A hydatidiform mole is removed by suction evacuation and curettage. Serum β-hCG is assayed weekly after evacuation and generally declines within 3 to 4 months to undetectable levels. Levels are followed for 6–12 months, and pregnancy should be avoided during this time. Patients with persistent β-hCG titers in the absence of a pregnancy may have gestational choriocarcinoma and should be worked up and treated as described in the following section.

Gestational Choriocarcinoma

Half of gestational choriocarcinomas arise in the context of a molar pregnancy. The remainder are seen following a normal, ectopic, or aborted pregnancy. Choriocarcinomas may be locally invasive or may metastasize through the circulation to the lungs, vagina, brain, GI tract, liver, and kidneys.

SIGNS & SYMPTOMS

Choriocarcinoma generally presents after metastasis has occurred, and the diagnosis may be missed unless onset follows a molar pregnancy. Vaginal bleeding, dyspnea, cough, hemoptysis, CNS findings, and rectal bleeding are possible signs of metastases and should prompt an evaluation of β-hCG levels in any woman who has recently been pregnant.

High β-hCG levels and a "snowstorm" on ultrasound indicate gestational trophoblastic disease. To evaluate for metastasis, CT scans of the abdomen, pelvis, and head and a cerebrospinal fluid β-hCG titer are necessary.

Chemotherapy with methotrexate is initiated, but multiagent chemotherapy and radiation may be needed for persistent disease. Frequent follow-up β-hCG titers confirm remission in the majority of patients. If β-hCG levels do not fall to a normal level, a hysterectomy is indicated. Cure rates are greater than 90%.

Obstetric Complications of Pregnancy

Ectopic Pregnancy

In ectopic pregnancy, the fertilized ovum implants outside of the uterus. The most common site of implantation is the fallopian tube, usually in the ampulla, but implantation may occur on the ovary, outside the tube, on the pelvic wall, or even on the omentum. Ectopic pregnancy is often related to prior tubal infection and scarring. Risk factors for ectopic pregnancy include history of sexually transmitted diseases (STDs); intrauterine device (IUD) use; prior tubal surgery, including tubal ligation; prior ectopic pregnancy; and any risk factor for STDs, including multiple sex partners. Rupture of an ectopic pregnancy can cause life-threatening intra-abdominal hemorrhage.

Patients are often unaware of their pregnancy, and ectopic pregnancies sometimes reabsorb without causing clinical symptoms. With an unruptured ectopic pregnancy, signs of early pregnancy (amenorrhea, nausea) may accompany light vaginal bleeding ("spotting") and crampy lower abdominal pain. Physical examination shows abdominal tenderness, adnexal tenderness, and an adnexal fullness or mass in 50% of patients. A ruptured ectopic pregnancy usually presents during weeks 6 to 8 of gestation, with sudden, sharp abdominal or pelvic pain accompanied by guarding, rigidity, and rebound tenderness. Rapid intra-abdominal hemorrhage may result in hypotension and shock.

An elevated urine or serum β-hCG level confirms the pregnancy, but it does not confirm that the pregnancy is ectopic. During an ectopic pregnancy, β-hCG levels do not rise as rapidly as in normal pregnancies, in which β-hCG levels should double every 48 hours. In a stable patient with suspected ectopic pregnancy, the rate of rise of β-hCG over several days can assist in the diagnosis. In an unstable patient, however, immediate action is required. When the β-hCG titer reaches 6,500 mIU/mL, a gestational sac is normally visible on transvaginal or transabdominal ultrasound. Its absence at high β-hCG levels strongly suggests ectopic pregnancy. Ultrasound can also show hemoperitoneum, consistent with rupture. Laparoscopy confirms the diagnosis, if necessary.

Treatment options for an unruptured ectopic pregnancy include surgical removal or methotrexate, which is used only for early presentations. A ruptured ectopic pregnancy is treated with immediate fluid resuscitation and surgery. Surgical intervention may involve an attempt to remove the products of conception while preserving the fallopian tube.

OBSTETRICS

Spontaneous Abortion

Commonly called "miscarriage," spontaneous abortion (SAB) is the loss of the products of conception before 20 weeks of gestation. It is a frequent complication, occurring in approximately 20% of all pregnancies. The majority of SABs occur during the first trimester, and fetal causes (e.g., chromosomal abnormalities) are generally responsible. Parental karyotypes are checked only in cases of repeated SABs. Second-trimester SABs are more often due to maternal causes, such as infections, cervical abnormalities (e.g., incompetence), uterine abnormalities, medical disease, and cocaine use. In these late abortions, a more mature placenta increases the risk of maternal bleeding, and more advanced fetal bone formation increases the risk of uterine perforation. The different types of SABs are discussed in the following list.

- **Threatened abortion** refers to any uterine cramping or bleeding in the presence of a closed cervix during the first 20 weeks of pregnancy. In addition to inspection of the cervix, diagnosis requires ultrasonography to confirm cardiac activity and a viable fetus. If the fetus appears viable, maternal bed rest and pelvic rest are the only available treatment. At least one-fourth of threatened abortions will progress to complete abortion.
- **Inevitable abortion** involves uterine bleeding or pain when the cervix is beginning to efface or dilate. Prevention of the abortion is not possible. A dilation and curettage (D&C) is often performed to ensure that no products of conception are retained.
- **Incomplete abortion** is the term used to describe the passage of part of the products of conception through the cervix. The cervix is dilated, and fetal tissue may be visible on examination. Bleeding from the uterus is present and may be severe. Again, a D&C is not always necessary but will remove any remaining products of conception from the uterus.
- **Complete abortion** refers to passage of all of the products of conception, with subsequent closure of the cervix and return of the uterus to its normal size. Complete abortions do not require any treatment.
- A **missed abortion** refers to the death of a fetus and its retention in utero for 4 weeks or longer. A D&C is indicated.

Therapeutic Abortion

Elective termination of a pregnancy may be performed during the first and second trimesters. First-trimester elective abortions are currently legal throughout the United States, although the practice is controversial. D&C and vacuum curettage are the primary methods used. Very early abortions can be induced medically using the progesterone antagonist mifepristone (RU 486) or the antifolate methotrexate. Limitations on second-trimester abortions are determined by the individual states. The most common procedure used for second-trimester abortions is dilation and evacuation, although prostaglandins or intra-amniotic saline injection are sometimes used to induce labor. Bleeding, infection, retained products of conception, and perforation of the uterus are the major complications.

Septic Abortion

Septic abortion refers to infection of the uterus before, during, or after an abortion. It may be caused by an improperly performed therapeutic abortion.

OBSTETRICS

OBSTETRICS

Patients present with acute infection involving fever, chills, and peritoneal signs. In severe cases, septic shock can occur, with hypotension, hypothermia, oliguria, and respiratory distress.

History and clinical presentation. Leukocytosis is present.

Stabilization, antibiotics, and evacuation of the uterus are indicated.

Intrauterine Fetal Death

Intrauterine fetal death is defined as death of a fetus after 20 weeks of gestational age but before onset of labor. Common etiologies include placental and cord complications, hypertensive states, erythroblastosis fetalis, congenital anomalies, infections, and autoimmune diseases.

A uterus small for gestational age, absence of fetal movements, and absence of fetal heart tones may be noted by the mother and on examination.

Ultrasonography confirms the absence of heart activity.

Management varies depending on gestational age. Fetal demise prior to 24 weeks can be treated with dilation and evacuation (D&E). Fetal demise before the twenty-eighth week of pregnancy can be treated by induction of labor or by waiting for spontaneous labor to begin. Spontaneous labor occurs within 3 weeks of fetal death in 80% of cases. Fetal death after 28 weeks of gestation is generally treated by induction of labor. If labor is not induced, weekly fibrinogen, hematocrit, and platelet counts are important for early detection of DIC, which occurs in a minority of patients.

Rhesus Isoimmunization

Rh blood group incompatibility arises when an Rh-negative woman conceives an Rh-positive fetus. RBCs from the fetus can enter the woman's circulation during pregnancy or, more commonly, during birth. These "foreign" RBCs stimulate the production of maternal antibodies against the Rh factor. Spontaneous or induced abortions of an Rh-positive fetus can also result in isoimmunization. In subsequent pregnancies, transplacental transmission of the maternal anti-Rh antibody leads to hemolytic anemia in the fetus or neonate. The resulting disease, called **erythroblastosis fetalis,** may be fatal (see Chapter 8). Unless a woman was previously sensitized by an incompatible transfusion, a first pregnancy rarely leads to erythroblastosis fetalis. The highest frequency of the Rh-negative genotype occurs in whites, and one in eight white couples is Rh incompatible. In addition to the major Rh antigen, designated D, that causes most cases of erythroblastosis fetalis, there are a number of other minor antigens that can cause incompatibility as well.

Isoimmunization does not have signs or symptoms during pregnancy, although hydrops fetalis and fetal demise may occur in severe cases. In less severe cases, bilirubin levels in the newborn can increase dramatically because of the hemolytic anemia. This can lead to kernicterus, characterized by decreased tone, poor feeding, apnea, seizures, and death. Survivors of kernicterus can be left with mental retardation, choreoathetosis, and hearing loss. High maternal anti-Rh antibody titers, checked in Rh-negative women at the first prenatal visit and at week 26, suggest sensitization of the mother. Amniocentesis showing high bilirubin levels in the amniotic fluid suggests more severe disease and potential for fetal death.

Amniocentesis results are followed throughout the pregnancy. If bilirubin levels are very elevated, intrauterine transfusions to the fetus can be performed at 2-week intervals. Early delivery may be needed. In the neonate, hyperbilirubinemia may necessitate phototherapy or an exchange transfusion.

At the first prenatal checkup, all patients should be screened for Rh type. If the patient is Rh-negative, maternal Rh antibody titers should be checked early in the pregnancy and repeated at the twenty-sixth week of gestation. A previously unsensitized mother will not normally produce anti-Rh antibody until after delivery, when mixing of the maternal and fetal blood occurs. Rh isoimmunization can be prevented by injecting the mother with anti-Rh immunoglobulin (RhoGAM) at 28 weeks and within 3 days after delivery. RhoGAM binds the fetal Rh factor and prevents the mother from developing anti-Rh antibodies, but it is too large to pass through the placenta to the Rh-positive fetus. RhoGAM should be given at the termination of each pregnancy, whether a delivery, ectopic pregnancy, or abortion, as well as any other time feto-maternal hemorrhage may occur (e.g., trauma).

Oligohydramnios

Oligohydramnios is a deficiency of amniotic fluid volume. Many cases are associated with IUGR and with a poor fetal outcome. Fetal stress may promote oligohydramnios because the fetal stress hormones increase fetal swallowing of amniotic fluid. Renal agenesis, ureteral or bladder anomalies, pulmonary hypoplasia, and other malformations can result in insufficient fluid secretion.

Very low amniotic fluid in the first trimester can cause severe structural abnormalities, such as facial distortion, limb contracture, poor lung development, and defects in the abdominal wall. In the third trimester, oligohydramnios can produce fetal hypoxia because of umbilical cord compression.

The condition is usually asymptomatic, although evidence of growth retardation or fetal distress may be present.

Ultrasound confirms oligohydramnios and evaluates for fetal abnormalities as well.

Hydration and rest may improve fluid volume. Induction of labor may be necessary if oligohydramnios is severe.

Polyhydramnios

Polyhydramnios—excess amniotic fluid volume—may develop gradually during pregnancy as a result of several possible causes. Fetal anomalies (e.g., duodenal atresia, tracheoesophageal fistula, or anencephaly) can lead to decreased swallowing and therefore decreased resorption of amniotic fluid. Pulmonary system anomalies (e.g., cystic malformations of the lung) can also lead to polyhydramnios because of excessive secretion. Other risk factors include diabetes, multiple gestation, and isoimmunization.

This complication is usually asymptomatic, although fundal height may be greater than expected. Preterm labor due to overdistention of the uterus may be the initial presentation.

Ultrasonography confirms polyhydramnios and evaluates fetal malformations. The mother should be tested for diabetes, anti-Rh antibody, and hemoglobinopathies.

Rest, tocolytics, and careful monitoring of the fetus may be of value for preterm labor. In an acute presentation because of multiple gestation, induction of labor may be necessary.

Multiple Gestation

Dizygotic twins arise through fertilization of two eggs by two sperm, resulting in two amnions and two chorions. Monozygotic twins develop through abnormal division of one fertilized egg. Multiple gestations are becoming more common after the recent introduction of fertility drugs that induce ovulation.

Multiple gestation has a higher risk of complications and higher rates of morbidity and mortality than singleton gestations. Women are at increased risk for gestational diabetes and preeclampsia, as well as preterm labor. The average gestational age at delivery is 36 weeks in twins versus 39 weeks in singletons. Prematurity leads to a high risk of respiratory distress syndrome, which is responsible for approximately half of the perinatal mortality of twins. Twin-twin transfusion syndrome, in which umbilical venous blood is unevenly shared between monochorionic twins, can cause severe complications.

Signs of multiple gestation include large size for dates (i.e., the uterus is larger than expected for the gestational age) and the auscultation of more than one fetal heart.

Ultrasound shows separate gestational sacs as early as week 6 of gestation.

Antepartum management can prolong gestation, decrease perinatal mortality, and decrease perinatal and maternal morbidity. Weekly visits starting after week 20 allow evaluation of cervical changes to detect preterm labor and blood pressure measurement to detect preeclampsia. Monthly ultrasound is useful to assess fetal growth and amniotic fluid volume.

Aggressive treatment of preterm labor is appropriate. Vertex-vertex twin presentations are most common and can be delivered vaginally. Otherwise, delivery is usually by cesarean section.

Preterm Labor

The onset of labor before the thirty-seventh week of gestation occurs in approximately 10% of all pregnancies in the United States. Risk factors include multiple gestation, infection, premature rupture of membranes, uterine anomalies, previous preterm labor or delivery, polyhydramnios, and cervical incompetence. Lower socioeconomic status and poor maternal nutrition are associated with a higher incidence of preterm labor.

Patients may report contractions, low-back pain, vaginal discharge, or bleeding.

Regular uterine contractions (at least six per hour) and concurrent cervical change occurring before the thirty-seventh week of gestation are the criteria for diagnosis. Cultures for chlamydia and group B streptococcus are taken to evaluate presence of infection. Ultrasound can rule out fetal or uterine anomalies, verify gestational age, and assess amniotic fluid volume. Amniocentesis may be performed to rule out infection and assess pulmonary maturity.

Preterm labor is relieved in half of patients simply with hydration and bed rest. Tocolytic agents should be administered unless chorioamnionitis, maternal compromise, or fetal distress requires immediate delivery. The beta-adrenergic agonists ritodrine or terbutaline are used for tocolysis with a high success rate. Magnesium, prostaglandin synthetase inhibitors, and calcium channel blockers are also used to arrest labor. Corticosteroids may be administered to accelerate maturation of the fetal lungs. Cervical cerclage (sewing the cervix closed) is never used to treat preterm labor. It may be performed in cases of incompetent cervix, when cervical dilation occurs in the absence of contractions.

OBSTETRICS

Premature Rupture of Membranes

When spontaneous rupture of membranes occurs before the onset of labor, it is called premature rupture of membranes (PROM). Vaginal or cervical infections, abnormal membrane physiology, and cervical incompetence may precipitate this event. If PROM occurs before the thirty-seventh week of gestation, it is referred to as **preterm PROM** (P-PROM) and has a high associated risk of preterm delivery.

SIGNS & SYMPTOMS

Patients note leaking vaginal fluid, which is generally clear but may be tinged with blood or meconium. Some uterine contractions may be present.

DIAGNOSIS

Vaginal fluid loss suggests PROM. The pooling of amniotic fluid in the vagina, a positive Nitrazine test, and ferning of dried amniotic fluid seen under a microscope confirm the diagnosis.

TREATMENT

Digital vaginal examinations should not be performed, to minimize the risk of introducing infection. A sterile speculum examination can confirm rupture, allow a visual cervical assessment, and permit cervical culture and amniotic fluid sampling for lung maturity tests. If the lungs are immature, delivery should be delayed, with bed rest and tocolysis if necessary, to provide time for lung maturation. Corticosteroid administration is recommended to speed lung maturity if P-PROM occurs before 34 weeks gestation. If the patient develops chorioamnionitis, antibiotics should be given and labor induced.

Third-trimester Bleeding

Before 20 weeks' gestation, bleeding is referred to as a threatened abortion. After 20 weeks, the term third-trimester bleeding is used, although the third trimester does not actually begin until week 26. Third-trimester bleeding complicates approximately 5% of pregnancies. Placental abruption and placenta previa are the most common causes of life-threatening hemorrhage and are discussed in detail in the following sections. Less severe third-trimester bleeding results from many extrauterine sources, such as cervical trauma (usually due to sexual activity); cervical inflammation or infection; cervical dilatation; coagulation disorders; and vaginal, vulvar, or rectal lesions. The most common cause of bleeding late in pregnancy is called "bloody show" and is due to the normal extrusion of the cervical mucus plug.

Abruptio Placenta

Early detachment of a normally implanted placenta can cause severe hemorrhage because this area is so highly vascularized. Risk factors for placental abruption include trauma, hypertension, cigarette smoking, cocaine use, and a history of prior abruption.

OBSTETRICS

Bleeding from an abruption is generally painful. The patient may report unremitting uterine or low-back pain associated with a tender and tonically contracted uterus. The symptoms depend on the degree of placental separation, the location of the placenta, and the subsequent loss of blood. Abruption leads to external bleeding in 90% of cases. In the remainder, the blood collects in the retroplacental space and can be detected from postpartum examination of the placenta. Maternal shock, DIC, and fetal distress or death may occur.

Abruptio placenta is primarily a clinical diagnosis, as ultrasonography shows the separation in less than one-half of patients. Vaginal examination should not be performed unless the diagnosis of placenta previa has been conclusively ruled out (see following section). The amount of vaginal bleeding gives minimal indication of the total blood loss. Uterine irritability may be evident on the tocometer.

If the abruption does not threaten fetal or maternal well-being, bed rest may reduce the bleeding. If the hemorrhage does not improve or if fetal or maternal well-being is compromised, immediate delivery should be performed.

Placenta Previa

In placenta previa, implantation of the placenta occurs over or near the cervical os. In total previa, the placenta completely covers the internal os, and in partial previa, the os is partially covered. Placenta previa is not uncommon early in pregnancy, but most cases resolve spontaneously as the placenta and uterus enlarge. Risk factors include multiparity, advanced maternal age, previous cesarean section, history of abortions, and uterine fibroids.

Painless, bright-red vaginal bleeding begins suddenly, usually early in the third trimester. The amount of blood loss varies from "spotting" to severe hemorrhage. It often resolves spontaneously, with another, heavier episode a few days later.

Ultrasound demonstrates the placement of the placenta in most cases. Manual vaginal examination is contraindicated because it can precipitate greater hemorrhage.

For minor bleeding early in pregnancy, bed rest is recommended. Tocolytics can be given to reduce uterine contractions, if present. Delivery must be by cesarean section. For severe bleeding, stabilization of the mother is critical, followed by cesarean delivery of the infant. Preterm delivery results in the high perinatal mortality associated with this complication.

Labor and Delivery

During the last 1 to 2 months of pregnancy, Braxton-Hicks ("false") contractions may be noted. These contractions are irregular, usually painless, and not associated with progressive cervical effacement and dilatation.

Stages of Normal Labor and Delivery

Normal labor begins between gestational weeks 38 and 42. It occurs in three stages. The first stage extends from the onset of labor to complete dilatation of the cervix. The second stage is from cervical dilatation until the birth of the infant, and the third stage lasts until delivery of the placenta. Some include a fourth stage, which extends from the end of placental delivery until the mother is stable, usually approximately 6 hours.

Stage 1: Cervical Dilatation

The first stage of labor is divided into a latent and an active phase. During the **latent phase,** the cervix softens and effaces (thins out), but it only dilates slightly. The latent phase normally lasts up to 20 hours in primiparas but is shorter in multiparas. The **active phase** of labor begins when the cervix has dilated to 3 to 4 cm and the uterus has begun contracting regularly. The rate of cervical dilatation increases during active labor, with minimal normal rates of 1 cm per hour in primiparas and 1.2 cm per hour in multiparas (Figure 7-1). During this time, the fetal head engages in the pelvis and begins its descent.

Fetal heart rate and uterine contractions should be monitored periodically during this stage of labor. Manual vaginal examinations should be minimized through the latent phase to prevent additional risk of infection and discomfort to the patient. During the active phase, regular examinations assess the progress of labor, including cervical dilatation and fetal descent.

Stage 2: Birth

The second stage of labor typically lasts 30 minutes to 3 hours in primiparas and 5 to 30 minutes in multiparas. The mother's efforts to bear down during regular uterine contractions increase her abdominal pressure and help to deliver the infant. The infant's head molds to fit the pelvis, then undergoes a series of typical movements (flexion, internal rotation, extension, and external rotation) to pass through the birth canal. Monitoring of the fetal heart rate and fetal descent should continue. Delivery of the fetus may be assisted by an episiotomy to prevent uncontrolled vaginal trauma.

Stage 3: Delivery of the Placenta

The third stage of labor involves separation of the placenta from the uterus, which occurs 5 to 30 minutes after birth of the child. Signs of separation include a sudden gush of blood from the vagina, lengthening of the umbilical cord, and firming of the uterine fundus. Af-

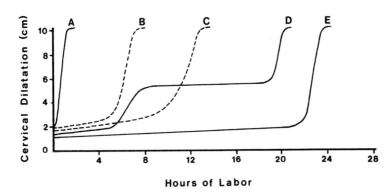

Fig. 7-1. Normal and abnormal labor curves. *A:* precipitate labor; *B:* normal multiparous labor; *C:* normal primigravida labor; *D:* protracted active phase because of arrest of dilatation; *E:* prolonged latent phase. (Reprinted with permission from Coustan D, Haning Jr. R, Singer D: *Human Reproduction: Growth and Development.* Boston, Little, Brown, 1995.)

ter delivery of the placenta, uterine massage and oxytocin will reduce excessive uterine bleeding. The placenta should be examined to verify that it is normal and that no placental fragments have been left in the uterus.

Stage 4: Recovery

The fourth stage of labor involves the stabilization of the mother. There is a risk of hemorrhage, particularly in the first hour after delivery. Close observation of the mother's uterine blood loss and vital signs is important. Perineal lacerations are repaired at this time. Lacerations are graded according to depth. First-degree lacerations involve the perineal skin or vaginal mucosa. Second-degree lesions extend into the submucosal tissue of the perineum or vagina. Third-degree lacerations involve the anal sphincter, and fourth-degree lacerations involve the rectal mucosa. After repair, a digital rectal examination is performed to rule out any additional rectal tears and any possibility that stitches have penetrated the rectal mucosa.

Fetal Heart Rate Monitoring

The normal fetal heart rate at term is 120 to 160 beats per minute. **Tachycardia** (>160 beats/min) may result from maternal or fetal infection, fetal anemia, hypoxia, or medications. **Bradycardia** (<120 beats/min), often caused by medications, congenital heart block, or fetal hypoxia, is generally threatening only if it is prolonged or associated with decreased variability. Normal **beat-to-beat variability** is approximately 5 beats per minute and reflects proper autonomic function. Increased variability may occur during mild hypoxia. Decreased variability is seen with fetal sleep, prematurity, some drugs, and hypoxia.

Fetal heart rate **accelerations** are generally reassuring signs of fetal well-being. An acceleration is a 15 beats per minute increase over baseline that lasts for at least 15 seconds. The fetal heart rate can be used to evaluate fetal well-being before labor, using either a nonstress test or contraction stress test. For a reassuring nonstress test, at least two accelerations and no decelerations should be detected in 20 minutes of monitoring. During a contraction stress test, uterine contractions are elicited, either with oxytocin administration or nipple stimulation. A reassuring test is a 10-minute interval with three contractions and no heart rate decelerations.

Decelerations are transitory episodes of a decreased fetal heart rate. Three types exist (Figure 7-2):

- **Early decelerations** occur synchronously with contractions. They arise because of head compression and do not suggest fetal distress.
- **Late decelerations** begin after onset of a uterine contraction and do not end until well after the contraction has stopped. They may indicate fetal hypoxia, especially if a loss of variability or an altered baseline fetal heart rate is associated. They are usually due to placental insufficiency, maternal venacaval compression, maternal hypotension, or uterine hyperactivity. Scalp sampling for fetal blood pH can confirm fetal hypoxia and acidosis.
- **Variable decelerations** are not consistent in intensity, duration, or onset relative to the contraction of the uterus. They are secondary to transient umbilical cord compression and suggest fetal distress only if variability is also decreased. If the woman changes position, cord compression is often relieved.

OBSTETRICS

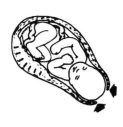

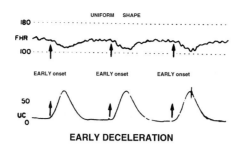

HEAD COMPRESSION

EARLY DECELERATION

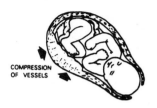

UTEROPLACENTAL INSUFFICIENCY

LATE DECELERATION

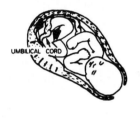

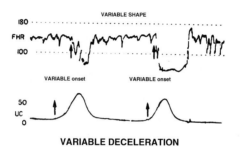

UMBILICAL CORD COMPRESSION

VARIABLE DECELERATION

Fig. 7-2. Fetal heart rate decelerations. FHR, fetal heart rate; UC, uterine contractions. (Reprinted with permission from Hon E: *An Introduction to Fetal Heart Rate Monitoring.* Los Angeles, University of Southern California, 1973.)

Intrapartum Fetal Stress

Fetal distress may be caused by the stress of labor. During uterine contractions, the fetal blood supply is repeatedly interrupted. Because the oxygen reserve of a healthy fetus will last 1 to 2 minutes, a normal fetus does not become hypoxic. A fetus with a decreased supply of oxygen, however, may become hypoxic during labor. Results of stress are demonstrated by fetal heart rate late decelerations and by decreases in fetal blood pH.

Meconium in the amniotic fluid is another sign of fetal distress and is detected in the amniotic fluid when the membranes rupture. Neonates with moderate to thick meconium should be aggressively managed (see Meconium Aspiration Syndrome, Chapter 8).

Abnormal Labor

Cephalopelvic Disproportion

In some deliveries, cephalopelvic disproportion—in which the fetal head cannot mechanically pass through the maternal bony pelvis—is evident. Contraction of the midpelvis is the most common cause. Disproportion at the pelvic inlet prevents engagement and descent of the fetal head.

Protracted or arrested labor. A decreased rate of cervical dilatation, or descent may be noted before arrest of descent.

Lack of progression of labor and manual evaluation of the bony pelvis establish the diagnosis.

Depending on the stage at which descent is blocked, an assisted delivery or cesarean section is necessary.

Fetal Malpresentations

Breech presentation is the most common malpresentation and involves the presentation of the fetal lower extremities or buttocks into the maternal pelvis. Other malpresentations include face and brow presentation, in which the fetal head fails to progress through the normal movements required for labor. Although one-fourth of fetuses are in a breech presentation before 28 weeks gestational age, few fetuses remain breech by 34 weeks.

Prematurity is a major risk factor for breech presentation, and breech babies often have low birth weight. Fetal anomalies, such as hydrocephalus and anencephaly, also predispose to breech, as do multiple gestation, uterine anomalies, polyhydramnios, and a contracted maternal pelvis. Breech presentations, particularly footling and double footling breeches, are at increased risk for cord prolapse.

Abdominal palpation reveals the fetal head in the fundal region. Vaginal examination permits palpation of the presenting part. Ultrasound confirms the presentation and can sometimes identify the cause.

External version at 37 weeks of gestation is successful in rotating the fetus in some patients, but placental abruption and cord compression are associated risks. Cesarean section is often indicated. Vaginal deliveries of breech infants increase the risk of cord prolapse, head entrapment, asphyxia, and birth injury.

Assisted Delivery

Obstetric forceps aid in fetal descent by providing traction and rotation. The most common indication is a prolonged second stage of labor that is due to failure of head rotation, inadequate uterine contractions, or cephalopelvic disproportion. **Vacuum extraction** may also be used when the uterus alone is not providing sufficient power for delivery. Fetal complications of assisted delivery (particularly forceps) include serious face, scalp, or head injuries and brain damage. Maternal complications include soft-tissue trauma and subsequent heavy bleeding.

Indications for Cesarean Section

The decision to perform a cesarean section is only rarely obvious. A history of previous "classic" cesarean section, in which a vertical incision was made in the uterus, is one absolute indication for repeat cesarean section because there is a high rate of uterine rupture in vaginal delivery after this procedure. The more common cesarean section technique, in which a low transverse incision into the uterus is made, is not necessarily an indication for repeat cesarean section. Vaginal birth may be attempted after this procedure, with a 60% to 80% success rate. The most common reason for cesarean section is failure to progress. In general, indications for cesarean section involve a threat to fetal health, maternal health, or both. These decisions are seldom clear-cut, but a list of relative indications is given in Table 7-3.

Postpartum Hemorrhage

Postpartum hemorrhage is defined as blood loss exceeding 500 mL during vaginal delivery or 1,000 mL during cesarean section. It is the second leading cause of maternal mortality. Uterine atony is responsible for the majority of cases, with risks from an overdistended uterus (e.g., multiple gestation), "grand multiparity," prolonged or augmented labor, or chorioamnionitis. Trauma to the cervix or vaginal tract, commonly a result of macrosomia or an instrumented vaginal delivery, can also cause hemorrhage. Most serious bleeding occurs immediately, but delayed postpartum hemorrhage may be due to retained placental tissue.

SIGNS & SYMPTOMS

Excessive blood from the uterus or vaginal tract.

Table 7-3. Relative indications for cesarean section

Fetal issues	Maternal issues	Fetal and maternal issues
Distress	Classic cesarean section	Placenta previa
Malpresentation	Prior uterine rupture	Placental abruption
Cord prolapse	Eclampsia	Cephalopelvic disproportion
Macrosomia	Failed induction of labor	
	Severe preeclampsia	
	Diabetes mellitus	
	Cardiac disease	

OBSTETRICS

Careful examination will determine the source of bleeding. In uterine atony, a large or boggy uterus is palpated through the abdominal wall. Vaginal and cervical inspection identify any lacerations. Manual exploration of the uterine cavity can diagnose uterine lacerations, retained products of conception, or partial inversion of the uterus.

Uterine massage and oxytocin help maintain uterine tone. Lacerations must be sutured. The delivered placenta should be examined to ensure that it is complete. In refractory hemorrhage, blood replacement is indicated. If the uterus remains atonic, hypogastric artery ligation, uterine embolization, or hysterectomy will save the patient's life.

Puerperium

Immediate Care of the Newborn

The following procedures are performed after the birth of a normal infant:

- **Clearing the airway.** Suctioning the mouth and nose clears excess fluid and prevents aspiration, which is a particular danger if meconium is present in the amniotic fluid.
- **Drying the baby.** This stimulates respiration and prevents heat loss.
- **Clamping the cord.** Delayed clamping results in significantly increased blood volume, increasing the risk of neonatal jaundice and tachypnea. Failure to clamp also prevents an accurate cord-gas measurement.
- **Verifying onset of respiration.** Delay of onset for up to 1 minute is acceptable. Respirations are generally induced by stimulation of the neonate. If unsuccessful, rapid resuscitation is critical.
- **Apgar scoring.** Heart rate, respiratory effort, muscle tone, cry, and color are assessed 1 and 5 minutes after birth. Each factor is scored on a 2-point scale. A score of at least 7 at 1 minute and 9 or 10 at 5 minutes is normal.

Physiology of the Normal Puerperium

The puerperium is the period after delivery until about 6 weeks postpartum. During this time, the maternal physiology returns to its prepregnant state.

Pelvic Changes

The lochia (normal uterine discharge) is bloody during the first days postpartum. It grows paler after a few days because of increasing amounts of mucus, and by the tenth day it is white or yellowish-white in appearance and consists primarily of microbes and cellular debris. The uterus decreases in weight, from 1 kg at delivery to 50 g within 3 weeks. The muscles of the pelvic floor gradually regain most of their prepregnancy tone.

Cardiovascular Changes

Immediately after delivery, the maternal peripheral vascular resistance increases sharply because the low-pressure uteroplacental component is gone. Some weight loss occurs in the first week as the plasma volume and extracellular fluid levels return to normal. Cardiac functioning returns to its prepregnant state within 3 weeks.

Menstrual Cycle Changes

Nursing mothers generally do not ovulate for several months, but this is variable and is no guarantee of contraception. Women who opt not to nurse typically regain their menstrual flow by 6 to 8 weeks postpartum.

Lactation and Breast-feeding

During the first half of pregnancy, the ductal elements of the breast proliferate because of the influence of estrogen. The epithelial cells then develop their secretory ability. High prolactin levels promote milk production, but this is inhibited by estrogen and other hormones. After delivery, the drop in placentally derived estrogen permits lactation to occur. The baby's suckling evokes release of both prolactin, for production of milk, and oxytocin, which induces contraction of myoepithelial cells in the milk ducts and causes ejection of fluid. Colostrum, or "early milk," is initially secreted. It contains protein, fat, secretory immunoglobulin A, and minerals. Mature milk is present within a week, containing protein, fat, lactose, and water.

Mothers often worry during the first days that their milk production is insufficient. They should be reassured that early milk is thin and that it is normal for infants to lose weight in the first week. Breast engorgement in the first few days may cause pain, which is relieved by breast-feeding and by applying hot compresses. The advantages of breast-feeding are many, including complete and inexpensive nutrition for the infant, transmission of immunoglobulins for improved immunity, reduced incidence of allergies and asthma later in life, mother-child bonding, and weight loss for the mother. There are very few contraindications to breast-feeding; these include HIV infection, active hepatitis infection, and the use of certain medications—particularly tetracycline, chloramphenicol, and warfarin.

Mastitis

Breast feeding–related mastitis, a cellulitis of the periglandular tissue, is most often caused by *Staphylococcus aureus.*

Onset is usually 2 to 4 weeks after breast-feeding begins. Fever and chills can occur, in addition to painful erythema and induration of the breast.

Clinical presentation. Breast milk culture is rarely needed.

Begin a penicillinase-resistant penicillin immediately, before culture results. Breast-feeding is not contraindicated.

OBSTETRICS

Postpartum Sepsis

Infection in the postpartum period usually occurs in the uterus or urinary tract. It follows cesarean section more often than vaginal delivery. Other risk factors include anemia, preeclampsia, premature and prolonged rupture of membranes, extended labor, multiple vaginal examinations during labor, traumatic delivery, and postpartum hemorrhage. Anaerobic organisms cause most postpartum infections, and *Escherichia coli* is the most common aerobic pathogen.

Endometritis (infection of the uterine endometrium) is characterized by fever and uterine tenderness. Reduced lochia is often associated with a more severe sepsis. **Parametritis** (inflammation of connective tissue around the uterus) is characterized by a fixed, painful uterus and high fever. **UTIs,** as usual, present with increased urgency, frequency, and dysuria. **Pelvic thrombophlebitis** is a complication of postpartum sepsis that presents with a persistent, spiking fever that is not responsive to antibiotics.

Temperature of 38°C or higher, lasting 2 days and starting between the second and tenth day postpartum. Other sources of fever, particularly mastitis or deep venous thrombosis, must be excluded. Blood and urine cultures can establish the infecting organism.

Antibiotics with broad anaerobic coverage should be given early and continued for 2 days after the fever has resolved. A commonly used regimen of "triple therapy" includes ampicillin, gentamicin, and clindamycin. Heparin therapy is indicated if pelvic thrombophlebitis is suspected.

Postpartum "Blues" and Postpartum Depression

Postpartum "blues" is a common complication of the puerperium, usually occurring 3 to 10 days after delivery and resolving spontaneously. Unlike postpartum blues, postpartum depression will not resolve in the puerperium. It occurs most often in primipara patients with a history of depression and in patients who do not have good social support. Depressive symptoms may be associated with apathy toward the infant, hallucinations, psychotic behavior, and homicidal or suicidal ideation. Antidepressant medication is helpful.

Postpartum Psychosis

Postpartum psychosis is less common, more severe, and longer lasting than postpartum depression, and the psychotic aspects are more pronounced. Hospitalization and antipsychotic medications may be necessary to stabilize the patient.

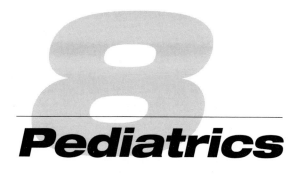

Pediatrics

(continued)

Infancy and Childhood

Normal Infant and Childhood Growth and Development

Growth and development in infants and children are rapidly occurring and constantly changing processes. Developmental landmarks in several different categories are listed in Table 8-1. Although specific ages are mentioned, keep in mind that these are guidelines that may vary from child to child. Slow development in any area may be hereditary; only

Table 8-1. Childhood developmental landmarks

Age	Gross motor	Fine motor	Language	Personal	Cognitive and social
2 mos	Lifts head to 45°	Eyes follow to midline	Vocalizes	Smiles	State of half-waking consciousness
4 mos	Lifts head to 90°	Eyes follow past midline	Laughs	Regards own hand	Slight awareness of caregiver
6 mos	Rolls over	Grasps rattle	Turns to voice	Feeds self	Separates world into "Mom" and "not Mom"
12 mos	Sits without support Pulls to stand	Pincer grasp	Babbles	Indicates wants	Stranger anxiety
18 mos	Walks well	Makes tower of two blocks	Says three words	Uses spoon and cup	Temper tantrums Rejects help Frequently brings objects to caregiver
2 yrs	Runs Climbs steps	Makes tower of four blocks	Combines words	Removes clothes	Develops concept of object permanence
4 yrs	Balances on one foot for 2 seconds	Copies a circle	Explains pictures Speech can be understood	Dresses self	Magical thinking Egocentric (only aware of own viewpoint) Symbolic play
6 yrs	Balances on one foot for 6 seconds	Draws a person with six parts	Defines words Knows opposites	Prepares cereal	Logical thinking begins Understands conservation of mass and volume

PEDIATRICS

significant delays in growth and development are likely to become cause for concern. Nonetheless, progress should be assessed at each pediatric visit to identify problems early and provide the child with any extra assistance necessary.

Newborns generally lose approximately 10% of their body weight in the first few days of life but gain it back within 10 days. Babies gain approximately 30 g (1 oz) per day for the first few months. Before 6 months of age, nutrition is the primary factor in infant weight gain. After 6 months, genetic factors predominate, so growth percentiles can change significantly. Each child's growth should be plotted on a standardized graph at every visit. Any deviation from the expected curve on the graph should prompt further investigation. In this manner, feeding problems, failure to thrive, metabolic abnormalities, and obesity can be identified and addressed as quickly as possible.

Child-Parent Interaction

As a child grows, the parent must adapt to the child's changing needs. Over time, the infant forms an attachment to the primary caregiver. If this attachment is a reliable one, the developing infant feels secure enough to explore the environment but keeps the parent within close distance and periodically returns for reassurance. Infants with less secure attachment may be clingy, agitated, and afraid to explore. Alternatively, a poorly attached infant may explore the world with independence, not looking back to the parent for security, because he or she has learned not to expect the parent to be there for support. This infant will tend to be very accident-prone. As a toddler begins to develop his or her own identity, the parent must encourage the child's individuation and exploration, while enforcing enough limitations to keep the child safe. In early childhood, the child begins to assume a role in the social structure, and the parent should gradually allow the child to accept more responsibility. In middle childhood, the child can exert more self-control and think more logically. The parent should respond by using reason in rule setting. In adolescence, the child moves toward even greater independence. This may cause conflict in the parent-child relationship until a new balance of mutual tolerance and respect is achieved.

Well-Child Care

In addition to administering immunizations, pediatric visits should be used to provide medical screening, developmental guidance, and accident-prevention advice.

Health Screening

- **Weight and height.** Measure and graph at every visit.
- **Vision.** Screen for strabismus (corneal light reflexes and cover test), retinoblastoma and cataracts (red reflex test), and basic vision (ability to follow toy) in infancy. Check visual acuity at school entry or earlier.
- **Hearing.** Hearing impairment should be detected before the age of 3 months to allow for early intervention. Screening can be done using auditory brainstem response or otoacoustic emissions testing.
- **Dental.** Check for caries. Encourage regular checkups. Discuss brushing and no bottles in bed.
- **Hematocrit.** Iron-deficiency anemia is most common between age 9 and 24 months, and a hematocrit should be checked at this time.

- **Lead.** Lead levels should be checked at age 9 and 24 months, especially in children who live in houses built before 1960 with peeling paint or restoration in progress.
- **Tuberculosis.** Check PPD at age 1 year and yearly thereafter in high-risk populations.

Anticipatory Guidance

- **Feeding.** Breast-fed infants nurse 8 to 10 times per day. Solids can be introduced at age 6 months. Iron fortification should begin at this time as well. Cow's milk should be avoided until 12 months of age because of an increased risk of developing an allergic response to the cow's milk protein.
- **Elimination.** A normal newborn may pass stool as often as 7 times a day or as seldom as once every 7 days. Children may be neurologically capable of toilet training as early as 18 months, but success is more common at 2–3 years of age. Training should take advantage of the child's natural pleasure in her own accomplishments and her desire to please and imitate her parents. If the child is resistant or disinterested, advise the parents to try again after several months. Accidents are normal throughout early childhood.
- **Development.** At 6 to 12 weeks of age, infants may cry several hours a day, frequently because of fatigue and overstimulation. Parents should be counseled to provide a soothing atmosphere for the baby and to accept crying as normal behavior. Later in infancy, babies respond well to games that help them practice new skills, such as reaching and babbling. Interactive play should be encouraged. Reading to children helps develop school readiness. TV should be limited to 1–2 hours a day, at most.
- **Discipline.** Excessive scolding, threats, and physical punishment should generally be avoided. Clear limits and consequences should be established. "Time-outs" (separation from the situation for several minutes) are often effective. Parents should not discipline behavior that is developmentally normal (e.g., the stubborn 2 year old). Positive reinforcement of desirable behavior should be encouraged.

Accident Prevention

- **Car seats.** By law, infants weighing less than 20 pounds must be placed in a rear-facing infant seat. Children weighing 20 to 40 pounds may face forward in a toddler seat.
- **Gun safety.** Weapons should be stored unloaded and locked out of reach of children.
- **Drowning prevention.** Toddlers can drown in bathtubs, wading pools, and even buckets. Supervision near water is essential.
- **Burn prevention.** Turn hot-water heaters to lower temperatures. Keep pot handles turned toward the back of the stove. Install and check smoke detectors.
- **Avoiding falls.** Some babies roll over at 2 months of age, much earlier than expected, so changing-table safety is imperative. Baby walkers are notoriously dangerous and should be avoided. Bicycle helmets can prevent serious injury when using any wheeled toy.
- **Poisoning prevention.** Medicines, cleaning agents, and insecticides should be kept in childproof locations. Syrup of ipecac and the telephone number for poison control should be kept handy.

Physician-Child-Parent Communication

When dealing with pediatric patients, physicians often have to participate in three-way communication and address issues concerning both the parent's and the child's interests. The following suggestions for communication may be helpful.

- Young children may be most comfortable undergoing examination while on a parent's lap. Ask older children, preferably when the parent is not around, if they would like to have a parent present in the room during the examination. For preteens and teens, try to see the patient without the parent so that you will have adequate privacy to address such issues as sexual behavior, drug and alcohol use, and depression or suicidal tendencies.
- Children and teens may feel intimidated by an excessively authoritarian manner. Try to communicate with them on an equal basis when possible, while maintaining your professional demeanor.
- Beware of countertransference on your part. This means that you should not overidentify with either the child ("The parents are being too strict and are the enemy") or with the parents ("This child's actions are bad and should be controlled").

Congenital and Perinatal Infections

TORCH Infections

TORCH is an acronym used for congenital and perinatal infections.

T	Toxoplasmosis
O	Other—Syphilis
	Varicella-zoster
R	Rubella
C	Cytomegalovirus
H	Herpes simplex
	Hepatitis B
	HIV

PEDIATRICS

Congenital Toxoplasmosis

Congenital toxoplasmosis, a transplacental infection by *Toxoplasma gondii,* occurs after primary maternal infection with the parasite, which is found in cat feces and raw meat. Fetuses of women with prior infections are not at risk of congenital toxoplasmosis unless the women are immunocompromised.

SIGNS & SYMPTOMS

The classic congenital toxoplasmosis syndrome includes chorioretinitis, intracranial calcifications, hydrocephalus, hepatosplenomegaly, and jaundice. Most infants are asymptomatic at birth but may have later sequelae that include mental retardation, seizures, blindness, and deafness.

DIAGNOSIS

Immunoglobulin M (IgM) titers and increasing IgG titers in the infant suggest infection. Stable IgG titers only suggest prior maternal infection and normal transfer of antibodies to the infant prenatally.

Little effective treatment is available for infants.

TREATMENT

Pregnant women should avoid undercooked meat and cat litter. Treatment of primary infections in pregnant women reduces congenital infections.

PREVENTION

Congenital Rubella

Transplacental rubella infection occurs when pregnant women become infected with the rubella virus. Rates of transmission to the fetus are as high as 80% during the first trimester. During these early weeks, the fetus is also at the greatest risk of developing abnormalities. Infected women may be asymptomatic or may experience upper respiratory symptoms, arthritis, and a telltale rash that begins on the face.

Fetal effects vary depending on the gestational age at the time of infection. Typical anomalies include a purpuric "blueberry muffin" rash, intrauterine growth retardation (IUGR), mental retardation, cataracts, retinopathy, cardiac defects, jaundice, and hepatosplenomegaly. Bony radiolucencies are demonstrated on x-ray. Hearing loss may be the only manifestation of infection late in pregnancy.

SIGNS & SYMPTOMS

Rising antibody titers and viral cultures.

DIAGNOSIS

No effective treatment exists.

TREATMENT

Prevention is crucial. Immunization typically occurs in childhood, but antibody titer levels should be verified in all women before pregnancy. Immunization is contraindicated during the pregnancy, but titers should be checked so that nonimmune women can be vaccinated after delivery. If a nonimmunized pregnant woman is exposed to rubella, immunoglobulin can be administered, and termination of the pregnancy may be considered.

PREVENTION

Cytomegalovirus

Cytomegalovirus (CMV) is the virus most commonly transmitted from mother to fetus. The infant's infection may be congenital (acquired from transplacental infection) or perinatal (acquired from contact with infected maternal secretions during delivery or breast-feeding). Mothers who are newly infected with CMV during pregnancy are more likely to transmit their infections than mothers who are asymptomatic carriers of the virus. Maternal primary infection is mild, however, and often goes unnoticed.

The majority of infected infants are asymptomatic at birth. Only 10% of congenitally infected infants have acute symptoms, which may include prematurity, IUGR, hepatosplenomegaly, jaundice, petechiae, microcephaly, periventricular calcifications, and chorioretinitis. The combination of jaundice and petechiae causes the infant to have a "blueberry corn muffin" appearance. Symptomatic CMV has a 20% mortality rate, and 90% of survivors have sequelae of mental retardation, seizures, hearing loss, and visual defects. Among asymptomatic infected infants, 10% will have neurologic sequelae, most often involving hearing loss. These infants are usually infected later in gestation. Infections at the time of delivery may cause pneumonitis.

Infant IgM antibodies against CMV suggest infection. Isolating the virus from urine, blood, CSF, amniotic fluid, or the placenta is confirmatory.

None available.

Neonatal Herpes Simplex Virus

Neonatal herpes simplex virus (HSV) infection, generally caused by HSV type 2, is usually transmitted by delivery through an infected vaginal tract. Transplacental and nosocomial spread also occur. Mothers may be unaware of their HSV infection, and the risk of transmission is higher during a primary maternal infection.

Within 1 to 4 weeks of birth, skin vesicles appear in approximately half of infected infants. Some have only localized disease, with skin, mouth, and eye involvement. Disseminated infection also occurs, however, including temperature instability, lethargy, respiratory difficulty, seizures, pneumonitis, hepatitis, and disseminated intravascular coagulation (DIC). Another form of localized disease, encephalitis, tends to occur in infants who do not develop skin lesions. Neurologic involvement results in severe neurologic sequelae in survivors.

Culture of CSF or scrapings from lesions may reveal the virus. Polymerase chain reaction (PCR) for HSV DNA in the CSF is more sensitive in encephalitis. Brain biopsy is the gold standard.

Vidarabine or acyclovir decreases mortality by 50% and decreases the sequelae of both localized and disseminated disease.

Cesarean section is recommended in women with active lesions at the time of delivery, especially if the lesions are due to primary infection.

PREVENTION

Neonatal Hepatitis B Infection

Neonatal hepatitis B (HBV) infection is generally acquired during delivery. Most infections come from mothers who are asymptomatic carriers of HBV; however, infants of women who are newly infected late in pregnancy are also at very high risk of becoming infected. Transplacental transmission is rare. The main risk to the infant is becoming an HBV carrier, with the resulting chronic hepatitis and an increased risk of hepatocellular carcinoma.

Most infants develop chronic hepatitis, which is generally subclinical. Some infants develop acute hepatitis that is self-limited and typically mild.

SIGNS & SYMPTOMS

HBsAg serology.

DIAGNOSIS

Acute hepatitis is treated symptomatically.

TREATMENT

Infants of infected women should receive hepatitis B immunoglobulin and hepatitis B vaccine as soon as possible after delivery. See Chapter 9 for specific recommendations.

PREVENTION

Congenital Syphilis

Risk of congenital syphilis, a transplacentally acquired infection, depends on the mother's stage of disease during pregnancy. Primary and secondary syphilis are usually transmitted, whereas latent and tertiary syphilis are not.

Most newborns are asymptomatic at birth and develop symptoms within a few weeks to months. A bright red maculopapular rash on the palms and soles is characteristic. Hepatosplenomegaly, jaundice, and anemia with an increase in nucleated red blood cells may develop. Later, the infant may exhibit failure to thrive. "Snuffles" (discharge due to nasal bone necrosis) in a young infant may be the presenting sign. Within 3 months, bone changes may result in bone inflammation or pseudoparalysis. Most infected infants remain in the latent stage throughout their lives, although some have late manifestations.

SIGNS & SYMPTOMS

PEDIATRICS

Dark-field microscopy from lesion scrapings, or rapid plasma reagin (RPR) and VDRL tests are diagnostic. Long bone x-rays will show characteristic radiologic abnormalities.

Penicillin is given to infected infants. Prognosis is good.

This disease is entirely preventable with adequate diagnosis and treatment of pregnant women.

Congenital Varicella

Varicella infection has only a 5% transmission rate across the placenta. Infants whose mothers develop chickenpox fewer than 5 days before delivery or less than 2 days after delivery are at risk for increased morbidity and mortality.

Transplacental exposure results in limb hypoplasia, microcephaly, cortical atrophy, chorioretinitis, and cutaneous scars. Perinatal exposure results in severe chickenpox.

Increasing maternal IgG titers, neonatal IgM, or viral culture.

Pregnant women exposed to varicella should receive varicella immunoglobulin (VZIG). Women with the disease can be treated with acyclovir. VZIG is given to infants whose mothers develop chickenpox within 5 days before and 2 days after delivery.

Neonatal Sepsis

Neonatal sepsis is defined as any systemic bacterial infection within the first 4 weeks of life. It occurs more frequently in low birth-weight infants, in males, and in infants with respiratory depression. Early-onset sepsis, apparent 6 to 72 hours after birth, is due to infection acquired in utero or during delivery, and its risk increases with many complications of labor and delivery. Late-onset sepsis is often nosocomial, usually presenting after approximately 4 days. The most common organisms are group B streptococci (see Chapter 7) and *Escherichia coli.* Others include *Staphylococcus aureus, Staphylococcus epidermidis, Listeria monocytogenes,* and *Enterococcus.*

Symptoms of sepsis are often subtle and nonspecific, with decreased activity, poor feeding, temperature instability (hyperthermia or hypothermia), apnea, and bradycardia. Early-onset sepsis causes respiratory failure, meningitis, shock, DIC, and acute tubular necrosis.

If bacterial infection is suspected, obtain a CBC and chest x-ray and culture the blood, CSF, and urine. The WBC count is considered abnormal and indicative of possible sepsis if it is less than 4,000/μL or greater than 25,000/μL.

Broad-spectrum antibiotics.

Substance-exposed Infants

Fetal Alcohol Syndrome

Fetal alcohol syndrome, an all-too-common result of alcohol ingestion during pregnancy, involves a dose-related spectrum of defects. Infants have IUGR and dysmorphic features, including microcephaly, short palpebral fissures, cardiac anomalies, and joint defects. Later manifestations include mental retardation and hyperactivity. Fetal alcohol syndrome is the leading cause of preventable mental retardation.

Narcotic Exposure

Infants exposed to heroin, methadone, and other narcotics in utero are at risk for a withdrawal syndrome after birth. Withdrawal symptoms include irritability, tremors, hypertonicity, high-pitched cry, sweating, stuffy nose, sneezing, and yawning. More severe withdrawal involves vomiting, diarrhea, and seizures. The symptoms from methadone withdrawal are generally more severe and prolonged than those from heroin withdrawal. Urine toxicology confirms the diagnosis only if the drug has been used within a few days of delivery. Swaddling the infant in a quiet environment is usually sufficient treatment. Otherwise, phenobarbital or tincture of opium may be administered and tapered slowly. These infants are at an increased risk of sudden infant death syndrome.

Cocaine Exposure

Cocaine use during pregnancy leads to an increased risk of preterm labor and placental abruption, as well as a range of fetal effects. Vascular disruption secondary to cocaine use may have early effects on the fetus, causing limb reduction malformations and intestinal atresias. Low birth weight, low Apgar scores, cerebral infarcts, and intraventricular hemorrhages are also found. Signs of exposure include irritability and jitteriness, which are treated by swaddling the infant and providing a quiet, low-stimulation environment.

Gastroenterology

Tracheoesophageal Fistula

Often associated with esophageal atresia (a blind pouch), tracheoesophageal fistula is a congenital malformation resulting in a tract between the trachea and the esophagus.

Neonates have coughing and cyanosis during feeding and will likely develop aspiration pneumonia. If the esophagus is patent, abdominal distention may develop when air travels through the fistula to the stomach.

X-ray after nasogastric tube placement identifies esophageal atresia. Excess gas in the stomach can indicate a tracheoesophageal fistula, and bronchoscopy confirms the diagnosis.

Surgical repair is needed.

Diaphragmatic Hernia

Diaphragmatic hernia, protrusion of parts of the GI tract through the diaphragm and into the thorax, generally occurs on the left side and may result in a hypoplastic left lung. Respiratory distress, a sunken abdomen, and bowel sounds over the left hemithorax indicate this disorder. X-ray is confirmatory. Large hernias are often fatal because of poor lung development. Small defects can be corrected surgically, although pulmonary effects persist.

Pyloric Stenosis

Pyloric stenosis is a muscular hypertrophy of the pyloric valve that causes obstruction. It occurs most often in boys. This hypertrophy begins at birth, and signs of obstruction begin to appear at age 2 to 4 weeks. Projectile vomiting after eating, visible peristaltic waves, poor weight gain, and constipation suggest this diagnosis. An olive-sized mass can be palpated in the right epigastrium, and a mass is visible on ultrasound. Barium swallow x-ray confirms the diagnosis, showing the "string sign" of a narrowed lumen. Surgery is curative.

Necrotizing Enterocolitis

Necrotizing enterocolitis and sloughing of the intestinal mucosa is the most common surgical emergency in neonates. Preterm and low birth-weight newborns, as well as full-term infants with malnutrition and diarrhea, are most commonly affected. Etiology is unknown.

Infants have bilious vomiting, abdominal distention, bloody stools, and lethargy. Peritonitis, acidosis, DIC, and shock may occur.

DIAGNOSIS

X-ray shows small-bowel distention and, later, pneumatosis (air in the bowel wall). Perforation, with free peritoneal air on x-ray, occurs in 20% of cases.

TREATMENT

Nasogastric suction, total parenteral nutrition, and IV antibiotics should be started immediately. Resection of the necrotic portion is usually necessary.

Meconium Ileus

Meconium ileus is an early sign of cystic fibrosis. Infants with this disorder have abnormally thick meconium containing undigested protein. Loops of intestine can often be palpated, and in utero volvulus may occur and infarct. Infarcted bowel segments often reabsorb, resulting in atresia or cyst formation. A positive sweat test or DNA testing confirms the diagnosis of cystic fibrosis.

Hirschsprung's Disease

Also called *congenital megacolon,* Hirschsprung's disease is caused by the absence of autonomic innervation in a portion of the bowel wall. Continuous smooth muscle spasm causes partial obstruction, and the proximal bowel segment becomes massively dilated. This condition is usually evident in early infancy, but diagnosis may be delayed by several months or years. Distention, obstipation, and late vomiting are key features, and barium enema x-ray shows a dilated proximal segment and a narrowed distal segment. Rectal biopsy, demonstrating the absence of nerve ganglia, is confirmatory. A colostomy is necessary for immediate management. Later, the aganglionic segment should be resected. Toxic enterocolitis is a complication of untreated disease.

Intussusception

Intussusception is the telescoping of one bowel segment into an adjacent segment. Usually, the terminal ileum slides into the right colon. Intussusception is the most common cause of bowel obstruction in children younger than 2 years of age. In 95% of patients, the etiology is unknown. Hypertrophied Peyer's patches may provide the leading edge, and there is an association with adenovirus infections. Ischemia of the bowel is a serious complication.

Children present with the sudden onset of abdominal pain that occurs in episodes lasting approximately 1 minute. Reflex vomiting may occur early, but vomiting that is due to the obstruction does not occur until later. "Currant jelly" stool is common because of blood and mucus. Pallor, sweating, and vomiting are the main symptoms in very small infants.

Leukocytosis with a left shift and hemoconcentration are generally present.

A palpable mass may be felt in the right upper quadrant with no cecum palpable in the right lower quadrant. Obstruction can be seen with barium enema.

Administration of the barium enema itself will reduce the intussusception in the majority of patients and should be repeated if unsuccessful. Surgical reduction is needed for the rest, with resection of any gangrenous portions.

Encopresis

Encopresis is an elimination disorder that involves the passage of feces at inappropriate times. Elimination is generally involuntary. It may be due to constipation with overflow incontinence, resistance to toilet training, or a disruptive behavior disorder.

In addition to inappropriate passage of feces, the child may experience embarrassment and avoidance of social situations. If constipation is present, the patient may have continuous fecal leakage and anal fissures.

For this diagnosis to apply, the child must be at least 4 years old and have had episodes of encopresis at least once a month for 3 months.

Complete bowel evacuation should be followed by establishment of regular bowel movements. Giving the patient mineral oil, roughage, laxatives, and regular toileting times throughout the day may help.

Glycogen Storage Diseases

Glycogen storage diseases belong to a group of rare, usually autosomal-recessive disorders with varying degrees of severity. Specific defects in carbohydrate metabolism lead to abnormal glycogen accumulation in the liver, muscle, nerves, heart, and other organs. Glycogen stores can be visualized on MRI. Tissue biopsy and enzyme assay confirm the diagnosis. Etiologies include:

- **Pompe's disease,** an alpha-1,4-glucosidase deficiency that is fatal by age 2 years, with glycogen buildup in many organs.
- **von Gierke's disease,** a glucose 6-phosphatase deficiency that leads to enlarged liver and kidneys, growth retardation, and electrolyte abnormalities.
- **McArdle's disease,** a milder disorder in which muscle phosphorylase is absent. Patients experience cramps and myoglobinuria after exercise. Limiting physical activity and increasing fluid intake help to minimize the symptoms, and diuresis after exertion prevents the myoglobinuria from progressing to renal failure.

Hyperbilirubinemia

Jaundice in the newborn may reflect increased production (often due to hemolysis) or decreased excretion of bilirubin. The most common type of hyperbilirubinemia is "physiologic" jaundice, in which levels of unconjugated (indirect) bilirubin are elevated because high RBC turnover occurs before the liver is mature enough to conjugate and excrete the bile. Approximately 50% of full-term infants and even more preterm infants experience this mild increase in bilirubin, which resolves in 1 to 2 weeks. Other causes of hyperbilirubinemia are listed in Table 8-2. Severe elevations of bilirubin are treated to avoid **kernicterus,** a rare syndrome that occurs when unconjugated bilirubin is deposited in the basal ganglia and hippocampus, causing nerve cell death and brain damage.

Table 8-2. Causes of hyperbilirubinemia

Overproduction from increased hemolysis
    Fetal-maternal blood group incompatibility (Rh, ABO)
    RBC abnormalities (hereditary spherocytosis, elliptocytosis)
    Enzyme abnormalities (G6PD deficiency, pyruvate kinase deficiency)
Overproduction without hemolysis
    Extravascular hemorrhage (hematoma, intraventricular hemorrhage)
    Polycythemia (maternal-fetal transfusion, delayed cord clamping)
    Increased enterohepatic circulation (GI obstruction, ileus)
Undersecretion
    Physiologic jaundice
    Familial jaundice (Crigler-Najjar syndrome)
    Gilbert syndrome
    Biliary atresia
Mixed
    Intrauterine infection
    Sepsis
    Respiratory distress syndrome

G6PD, glucose 6-phosphate dehydrogenase; Rh, rhesus.

PEDIATRICS

Jaundice develops from the head downward and has no other symptoms. Signs of kernicterus are lethargy, poor feeding, high-pitched cry, hypertonicity, seizures, apnea, and death. Developmental manifestations, including mental retardation, sensorineural hearing loss, athetoid cerebral palsy, and paralysis of upward gaze, are irreversible.

Nonphysiologic jaundice should be suspected if jaundice is seen in the first 24 hours of life or if the bilirubin rises above 15 mg/dL before day 3 of life. Workup includes CBC with peripheral smear and reticulocyte count, maternal and fetal blood typing, direct and indirect Coombs' tests, and bilirubin fractionation. Conjugated (direct) bilirubin greater than 2 mg/dL is always abnormal and the exact cause should be established to prevent liver damage.

Good hydration and frequent feeding promote bilirubin excretion in the GI tract. Phototherapy converts unconjugated bilirubin into a water-soluble form, which the infant can then excrete in the urine and bile. For elevations (>20–25 mg/dL) exchange transfusions can be considered.

Failure to Thrive

Failure to thrive (FTT) is the term used to describe infants and young children who are underweight (<80% of ideal weight for height or below the 3rd percentile for age) or who fail to gain weight at the expected rate. The etiology may be organic (i.e., due to underlying illness), nonorganic (i.e., due to neglect or other difficulties in the parent-child interaction), or mixed.

A complete history and physical should be done to search for signs of genetic, pulmonary, cardiovascular, gastrointestinal, or central nervous system disorders that could account for the low weight; however, be aware that chronically ill children are also at risk of neglect. The infant's behavior may suggest emotional or physical deprivation. The absence of smiling, lack of normal social interaction, or presence of self-stimulatory behavior (i.e., head banging) may indicate interactive problems within the family.

The search for organic etiologies should be guided by the history and physical. Hematocrit, urinalysis and urine culture, and electrolytes are all reasonable. Testing for HIV, tuberculosis, and cystic fibrosis should be considered. Calorie intake and weight gain should be monitored carefully. Occasionally, infants are hospitalized to assess their weight gain in a controlled setting.

Nonorganic FTT is treated with a high calorie diet, parental education, and other social support services. Foster placement is sometimes necessary.

Familial Short Stature and Constitutional Growth Delay

Undersized children whose parents are also smaller than average may have **familial short stature.** These children are normal in every other way (i.e., bone age, growth velocity, timing of pubertal growth spurt). Children with **constitutional growth delay** lag 2–4 years behind average in height, bone age, and onset of puberty. This condition occurs more frequently in boys, and there is often a family history of similar delay. The final adult height is normal.

Cardiovascular Disorders

Fetal Circulation

Fetal gas exchange occurs in the uteroplacental circulation. Fetal hemoglobin has a higher affinity for oxygen than does maternal hemoglobin, so it is able to withdraw oxygen from the maternal blood. The fetal *umbilical arteries* bring deoxygenated blood to the placenta, and the *umbilical vein* carries oxygenated blood from the placenta to the fetal portal system (Figure 8-1). Some of the blood from the umbilical vein passes through the liver and then into the inferior vena cava. The rest enters the *ductus venosus,* which leads directly from the umbilical vein into the vena cava. As the oxygenated blood enters the right atrium, one-third crosses the *foramen ovale* directly into the left atrium and travels via the aorta to the brain and upper body. Two-thirds enters the right ventricle, mixes with deoxygenated superior vena caval blood, and passes into the pulmonary trunk. Most of this blood bypasses the lungs via the *ductus arteriosus,* which leads to the descending aorta. Although some of this blood supplies the lower body, the majority enters the umbilical arteries and returns to the placenta.

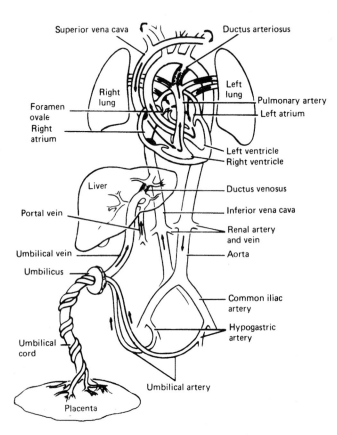

Fig. 8-1. Fetal circulation. (Reprinted with permission from DeCherney A, Pernoll M (eds): *Current and Gynecologic Diagnosis and Treatment,* 8th ed. Norwalk, Appleton & Lange, 1994, p 171.)

PEDIATRICS

At birth, lung expansion causes resistance of the pulmonary vascular bed to drop and pulmonary blood flow to increase, resulting in a decrease in flow through the ductus arteriosus. The ductus arteriosus closes soon after birth.

Congenital Heart Defects

Congenital heart defects occur in approximately 1% of all children. They may result in left-to-right shunts (in which blood that has been through the lungs is shunted back to the venous side of the heart and goes through the lungs again) or right-to-left shunts (in which blood that has not been oxygenated in the lungs goes directly into the arterial circulation). Intrauterine risk factors for congenital heart disease include maternal alcohol use, medications (estrogens, lithium, anticonvulsants), congenital infection (rubella), and pre-existing maternal diabetes. Patients with the heart defects described here should receive antibiotic prophylaxis against bacterial endocarditis prior to dental procedures. The exception is mild atrial septal defect, which requires no prophylaxis.

Atrial Septal Defect

An atrial septal defect (ASD) is an opening between the left atrium and right atrium, usually a result of a patent foramen ovale (Figure 8-2A,B). This condition usually results in a left-to-right shunt, so that blood volume is increased on the right side.

SIGNS & SYMPTOMS

The hallmark heart sound is a widely split, fixed S_2, because the increased right-sided blood volume delays closure of the pulmonic valve. A systolic ejection murmur is usually heard at the pulmonic area (second intercostal space to the left of the sternum), which results from increased blood velocity in the pulmonary artery.

DIAGNOSIS

ECG may show right ventricular conduction abnormalities (i.e., a right bundle branch block pattern). Echocardiography and cardiac catheterization are diagnostic.

TREATMENT

Very small defects may not need treatment. Larger ones require surgical correction to prevent pulmonary hypertension in adulthood.

Ventricular Septal Defect

A ventricular septal defect (VSD) is an opening between the left and the right ventricles (Figure 8-2C), and it is the most common type of congenital cardiac defect. It results in a left-to-right shunt because of the greater power of the left ventricle.

PEDIATRICS

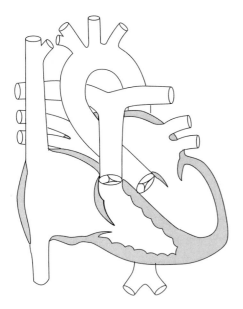

A. Normal Heart

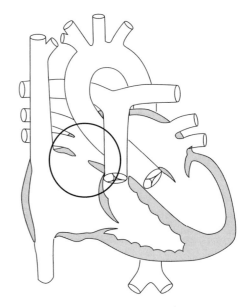

B. Atrial Septal Defect

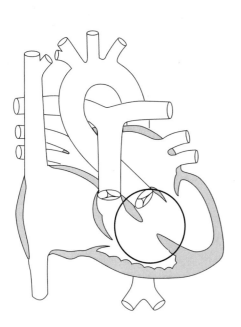

C. Ventricular Septal Defect

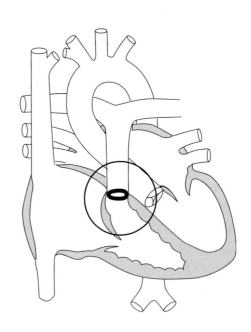

D. Pulmonary Stenosis

Fig. 8-2. Normal heart (**A**) and congenital heart defects (**B–G**). (Reproduced with permission from: Atrial Septal Defect, 1979. Ventricular Septal Defect, 1979. Patent Ductus Arteriosus, 1979. Transposition of the Great Arteries, 1979. Tetralogy of Fallot, 1979. Pulmonary Stenosis, 1979. c American Heart Association.)

SIGNS & SYMPTOMS

The hallmark heart sound is a harsh pansystolic murmur, heard best along the left sternal border. A thrill (vibration felt with a hand on the patient's chest) may be associated with the murmur. Infants with large defects have frequent respiratory infections and poor weight gain. Easy fatigability and congestive heart failure (CHF) are also typical.

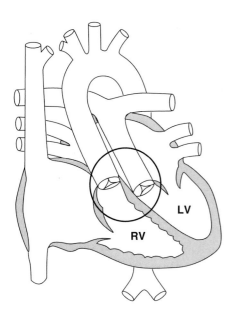

E. Transposition of the Great Arteries

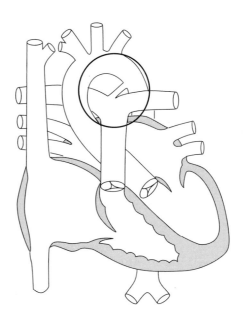

F. Patent Ductus Arteriosus

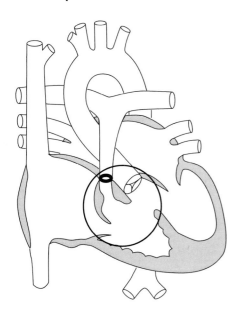

G. Tetralogy of Fallot

ECG may show left or right ventricular hypertrophy. Echocardiography and cardiac catheterization are diagnostic.

PEDIATRICS

Small ventricular septal defects may need no treatment and often close spontaneously. Larger defects require surgical repair or the patient risks developing **Eisenmenger's syndrome,** a condition in which the direction of the shunt becomes reversed (left-to-right shunt becomes right-to-left) because of increased pulmonary hypertension. This situation results in cyanosis and, eventually, heart failure.

Endocardial Cushion Defect

The endocardial cushions are embryonic structures necessary for normal development of the atrioventricular (AV) valves, the atrial septum, and the ventricular septum. Malformation of these cushions results in complex combinations of valvular and septal defects. The complete form of the defect results in a common AV canal, producing a two-chambered heart in which the atria are connected by an ASD, the ventricles are connected by a VSD, and only one AV valve exists. In the incomplete form, there is an ostium primum defect, in which an ASD is associated with minor AV valve abnormalities. These abnormalities are found in 20% of children with Down syndrome.

Patients with the incomplete defect have signs and symptoms of an ASD. The complete form causes CHF and recurrent pneumonitis. Murmurs vary depending on the defect.

ECG usually shows left axis deviation. Echocardiography and cardiac catheterization are diagnostic, revealing the valvular and septal abnormalities.

The need for treatment depends on the severity of the defect. Surgical treatment may be required to prevent CHF in later life. Patients who do not receive appropriate treatment may develop Eisenmenger's syndrome, in which severely increased pulmonary resistance results in a directional change of shunted blood.

Pulmonary Stenosis

Pulmonary stenosis results when the pulmonary valve cusps are fused together or the pulmonary trunk is very small and obstructive to blood flow (Figure 8-2D). There may be an associated ASD or VSD, which results in a right-to-left shunt.

Mild stenosis is asymptomatic. Severe disease causes cyanosis and right-sided CHF. The hallmark heart sound is a high-pitched systolic murmur at the left second intercostal space with a soft or absent S_2. Because the pulmonic valve is abnormal, the pulmonic component of S_2 is weak. There may be a pulmonic valve systolic ejection click. A parasternal lift and prominent thrill may also be noted as a result of right ventricular hypertrophy.

ECG shows right ventricular hypertrophy. Echocardiography and cardiac catheterization are diagnostic.

If mild, no treatment may be needed. Severe stenosis, however, can cause heart failure or sudden death. Treatment consists of balloon valvuloplasty or surgery to enlarge the pulmonic valve.

Transposition of the Great Vessels

In transposition of the great vessels, the aorta arises from the right ventricle and the pulmonary trunk arises from the left ventricle, resulting in a "transposition" of normal anatomy (Figure 8-2E). Without a septal defect allowing oxygenated and deoxygenated blood to mix, transposition of the great vessels is incompatible with life.

Newborns with transposition usually show extreme cyanosis immediately after birth.

Chest x-ray may show narrowing of the base of the heart, and the normal pulmonary artery markings may be absent. Diagnosis is confirmed with echocardiography or cardiac catheterization.

Immediate palliative treatment includes balloon septostomy to widen the septal defect, allowing for increased mixing of oxygenated and deoxygenated blood. Surgical correction is performed later in infancy.

Patent Ductus Arteriosus

Patent ductus arteriosus (PDA) occurs when the ductus arteriosus, a bypass that shunts blood from the pulmonary artery to the aorta during fetal life, does not close properly (Figure 8-2F). This state results in a left-to-right shunt because of the greater systemic blood pressure, but Eisenmenger's syndrome may develop later.

The characteristic heart sound is a continuous "machinery" murmur throughout systole and diastole. Pulses are bounding, and a widened pulse pressure is noted on blood pressure.

ECG may show left ventricular hypertrophy. Echocardiography and cardiac catheterization are diagnostic.

Indomethacin often induces closure in the first few days of life. If correction is necessary later in life, transcatheter occlusion or surgical ligation of the ductus may be performed.

Coarctation of the Aorta

Coarctation of the aorta is a localized narrowing of the aortic arch immediately distal to the origin of the left subclavian artery. A bicuspid aortic valve is present in 25% of cases.

In infants with severe disease, CHF develops as the ductus arteriosus closes. Older patients present with hypertension in the arms but not in the legs. Femoral pulses are weak and delayed when compared with upper-extremity pulses. Older patients may have leg claudication with exertion. On examination, a midsystolic or continuous murmur is heard best in the patient's back. A diastolic murmur caused by aortic insufficiency (due to bicuspid valves) may be present.

ECG reveals left ventricular hypertrophy. X-ray may show "scalloping" of ribs because of enlarged intercostal arteries. These vessels provide collateral circulation from the internal thoracic artery. Echocardiography and cardiac catheterization are used for definitive diagnosis.

In infants, keeping the ductus arteriosus open with prostaglandin infusion will maintain renal and lower extremity perfusion. Percutaneous balloon angioplasty may be used as a temporary measure to stabilize patients before surgery can be performed. All patients younger than age 20 years should undergo resection of the stenosed portion of the aorta. Patients younger than 40 years should have surgery if other cardiac risk factors are great (e.g., uncontrolled hypertension). Patients older than 50 years generally do not undergo surgery because the risks involved are high.

Tetralogy of Fallot

Tetralogy of Fallot is a classic syndrome that consists of four abnormalities: VSD, right ventricular hypertrophy, pulmonary stenosis, and an overriding aorta (Figure 8-2G). Because of the pulmonary stenosis, there is a right-to-left shunt through the VSD, with passage of deoxygenated blood from the right ventricle to the left ventricle and into the systemic circulation.

Depending on the severity of the pulmonary blood flow restriction, infants may develop cyanosis and a right ventricular ejection murmur at the left upper sternal border shortly after birth. Older children often squat during play to increase venous return and, therefore, cardiac output. Hypoxic spells, in which a child becomes increasingly agitated, hyperpneic, and cyanotic until he lapses into unconsciousness, occur and resolve spontaneously. They are due to an increase in the right-to-left shunt.

Chest x-ray may show right ventricular enlargement and a concave pulmonary artery segment. ECG shows right ventricular hypertrophy and right axis deviation. Diagnosis is confirmed with echocardiography and catheterization.

Prostaglandin injections may be given initially to maintain a PDA and preserve pulmonary blood flow. Surgical correction is the definitive treatment. Hypoxemic spells are treated by putting the child in knee-chest position to increase systemic vascular resistance.

PEDIATRICS

Respiratory Disorders

Meconium Aspiration Syndrome

Meconium is the neonate's first stool, consisting mostly of sloughed cells, mucus, and bile pigments. Some infants, particularly those who are post-term or suffer fetal hypoxia, pass meconium into the amniotic sac before birth. At birth, aspiration may occur, resulting in obstruction or chemical pneumonia. Complete blockage of the bronchi causes atelectasis, whereas partial obstruction causes air trapping with associated pneumothorax or pneumo-mediastinum. Persistent pulmonary hypertension may develop.

Tachypnea, retractions, cyanosis, and an overdistended chest are all characteristic signs. Meconium staining of the umbilical cord and nails shows that meconium has been passed into the amniotic fluid and indicates that aspiration may have occurred.

Chest x-ray demonstrates patchy atelectasis with areas of hyperinflation. Pneumothorax is common.

The infant's nose, mouth, and trachea should be suctioned at delivery before respiration has been established. Compromised infants require oxygen supplementation and may need mechanical ventilation.

Transient Tachypnea of the Newborn

Transient tachypnea of the newborn (TTN) results from delayed resorption of fetal lung fluid. Fluid is normally absorbed across the lung epithelium and expelled from the mouth when the thorax is compressed during vaginal delivery. Infants with TTN are full term but have typically been delivered by cesarean section.

The infant is tachypneic but appears comfortable. Grunting and retractions may be present. Cyanosis is rare. There are rales on auscultation.

Chest x-ray shows hyperinflated lungs with prominent vascular markings and fluid in the interlobar fissures.

Supplemental oxygen may be needed. Recovery is complete within 2 to 3 days.

PEDIATRICS

Respiratory Distress Syndrome of the Newborn

Also known as *hyaline membrane disease,* respiratory distress syndrome of the newborn is seen predominantly in preterm infants, especially those at less than 34 weeks of gestation. Decreased production of pulmonary surfactant results in atelectasis of the newborn lung, causing severe breathing difficulty.

SIGNS & SYMPTOMS

Within a few hours of delivery, the newborn develops rapid, labored breathing accompanied by grunting, intercostal retractions, nasal flaring, and cyanosis. Auscultation reveals crackles and decreased breath sounds. Symptoms worsen in the first 2–3 days of life.

DIAGNOSIS

Diagnosis is based on history, physical examination, and arterial blood gas data demonstrating high CO_2 and low O_2 levels. Chest x-ray shows diffuse atelectasis, causing a "ground glass" appearance, and air bronchograms.

TREATMENT

Administration of artificial surfactant is the current treatment of choice. Oxygen supplementation and the use of continuous positive airway pressure are also helpful. PaO_2 should be kept between 45 and 70 mm Hg because of the risk of retinopathy of prematurity with higher oxygen levels. Ventilator support may be necessary in severe cases.

PREVENTION

Fetal lung maturity can be assessed before delivery by determining the concentrations of lecithin (L), sphingomyelin (S), and phosphatidyl glycerol (PG) in the amniotic fluid. An L to S ratio higher than 2 accompanied by the presence of PG shows fetal lung maturity. If fetal lung maturity has not yet occurred, the mother may be given steroids, such as beclomethasone, 24 hours before delivery to hasten the production of pulmonary surfactant.

Neonatal Pneumonia

The infant's respiratory system may be infected in utero or during delivery. Infection is especially common if prolonged rupture of the membranes has led to amnionitis. Group B streptococci are the most frequent causative organisms, although gram-negative bacteria, *Mycoplasma hominis,* CMV, and HSV can also cause disease. Chlamydial pneumonia has a later onset (2 to 6 weeks postpartum) and is often preceded by conjunctivitis.

SIGNS & SYMPTOMS

Tachypnea, retractions, and cyanosis. Severe cases may involve respiratory failure and septic shock.

DIAGNOSIS

Chest x-rays show patchy infiltrates or consolidation. Cultures of blood and tracheal aspirate may help identify the causative organism.

TREATMENT

Broad-spectrum IV antibiotics and oxygen or mechanical ventilation as needed.

PEDIATRICS

Epiglottitis

Epiglottitis is a severe infection of the epiglottis and surrounding structures. It may become rapidly fatal as a result of sudden respiratory obstruction, particularly in young children with small airways. The causative organism is typically *Haemophilus influenzae* type b.

Rapid development of sore throat, fever, muffled voice, dysphagia, and drooling is characteristic. The patient may lean forward with neck extended and hands on knees (the "sniff" or "tripod" position) to improve breathing. Stridor (a harsh, high-pitched sound during inspiration) and retractions may also be noted.

Lateral neck films show a classic "thumbprint sign." Visualization of a red, swollen epiglottis is diagnostic but must be performed under controlled conditions to prevent airway obstruction. After an artificial airway is established, pharyngeal and blood cultures should be obtained.

Epiglottitis is a medical emergency. Patients suspected of epiglottitis should be kept calm, examined, and intubated. An IV cephalosporin should be administered.

Infants older than 2 months of age may receive *H. influenzae* type b vaccination. The vaccine need not be given after the age of 5 years because most individuals have immunity by that age.

Laryngotracheitis

Also known as *croup,* this disease of young children is usually caused by parainfluenza virus, but influenza and respiratory syncytial virus (RSV) may also be involved. This illness is often preceded by an upper respiratory infection, and seasonal outbreaks are common. Edema of the subglottic space causes symptoms.

A harsh, barking cough accompanied by hoarseness and inspiratory stridor is characteristic. Drooling is not common, in contrast to epiglottitis.

The symptoms and examination are generally diagnostic. Anteroposterior neck x-rays show narrowing of the subglottic space (the "church steeple" sign).

Mild cases may be managed on an outpatient basis; more severe cases require hospitalization. Humidified air oxygen, nebulized racemic epinephrine, and steroids may be helpful.

Bronchiolitis

Bronchiolitis, a viral disease of the bronchioles, primarily affects infants younger than 2 years of age and often occurs in epidemics in the winter and spring. Bronchiolitis is usually caused by RSV and may progress to RSV pneumonia.

Children generally have 1 to 2 days of fever, rhinorrhea, and cough, followed by signs of respiratory distress, including wheezing and tachypnea. A hacking cough and vomiting may develop. Physical examination reveals wheezing, crackles, prolonged expiration, and hyperresonance to percussion.

Chest x-ray shows hyperinflation of the lungs, interstitial infiltrates, and areas of atelectasis. The nasopharynx may be swabbed to do a rapid test for antigen to RSV.

Supportive care includes adequate hydration, humidification, nebulizers, and oxygen. Ribavirin may be effective against RSV in very ill or high-risk infants. Hospitalization is necessary in severe disease and in infants younger than 2 months of age. Many infants with bronchiolitis go on to develop asthma.

Cystic Fibrosis

Cystic fibrosis (CF) is an autosomal-recessive disorder that is more frequent in white populations and is the result of a defect in the chloride-pumping mechanism of exocrine glands. The resulting secretions are thick, sticky, and excessive. The classic triad of abnormalities includes chronic obstructive pulmonary disease, pancreatic enzyme insufficiency, and high concentrations of sweat electrolytes. Males are typically infertile. Life expectancy is 30 years.

Clinical course ranges from mild to severe. Newborns can present with GI obstruction because of meconium ileus. Most children will have inadequate weight gain. They present with recurrent respiratory infections (due to viscous lung secretions) and malodorous steatorrhea (due to lack of pancreatic enzymes). Ten percent of patients are not diagnosed until age 10.

The "sweat test," in which the electrolyte concentrations of the sweat are determined, shows elevated sodium and chloride. Because of this, parents often report that their children "taste salty." DNA testing may also be used for diagnosis.

Treatment is comprehensive and includes diet therapy, pancreatic enzyme replacement, chest physiotherapy, and antibiotic prophylaxis against respiratory infections. Gene therapy for CF is currently being studied but is not yet available.

PEDIATRICS

Urology

Circumcision

Circumcision is a surgical procedure to remove the foreskin from a boy's penis. This procedure is performed in the United States for a variety of religious and cultural reasons but is much less common in many other parts of the world. It may be medically indicated in cases of phimosis (inability to retract the foreskin after age 3 years) and paraphimosis (a painful condition in which the foreskin becomes stuck behind the corona of the glans). It may also reduce the incidence of penile cancer and urinary tract infections (UTIs) in boys, although these are rare conditions. It is absolutely contraindicated in infants with hypospadias (see next section) and may be contraindicated in boys with bleeding disorders. Risks include pain, infection, and various degrees of mutilation.

Hypospadias

Hypospadias is a congenital displacement of the urethral opening, toward the underside of the penile shaft. Other malformations, such as a dorsal hood (incomplete foreskin) and chordee (ventral curvature of the penis), are commonly associated with this defect. Therapy, when necessary, is surgical.

Cryptorchidism

One or both testes may lie in the abdominal cavity (true cryptorchidism) or in the inguinal canal (incomplete descent). Undescended testes have a higher potential for the later development of testicular carcinoma, and if not surgically lowered, will not be able to produce sperm. *Retractile testes* descend into the scrotum at times but then retract into the inguinal canal. This condition requires no treatment and usually resolves by adolescence.

SIGNS & SYMPTOMS

Scrotal sac without a testicle, even in relaxed situations such as a hot bath.

TREATMENT

Surgery to place the testicle in the scrotal sac is usually done before age 2 years and must be done before age 5 years if the potential for spermatogenesis is to be maintained. This surgery does not decrease the risk of testicular cancer.

Enuresis

Nocturnal bedwetting is normal in the first several years of life. Thereafter, voluntary control can be expected. Nocturnal enuresis occurs in 30% of 4 year olds and in 10% of 6 year olds. There is a familial tendency to late development of night-time control, and boys are more commonly affected than girls. Only 1% to 2% of cases in children have an organic etiology, but any suspicious findings on history, examination, urinalysis, or urine culture should prompt further workup. Treatment options include behavior modification strategies (e.g., awarding stickers for dry nights), enuresis alarms, and medications (desmopressin, imipramine). Care must be taken to maintain the child's self-esteem. Family therapy should be considered if stress seems to be a factor, particularly if enuresis recurs after a period of dryness.

Ureteral Reflux

Reflux of urine into the ureter usually occurs because of a congenital defect in the connection between the ureter and the bladder. The increased pressure in the ureter can cause hydrostatic damage in the kidney and creates the potential for bacteria to ascend in the ureter, placing the kidney at risk for infection as well.

Persistent UTIs in a child are the most common presentation.

A voiding cystourethrogram (VCUG) will demonstrate the reflux.

If the reflux is mild, the situation should be monitored because it may disappear with time. Infections should be aggressively treated and antibiotic prophylaxis should be considered. Surgical repair is necessary in severe cases.

Wilms' Tumor (Nephroblastoma)

Wilms' tumor (nephroblastoma) is the most common renal tumor in children, and most occur in children younger than age 4 years. Bilateral tumors are present in 10% of patients.

An asymptomatic abdominal mass is the most common presenting finding. Hematuria, hypertension, weight loss, and fever may also occur.

Ultrasound and CT scan define tumor extent and determine the presence of bilateral involvement or liver metastases. Chest x-ray will identify pulmonary metastases.

PEDIATRICS

Surgical resection and chemotherapy with vincristine and actinomycin D are typically used. Radiotherapy may be appropriate in some cases. Prognosis is generally good, especially with younger children.

Endocrinology

Congenital Hypothyroidism (Cretinism)

Congenital hypothyroidism (cretinism) is a rare deficiency of thyroid hormone that is due to severe iodine deficiency, thyroid dysgenesis, or inborn errors of thyroid hormone synthesis. If left untreated, mental and growth retardation occur.

Prolonged neonatal jaundice may be the first symptom. Large fontanelles, a thick tongue, a hoarse cry, poor feeding, and infrequent stools are other signs. Bone growth is delayed.

Routine newborn blood testing reveals low T_4 and high thyroid-stimulating hormone.

Levothyroxine must be started in the first few weeks of life to minimize developmental delay.

Hematology

Hemolytic Disease of the Newborn (Erythroblastosis Fetalis)

If Rhesus (Rh)-positive fetal cells enter the circulation of an Rh-negative mother, the mother may develop anti-Rh antibodies. This typically occurs during delivery, during a therapeutic abortion, during invasive procedures, such as amniocentesis, or during third-trimester bleeding. Once maternal anti-Rh antibodies form, they can then cross the placenta and cause massive hemolysis and death to this and any future Rh-positive fetuses. This is hemolytic disease of the newborn. Approximately 15% of whites are Rh-negative. The rate is lower for Asians and African-Americans.

Prevention consists of passive immunization with $Rh_o(D)$ immune globulin (RhoGAM) given within 72 hours of the delivery or abortion. RhoGAM acts by binding to all fetal Rh-positive cells in the mother's blood, preventing the mother from synthesizing anti-Rh antibodies. Rh-negative women are prophylactically given RhoGAM in the twenty-eighth week of pregnancy. RhoGAM does not pose any danger to the fetus because the immunoglobulin antibodies are too large to pass through the placenta. If erythroblastosis fetalis does develop, RBC transfusions may be necessary.

Musculoskeletal Disorders

Congenital Hip Dislocation

Congenital hip dislocation occurs when the femoral head is partially or completely displaced from the acetabulum. Risk factors include breech presentation and oligohydramnios. Dislocations may be unilateral or bilateral. Because dislocations may be difficult to detect at birth, periodic examinations should be performed throughout the first year of life.

SIGNS & SYMPTOMS

The thigh cannot be completely abducted to the surface of the examination table when the hip and knee are flexed. This maneuver causes a palpable "clunk" as the femoral head pops into the acetabulum. ("Clicks" are more common, less significant, and usually disappear within a few months.) If the dislocation is unilateral, the skin folds of the thighs may be asymmetric.

DIAGNOSIS

X-rays are difficult to interpret and are only helpful if they confirm the clinical suspicion.

TREATMENT

The hip must be splinted in an abducted, laterally rotated position. This position encourages the acetabulum to form normally. If treatment is delayed, permanent deformity can result.

Phocomelia

Phocomelia is a developmental anomaly characterized by the absence of the proximal portion of the arms or legs, so that the hands or feet are attached to the trunk by a small, irregularly shaped bone. The sedative thalidomide, which was prescribed in Europe in the 1950s and early 1960s, caused an epidemic of babies with this condition. This is a U.S. Food and Drug Administration success story, as thalidomide was never approved for use in the United States. (Why this topic remains on the United States Medical Licensing Examination topic list is beyond our comprehension!)

Osteochondritis

Osteochondritis is the inflammation of both bone and cartilage. Osteochondritis can vary greatly in location and etiology; however, a common presentation in active adolescents is

Osgood-Schlatter disease, an osteochondritis of the tibial tubercle. It is thought to be due to continuous traction of the patellar tendon on the immature epiphyseal insertion.

In Osgood-Schlatter disease, pain, swelling, and tenderness occur at the site of the patellar tendon insertion.

X-ray may show fragmentation of the tibial tubercle.

Patients should avoid excessive activity, particularly deep knee bends, until the condition resolves. The course is usually several weeks to months. Immobilization and surgery are necessary only in extreme cases.

Slipped Capital Femoral Epiphysis

In slipped capital femoral epiphysis, the femoral head literally slips with respect to the femoral shaft. The condition is most common in overweight teenagers.

The onset of symptoms is gradual. Hip stiffness leads to limping, which is followed by hip pain that radiates down the anteromedial thigh to the knee. The leg is externally rotated, and there is limitation of internal rotation and abduction of the hips.

X-rays show displacement of the femoral head.

Surgery is required to pin the head and prevent further slippage. Even with optimal treatment, there is a high incidence of arthritis and avascular necrosis.

Neurology and Special Senses

Neonatal Conjunctivitis

Neonatal conjunctivitis is a common eye inflammation with several etiologies. Bacteria (particularly *Streptococcus pneumoniae, H. influenzae,* and *Neisseria gonorrhoeae*) and viruses (such as HSV) are common agents. Chemical injury can result from silver nitrate drops used for prophylaxis against gonorrheal infection. Chlamydial conjunctivitis is acquired during delivery in one-half of infants born to infected mothers.

Injected conjunctivae and eyelid edema are common. Discharge may be present. Chemical conjunctivitis presents 1 to 2 days after birth. Bacterial etiologies cause symptoms in 2 to 5 days. Chlamydial infection presents 5 to 10 days after birth, and herpes simplex conjunctivitis may be delayed by 2 weeks.

Gram's stain and culture of discharge.

Chemical conjunctivitis resolves completely within 1 to 2 days. Most bacterial infections are treated with topical preparations. Chlamydial disease is treated with oral erythromycin, because systemic antibiotic treatment will prevent chlamydial pneumonia, a later complication of intrapartum chlamydial infection. Gonorrheal disease requires hospitalization and ceftriaxone.

Silver nitrate drops applied at birth protect against gonorrheal disease but risks chemical conjunctivitis. Topical erythromycin protects against bacteria and has few side effects.

Retinoblastoma

Retinoblastoma is a childhood malignancy of the immature retina that is often hereditary and may be associated with other malignancies, such as osteosarcoma, in later life. On examination, these children have a white reflex, or "cat's eye" instead of the normal red reflex. Ophthalmologic surgery may be curative if the tumor is caught in its early stages.

Otitis Media

Otitis media, infection of the middle ear, typically occurs in infants and young children because of the short length and horizontal position of their eustachian tube. Symptoms are preceded by a viral respiratory infection that causes obstruction of the eustachian tube and allows bacteria to multiply in the middle ears. Common organisms include *S. pneumoniae*, *H. influenzae*, *Moraxella catarrhalis*, *Streptococcus pyogenes*, and *S. aureus*.

Persistent ear pain and fever are typical. Temporary hearing loss may occur. On examination, the tympanic membrane is red and bulging, with loss of tympanic bony landmarks, light reflex, and mobility. Bloody or purulent discharge may be present if the tympanic membrane has perforated.

Diagnosis is based on the clinical presentation and examination.

Antibiotics, such as amoxicillin, are usually effective, but resistance may develop. Antibiotic prophylaxis and tympanic tubes may be considered in children with recurrent infections. Serious complications of inadequately treated infections include mastoiditis, meningitis, and permanent hearing loss.

Mastoiditis

Infection of the mastoid process may occur several weeks after inadequately treated otitis media. *S. pneumoniae,* group A streptococcus, *S. aureus,* and *H. influenzae* are common organisms.

Redness and swelling of the mastoid process, accompanied by pain, tenderness, and fever is the typical presentation. Hearing loss also may occur.

X-ray reveals destruction of the mastoid air cells and fluid in the air pockets. CT scan may provide a definitive diagnosis.

IV antibiotics are necessary. If complete resolution does not occur, surgical drainage may be required.

Perinatal Intracranial Hemorrhage

Bleeding in or around the brain may occur in three locations:

1. Preterm infants are particularly at risk for **intraventricular hemorrhage,** which is caused by hypoxia and by mechanical pressure on the infant's head at birth. As many as 40% of preterm infants have these intraventricular hemorrhages, which are often bilateral and occur in the germinal matrix (developing periventricular tissue that is seen in the fetus and is still present in preterm babies). Neonates may be asymptomatic but can have apnea and cyanosis. The prognosis varies with the extent of bleeding, but severe neurologic sequelae may result.
2. **Subarachnoid hemorrhages** are more often seen in full-term infants. They may be related to birth trauma or to germinal matrix bleeding. Seizures are common and are typically brief. Patients usually do well, with no long-term sequelae.
3. **Subdural hemorrhages** result from traumatic tears in the bridging veins, which cause bleeding in the subdural space. They are often seen after difficult deliveries or in large infants. Seizures, vomiting, irritability, and a rapidly enlarging head are seen. The majority of infants survive without any sequelae.

The CSF may contain RBCs or gross blood, particularly with a subarachnoid hemorrhage. Metabolic studies should be performed to rule out other sources of neurologic disturbances.

Ultrasound and CT scan will show blood.

Supportive care. Small subdural taps may be helpful to treat subdural hemorrhages.

Neonatal Meningitis

Neonatal meningitis is a bacterial infection of the meninges that occurs within 4 weeks of birth. It is more common in males and low birth-weight infants. Meningitis accompanies 25% of neonatal sepsis cases, usually resulting from bacteremia. Infections are commonly the result of group B streptococcus, *E. coli,* and *Listeria.* One-third of survivors have significant neurologic sequelae.

Sepsis is usually more apparent than meningitis, but infants may have some CNS signs such as lethargy, focal seizures, and vomiting. A full fontanelle and nuchal rigidity are apparent in only a minority of patients.

Blood cultures are positive in 85% of cases. CSF examination provides a definitive diagnosis.

Even with broad-spectrum antibiotics, mortality is approximately 25%. Antibiotics should be tailored to the specific organism.

Tay-Sachs Disease

Tay-Sachs disease is an autosomal-recessive disorder that is most common in Eastern European Jews and French Canadians. It involves the absence of hexosaminidase A, which is needed for metabolism of lipid gangliosides, so gangliosides accumulate within the brain.

Presenting symptoms are a loss of alertness and excessive response to noise (hyperacusis) in the first year of life. Cherry-red spots may be observed on the retina. Infants have early and progressive developmental delay, paralysis, blindness, and dementia. Death occurs by age 4 years.

Decreased hexosaminidase A activity can be detected in the serum.

No treatment exists for the affected infant.

Genetic screening identifies carriers of the Tay-Sachs gene, who should undergo counseling before pregnancy. Prenatal diagnosis of infants is also possible, and prospective parents may choose to terminate affected pregnancies.

Cerebral Palsy

Cerebral palsy (CP) is primarily a disease of movement that results from CNS damage before the age of 5 years. Risk factors include in utero complications, IUGR, prematurity, birth trauma, and asphyxia.

Most patients have spastic syndromes, with any or all limbs affected. Affected limbs show increased deep tendon reflexes, increased tone, weakness, and underdevelopment. Toe-walking and a scissors gait are characteristic. Some patients develop syndromes involving choreoathetoid movement of the extremities or trunk, and these patients often have severe dysarthria. A minority of patients have ataxic syndromes because of cerebellar damage. Some affected children have normal intelligence, while others are mentally disabled. Hyperactivity and short attention spans are common. Seizures are present in one-fourth of patients with CP.

CP may be hard to identify early in infancy, but the clinical syndrome in a child at risk becomes apparent over time.

CP has no cure, but early intervention can maximize future independence. Physical therapy, speech training, bracing, orthopaedic surgery, and occupational therapy may all be useful. Special schooling is needed only with severe mental or physical deficits.

Duchenne's Muscular Dystrophy

Progressive painless muscular weakness and atrophy, together called muscular dystrophy, may occur in a number of inherited disorders. Duchenne's muscular dystrophy (DMD) is the most common type. It is an X-linked, recessive disease caused by a mutation in the dystrophin gene.

By age 5 years, patients present with toe-walking, a waddling gait, and difficulty running. The proximal legs are affected first, and then the proximal arms become involved. Pseudohypertrophy of the calves due to fatty infiltration of the muscle is classic, as is Gower's sign, in which a child pushes up off the floor and walks his hands up his legs to get to a standing position. By age 11 years, patients are usually no longer able to walk, and IQ testing eventually shows mental retardation. Heart involvement, scoliosis, and flexion contractures follow as the disease progresses. Death usually occurs by 25 years of age.

The clinical presentation is suggestive. Muscle necrosis and variation in muscle fiber size can be seen on muscle biopsy, and dystrophin is absent from the muscle specimen. Serum creatine kinase levels are elevated even before the onset of symptoms.

No treatment exists. Exercise is encouraged and corrective surgery is helpful. Physical therapy and braces can prevent or treat contractures.

Brain Neoplasms

The most common primary brain tumors of childhood are cerebellar astrocytoma and medulloblastoma (see Chapter 13 for a more complete discussion).

Psychiatric Disorders

Mental Retardation

Mental retardation, generally defined as an IQ of 70 or less, can be due to chromosomal abnormalities (Down syndrome, Prader-Willi syndrome), teratogens (fetal alcohol syndrome), infection (congenital rubella), hypoxia, trauma, and toxic exposure (lead poisoning).

The child is significantly delayed in reaching social and developmental milestones. Physical examination has related findings only in certain syndromes, such as Down syndrome and fetal alcohol syndrome.

IQ can be assessed by several standardized intelligence tests. Adaptive functioning (i.e., the ability to communicate and care for self) can be assessed by questioning the patient's caregivers, as well as by using several available scales.

PEDIATRICS

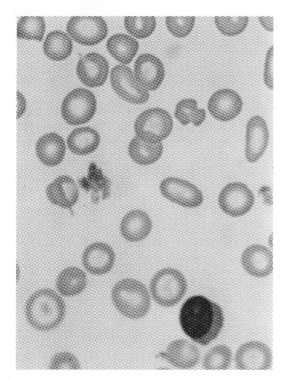

Fig. 10-1. Iron-deficiency anemia. Note the increased central pallor of the RBCs as well as a target cell in the lower left-hand corner. (Reprinted with permission from Kapff C, Jandl J: *Blood: Atlas and Sourcebook of Hematology,* 2nd ed. Boston, Little, Brown, 1991, p 27.)

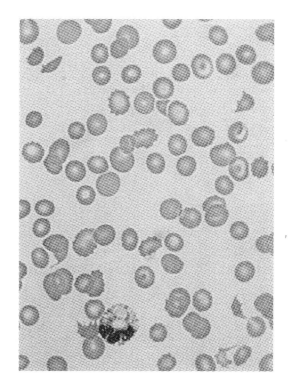

Fig. 10-2. Hemolytic anemia. Note the numerous helmet cells, burr cells, and fragments as well as lack of platelets. (Reprinted with permission from Kapff C, Jandl J: *Blood: Atlas and Sourcebook of Hematology,* 2nd ed. Boston, Little, Brown, 1991, p 39.)

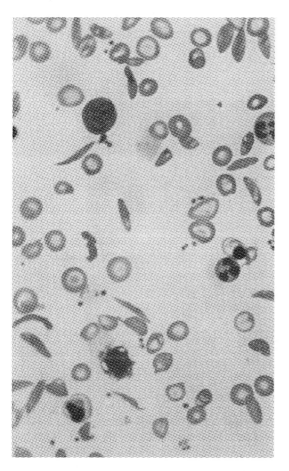

Fig. 10-3. Sickle cell anemia. Note the sickle-shaped cells. (Reprinted with permission from Kapff C, Jandl J: *Blood: Atlas and Sourcebook of Hematology,* 2nd ed. Boston, Little, Brown, 1991, p 49.)

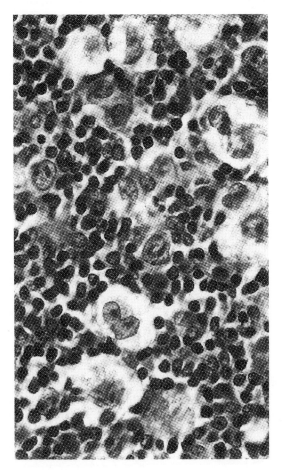

Fig. 10-6. Hodgkin's lymphoma. The classic "owl-eyes" Reed-Sternberg cells are present. (Reprinted with permission from Kapff C, Jandl J: *Blood: Atlas and Sourcebook of Hematology,* 2nd ed. Boston, Little, Brown, 1991, p 119.)

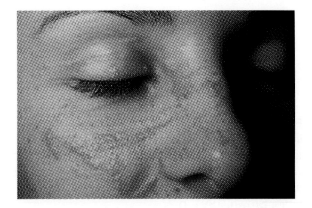

Fig. 11-1. Contact dermatitis from poison ivy. (Reprinted with permission from Hall J: *Sauer's Manual of Skin Diseases,* 8th ed. Philadelphia, Lippincott Williams & Wilkins, 2000, p 67.)

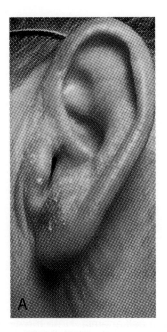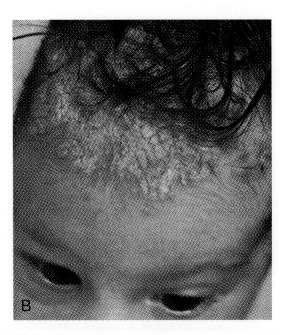

Fig. 11-2. Seborrheic dermatitis. **(A)** Adult. **(B)** Infancy. (Reprinted with permission from Hall J: *Sauer's Manual of Skin Diseases,* 8th ed. Philadelphia, Lippincott Williams & Wilkins, 2000, p 115, 116.)

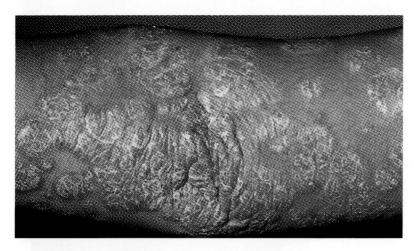

Fig. 11-3. Psoriasis on the elbow. (Reprinted with permission from Hall J: *Sauer's Manual of Skin Diseases,* 8th ed. Philadelphia, Lippincott Williams & Wilkins, 2000, p 128.)

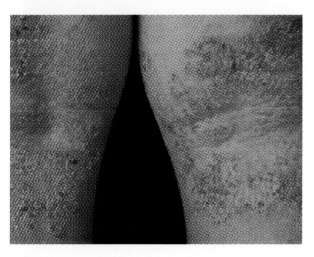

Fig. 11-4. Atopic dermatitis on the popliteal folds. (Reprinted with permission from Hall J: *Sauer's Manual of Skin Diseases,* 8th ed. Philadelphia, Lippincott Williams & Wilkins, 2000, p 77.)

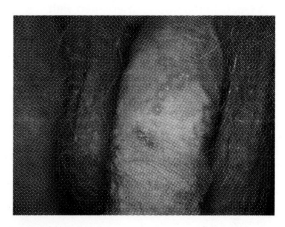

Fig. 11-5. Herpes simplex lesions. (Reprinted with permission from Hall J: *Sauer's Manual of Skin Diseases,* 8th ed. Philadelphia, Lippincott Williams & Wilkins, 2000, p 177.)

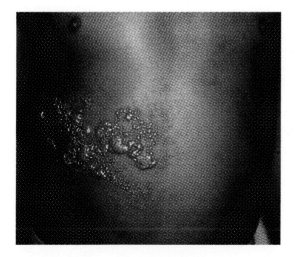

Fig. 11-6. Herpes zoster. (Reprinted with permission from Hall J: *Sauer's Manual of Skin Diseases,* 8th ed. Philadelphia, Lippincott Williams & Wilkins, 2000, p 261.)

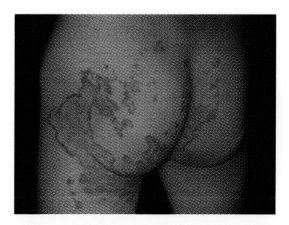

Fig. 11-7. Tinea corporis. (Reprinted with permission from Hall J: *Sauer's Manual of Skin Diseases,* 8th ed. Philadelphia, Lippincott Williams & Wilkins, 2000, p 211.)

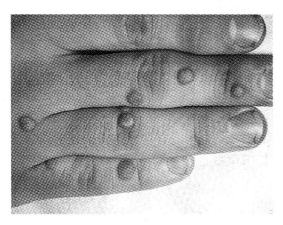

Fig. 11-8. Common warts. (Reprinted with permission from Hall J: *Sauer's Manual of Skin Diseases,* 8th ed. Philadelphia, Lippincott Williams & Wilkins, 2000, p 183.)

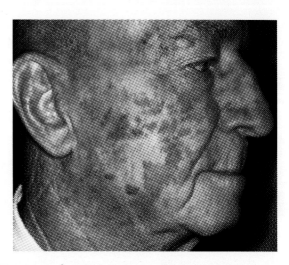

Fig. 11-9. Actinic keratosis. (Reprinted with permission from Hall J: *Sauer's Manual of Skin Diseases,* 8th ed. Philadelphia, Lippincott Williams & Wilkins, 2000, p 330.)

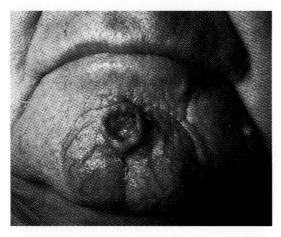

Fig. 11-10. Squamous cell carcinoma. (Reprinted with permission from Hall J: *Sauer's Manual of Skin Diseases,* 8th ed. Philadelphia, Lippincott Williams & Wilkins, 2000, p 337.)

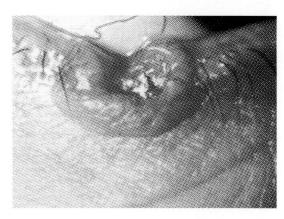

Fig. 11-11. Basal cell carcinoma. Note telangiectasia on the rolled edge of the ulcer. (Reprinted with permission from Hall J: *Sauer's Manual of Skin Diseases,* 8th ed. Philadelphia, Lippincott Williams & Wilkins, 2000, p 334.)

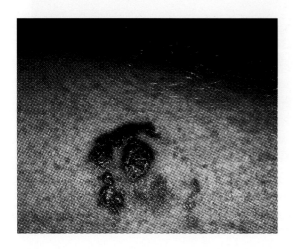

Fig. 11-12. Malignant melanoma. (Reprinted with permission from Hall J: *Sauer's Manual of Skin Diseases,* 8th ed. Philadelphia, Lippincott Williams & Wilkins, 2000, p 346.)

Appropriate environments for patients with mental retardation depend on the severity of the disorder. Patients with mild retardation and good support may live in the community, but more severe disease generally requires a supervised setting.

Communication Disorders

Communication disorders include a variety of defects in speech and language, such as stuttering and difficulties in pronunciation, understanding, or expression. The disorder may interfere with social communication. Standardized tests are available to evaluate the defects. Speech therapy may be helpful. As many as 80% of patients who stutter recover before the age of 16 years.

Learning Disorders

Academic functioning below what would be appropriate for the patient's age, IQ, and education is the primary feature of learning disorders, which include disorders of reading (dyslexia), mathematics, and written expression.

A history of delayed language development can be obtained in many cases. There may be clumsiness, right-left confusion, and difficulty naming objects or colors. Poor academic achievement may be accompanied by low self-esteem and problems in social skills. Patients have a high drop-out rate from school. Patients may also have attention-deficit hyperactivity disorder (ADHD) or major depressive disorder.

The patient's scores on certain standardized tests are at least two standard deviations lower than expected on the basis of general intelligence. Vision and hearing problems must be ruled out.

When learning disorders are identified early, intervention with direct and individualized instruction can improve functioning significantly.

Attention-deficit Hyperactivity Disorder

ADHD is a disorder of inattention and hyperactivity that is four times more prevalent in males than in females. It is most often diagnosed in elementary school-age children, and symptoms tend to remit as the patient matures. Some patients continue to have symptoms, particularly low self-esteem and academic failure, into adolescence and adulthood. Personality disorders may arise in adults.

Lack of attention in school work and play causes children to be easily distracted, make careless mistakes, and have difficulty finishing a task. Hyperactivity may involve fidgetiness, excessive talkativeness, or feelings of restlessness. Impulsivity is also a hallmark of ADHD, characterized by impatience, interrupting, and involvement in potentially dangerous activities.

PEDIATRICS

The patient's symptoms must begin before age 7 years and must be present in at least two separate settings.

DIAGNOSIS

Psychostimulant medications and behavioral therapies can control the disorder. Methylphenidate (Ritalin) is most effective, but side effects include insomnia, depression, headaches, stomachaches, and high blood pressure. Growth reduction may occur with high doses.

TREATMENT

Conduct Disorder

Conduct disorder consists of disruptive behavior patterns that violate basic societal norms. It is more common in boys than in girls.

Patients act aggressively, fight often, use weapons, act cruelly, or are sexually aggressive. Destruction of others' property and theft are also common.

SIGNS & SYMPTOMS

For this diagnosis to apply, the behavior patterns must persist for at least 1 year. The four subtypes include:

1. Aggressive behavior toward others or toward animals
2. Behavior resulting in property damage (e.g., arson)
3. Theft or deceit
4. Serious violations of societal rules

DIAGNOSIS

Psychotherapy, family therapy, and special schooling. Children with this disorder are at increased risk for developing antisocial personality disorder and substance abuse as adults.

TREATMENT

Oppositional Defiant Disorder

Oppositional defiant disorder is a disruptive behavior disorder characterized by negativity, hostility, and defiance. Before puberty, the diagnosis is more common in boys, but girls and boys have equal rates of developing this disorder after puberty.

Children lose their temper often, argue with authority figures, actively annoy others, blame others for mistakes, and are frequently angry, annoyed, or vindictive.

SIGNS & SYMPTOMS

For this diagnosis to apply, patients must display the preceding behaviors more frequently than is typical for their age over a period of at least 6 months.

DIAGNOSIS

Psychotherapy, family therapy, and special schooling.

Tic Disorders

A tic is an involuntary but sometimes suppressible motor movement or vocalization that is sudden, repeated, and stereotypical for the individual. **Tourette's syndrome** is a tic disorder that involves multiple, severe tics, both motor and vocal, which change over time. Contrary to popular perception, *coprolalia,* a complex tic involving involuntary utterance of obscenities, is seen in less than 10% of Tourette's patients. Patients have periods of remission, and symptoms lessen throughout adolescence and adulthood, but the disease usually lasts a lifetime. A genetic predisposition to Tourette's disorder has an autosomal-dominant pattern of inheritance.

Simple motor tics are eye blinking, grimacing, or shrugging, whereas complex motor tics can be gestures, jumping, or twirling when walking. Simple vocal tics, such as throat clearing or barking, are common. Complex vocal tics include repeated phrases, coprolalia, and echolalia (i.e., echoing another person's words). Stress tends to worsen tic disorders, and sleep or involvement in an activity generally diminishes tic activity.

Diagnosis requires frequent tics for at least 1 year, beginning before age 18 years.

Haloperidol or pimozide.

Separation Anxiety Disorder

In separation anxiety disorder, children are extremely anxious about being away from home or loved ones. The disorder usually develops before adolescence and may follow a traumatic event.

Patients may be homesick and extremely worried that something bad may happen to them or to their loved ones when they are away. Children cling to parents and refuse to attend activities away from home. They often have difficulty sleeping and may have nightmares.

Symptoms must persist for at least 4 weeks for this diagnosis to apply.

Separation anxiety disorder resolves within several years. Counseling may be useful.

Autistic Disorder

Autistic disorder involves deficits in communication, social involvement, and participation in activities, often coexistent with mental retardation or uneven intellectual ability. Males are affected four to five times more frequently than females. Patients may develop schizophrenia or seizure disorder as they age.

Language is delayed or altogether absent. Nonverbal communication is impaired, peer relationships are deficient, and social skills are poorly developed. Patients may be unaware of others around them. Stereotyped behaviors and activities are present, often with an insistence on regular routine. Patients may be impulsive, hyperactive, or aggressive, with inappropriate emotional responses. Nonspecific neurologic signs and symptoms may be present in addition to seizure disorder. **Asperger's syndrome** is a variant of autism in which severe social impairment and stereotyped behaviors occur without cognitive or language deficits. (Remember Dustin Hoffman in Rain Man?)

Signs and symptoms begin when the child is younger than 3 years old, but a normal period may precede onset. **Pervasive developmental disorder** is a term applied to patients who meet many, but not all, of the criteria for autism.

Behavior therapy and speech therapy may help, although no truly effective treatment is known. Haloperidol may somewhat reduce aggressive or self-destructive patterns.

Adolescence

Physical Changes of Puberty

The physical changes that occur during adolescence are divided into **Tanner stages,** which chronicle the development of pubic hair, breasts, and male genitalia (Tables 8-3 and 8-4). Onset of puberty varies widely. Puberty is considered precocious if it begins before age 8 years in girls or age 9 years in boys. It is considered delayed if there is no sign of development by age 13 years in girls or age 14 years in boys. Teens who are maturing appropriately but either earlier or later than their peers should be reassured that their bodies are normal.

Sexuality in Adolescence

Sexual feelings begin to emerge in early adolescence, before a teen is psychologically mature enough to handle intimate relationships or the repercussions of sexual activity. Mas-

Table 8-3. Tanner stages: female

Stage	Pubic hair	Breast development	Notes
1	None	Preadolescent	—
2	Minimal straight hair on labia	Breast budding with areola enlargement	Average age 11 yrs
3	Hair starts to darken and curl; increased amount	Breast and areola enlargement; areola level with rest of breast	Growth spurt, average age 12 yrs (scoliosis can worsen)
4	Adult (curly, dark, thick) hair but not on thighs	Areola forms secondary mound on breast; further enlargement	Menarche
5	Adult quality and distribution	Areola skin is level with the rest of breast again; adult size and form	—

turbation is a common behavior that allows teens to release their sexual tensions safely. Psychological damage can be done when a teen is made to feel guilty, embarrassed, or afraid about the effects of masturbation. Sexually impulsive behavior puts teens at risk for sexually transmitted diseases (STDs) and unintended pregnancy. Homosexual experimentation among teens is not uncommon and does not, by itself, lead to adult homosexuality. Teens who are struggling with an emerging homosexual identity typically face enormous familial and societal pressure and frequently experience periods of depression, substance abuse, homosexual or heterosexual promiscuity, and attempted suicide. These teens should be approached nonjudgmentally and offered the necessary support and assistance. All teens should be educated about their safer-sex options (including abstinence) and reminded that STDs (including AIDS) and unintended pregnancy *can* happen to them. Guiding teens to make conscious, healthy decisions about their sexual behavior can help establish a lifelong pattern of sexual responsibility.

Table 8-4. Tanner stages: male

Stage	Pubic hair	Penis	Scrotum and testes	Notes
1	None	Preadolescent	Preadolescent	—
2	Minimal fine, straight hair at base of penis	Slight enlargement	Testes enlarge; scrotal skin reddens and coarsens	Average age 12 yrs
3	Hair starts to darken, curl, and spread	Penile "growth spurt"	Increased size	Nocturnal emissions common
4	Adult (curly, dark, thick) hair but not on thighs	Increased length and width	Increased size and pigment	Growth spurt, average age 14 yrs; Gynecomastia common, age 14 yrs; Facial hair, average age 16 yrs
5	Adult quality and distribution	Adult	Adult	—

Psychological Changes of Adolescence

Early adolescence begins with the onset of puberty, usually between ages 10 and 13 years. At this age, children are frequently preoccupied with their rapidly changing bodies. Self-image and self-esteem are fragile. Although sexual feelings begin to emerge, most early adolescents feel more comfortable with their same-gender peers. New independence allows ties to family to loosen as focus shifts to the social group. Still, thought processes continue to be quite concrete, and teens of this age may have unrealistic career goals, such as being professional ball players or movie stars.

During **middle adolescence,** ages 14 to 16 years, rapid cognitive changes dominate development. As teens develop the ability to think abstractly, they start to see themselves as others see them. They typically become quite self-absorbed, and many try out several images, much to the dismay of their parents. Parental conflict increases as teens struggle for independence and a sense of self. Intoxicated with their newfound cognitive abilities, teens may feel a sense of omnipotence. They can solve the world's problems, they know all the answers, and nothing bad will ever happen to them. This attitude, besides being infuriating, is dangerous and leads to high rates of motor vehicle accidents and unintended pregnancies.

During **late adolescence,** ages 17 to 21 years, teens become more comfortable with their maturation and their relationships and more able to discuss roles and goals. As they become less self-centered, intimate relationships become more fulfilling and begin to supersede peer group interactions in importance. A dose of experience and the ability to think abstractly allow the late adolescent to more realistically plan for the future. Conflict lessens as the new young adult takes his or her place in the family structure.

As teens grapple with emotional and social issues, their difficulties in adaptation may be expressed in potentially damaging ways. Major causes of mortality in this age group include accidents, suicide, and homicide. Alcohol is often involved. Mortality rates for boys are about twice that for girls. Other important issues include the following:

- **Risk-taking behaviors,** such as drug and alcohol use, are common. Alcohol use has been reported in more than 90% of teens. Tobacco use (66%) and drug use (43%) are also common. Health education is sometimes ineffective because many teens have a feeling of immortality ("It can't happen to me").
- **Psychiatric disturbances,** such as depression and suicide, may become more frequent. More than 30% of adolescent girls and 15% of adolescent boys are reported to have symptoms of major depression. Homosexual teens are more likely to attempt suicide than their heterosexual peers, perhaps because of fears of social rejection. Clinical suspicion of depression should be explored, and the physician should ask about suicidal ideation in a straightforward manner. Contrary to a common fear, teens whose doctors discuss this topic are not more likely to commit suicide because "the doctor gave me the idea."
- **Eating disorders,** such as bulimia and anorexia, become more prevalent. Female adolescents are at special risk of developing distorted body images and eating disorders; more than 20% of teenage girls have manifestations of either anorexia or bulimia. In a clinical setting, physicians should openly discuss physical development with adolescents and reassure their anxieties about normalcy.

Physician-Patient Communication in Adolescence

Adolescents may be hesitant to discuss personal issues with physicians because they fear that their parents will be getting a "report." The physician is justified in maintaining confidentiality with teenage patients in most situations, although this agreement should be discussed in advance among all people involved. Such an agreement provides the teen with a nonparental adult to confide in and obtain advice from, and most parents will feel reassured by this. Many states allow teens to obtain treatment for health problems related to sexual behavior and drug use without requiring parental permission. If life-threatening behavior is suspected, however, a physician is required to break confidence and discuss the situation with the patient's parents or guardian.

PEDIATRICS

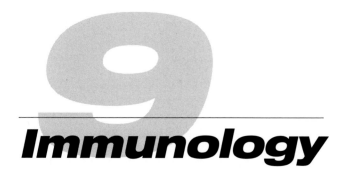

Immunology

Immunizations

Immunizations for normal, healthy children are shown in Table 9-1. Immunizations for adults and children with special circumstances are shown in Table 9-2.

General Notes

- Vaccinations may be started at 6 weeks of age, except for the hepatitis B vaccine series, which can be started at birth.
- Vaccinations need not be delayed when the child has a minor illness, a low-grade fever, or is taking antibiotics. Moderate or severe illness is a contraindication to vaccination.
- Vaccination schedules need not be changed for preterm infants. (See Hepatitis B for an exception.)
- If vaccination status is unknown, assume that no vaccinations have been given. There is generally no harm in extra doses.
- When immunizations fall behind schedule, there is no need to restart any series, no matter how much time has elapsed since the previous dose.
- The live-virus vaccines [measles-mumps-rubella (MMR), oral polio vaccine (OPV), varicella] should be avoided in immunosuppressed patients and pregnant women (due to the theoretical risk of transmission to the fetus). An exception is that MMR may be given to HIV patients who are not severely immunocompromised.

IMMUNOLOGY

Table 9-1. Recommended childhood immunization schedule*

Age ▶ Vaccine ▼	Birth	1 mo	2 mos	4 mos	6 mos	12 mos	15 mos	18 mos	24 mos	4–6 yrs	11–12 yrs	14–16 yrs
Hepatitis B	Hep B											
		Hep B			Hep B							
Diphtheria, Tetanus, Pertussis			DTaP	DTaP	DTaP		DTaP			DTaP	Td	
H. influenzae type b			Hib	Hib	Hib	Hib						
Polio			IPV	IPV	IPV					IPV		
Measles, Mumps, Rubella						MMR				MMR		
Varicella						Varicella						
Pneumococcal			PCV	PCV	PCV	PCV						

DTaP, diphtheria-tetanus-acellular pertussis; Hep B, hepatitis B; Hib, *Haemophilus influenzae* type b; IPV, inactivated poliovirus vaccine; MMR, measles-mumps-rubella; Td, tetanus-diphtheria toxoid (adult type); PCV, pneumoccocal vaccine.

*Approved by the Advisory Committee on Immunization Practices, the American Academy of Pediatrics, and the American Academy of Family Physicians. Vaccines are listed under the routinely recommended ages. Bars indicate range of acceptable ages for vaccination.

Table 9-2. Immunizations for adults and for children with special circumstances

	Tetanus & diphtheria toxoids (Td)	Influenza	Pneumococcal polysaccharide vaccine	Hepatitis A vaccine	Hepatitis B vaccine
Indications	All adults	a. Adults >50 yrs b. Nursing home residents c. Persons >6 mos old with chronic conditions (i.e., asthma, diabetes, immune deficiency, renal dysfunction) d. Women in their 2nd and 3rd trimester during flu season e. Close contacts of high-risk persons	a. >65 years b. >2 years with CHF or chronic heart disease, diabetes, liver disease, alcoholism, COPD or chronic pulmonary disease, sickle cell disease or asplenia, hematologic malignancy, renal failure, organ transplantation, HIV, immunosuppression, and CSF leaks c. Alaskan Natives and some American Indian populations	a. Travelers to countries with endemic infection b. Men who have sex with men c. IV and non-IV illegal drug users d. Persons with chronic liver disease or clotting factor problems e. Food handlers	a. Persons with occupational risk of exposure to blood or blood-contaminated body fluids b. Clients and staff of institutions for the developmentally delayed c. Hemodialysis patients d. Recipients of clotting factors e. Household contacts of those with HBV infection, including family of international adoptees who are HbsAg + f. IV drug users g. Men who have sex with men h. Anyone with multiple sex partners or a recent STD i. Prison inmates j. Unvaccinated teens *continued*

IMMUNOLOGY

IMMUNOLOGY

Table 9-2. Immunizations for adults and for children with special circumstances (continued)

	Tetanus & diphtheria toxoids (Td)	Influenza	Pneumococcal polysaccharide vaccine	Hepatitis A vaccine	Hepatitis B vaccine
Schedule	If previously unimmunized: 3 doses; 2nd 1–2 mos after first; 3rd 6–12 mos after second Booster every 10 years for life	Yearly each fall	One dose if >65; give booster at age 65 if 1st dose was given before age 60 High-risk children under 5 years of age and adult patients with asplenia, kidney disease, HIV, and other immuno-deficiencies should get a booster dose 5 years after the first	2 doses separated by 6–12 months	3 doses; second 1–2 mos after first, 3rd 4–6 mos after second
Contraindications		Acute febrile illness Anaphylactic allergy to eggs			Anaphylactic allergy to yeast

	Measles and mumps	Rubella	Polio	Varicella
Indications	Adults born after 1956 without written documentation of vaccination after first birthday	Persons (especially women) who are seronegative or have no history of vaccination after 1 year of age	Vaccination of adults is only necessary if they will be exposed to wild polio virus (travelers to endemic regions) or OPV (unvaccinated adults whose children will be receiving OPV)	Persons of any age without a reliable history of chicken pox, vaccination, or seropositivity, particularly teachers, health care workers, nonpregnant women of child-bearing age, persons in institutional settings, and those living with children or immuno-compromised adults
Schedule	At least 1 dose; 2nd dose of measles vaccine required 1 month later for those in college, health care professionals, and travelers	1 dose	If previously vaccinated, give 1 booster dose of IPV. If unvaccinated, 3 doses: 2nd dose 1–2 mos after 1st, 3rd 2–12 mos after 2nd	For persons <13, 1 dose. For those >13, 2 doses, separated by 4 weeks
Contraindications	a. Pregnancy (pregnancy should also be avoided for 1 mo following vaccination) b. Immunosuppressive therapy c. Severe HIV disease/AIDS d. IgG or blood products in previous 11 mos e. Anaphylactic allergy to neomycin	Same as for measles and mumps (pregnancy should be avoided for 3 mos following vaccination)	Pregnancy (but no adverse effects have ever been reported). OPV is no longer routinely recommended in the U.S. and is specifically contraindicated in patients with HIV and their household contacts	a. Anaphylactic allergy to gelatin or neomycin b. Untreated active TB c. Immunosuppression or HIV d. IgG or blood products in preceding 5 mos e. Pregnancy (pregnancy should also be avoided for 1 month following vaccination)

IMMUNOLOGY

Hepatitis B

- Infants of mothers who test positive for the hepatitis B virus surface antigen (HBsAg) should receive hepatitis B immunoglobulin (HBIG) and the first dose of the hepatitis B vaccine within 12 hours of birth. The second dose should be given at 1 month and the third dose at 6 months of age.
- Infants of mothers whose HBsAg status is unknown should receive hepatitis B vaccine within 12 hours of birth. The mother's blood should be drawn to determine the hepatitis B status. If HBsAg positive, the infant should receive HBIG as soon as possible (no later than 1 week of age).
- Premature infants weighing <2 kg whose mothers are HBsAg negative should not begin the series until they weigh 2 kg or are 2 months old. If the mother is HBsAg positive or unknown, administer hepatitis B vaccine at birth but do not count this vaccination as part of the three-dose series. Administer HBIG as soon as the mother is known to be HBsAg positive.

Diphtheria-Tetanus-Pertussis

The diphtheria–tetanus–acellular pertussis (DTaP) vaccine is associated with fewer side effects than the diphtheria tetanus–pertussis (DTP) vaccine. Vaccination may cause fever and brief, generalized seizures. Children with a family or personal history of seizures are at increased risk, but this is not a contraindication to vaccination. Acetaminophen may be given to decrease risk of fever and seizures. The only true contraindication to DTP/DTaP is a history of encephalopathy within 7 days of a previous dose. Relative contraindications include high temperature (greater than 105°F), continuous crying for more than 3 hours, collapse, or convulsion within 2 to 3 days after a previous DTP or DTaP vaccination. These children should receive diphtheria–tetanus (DT) unless there is a pertussis outbreak in progress. Pertussis vaccine is not indicated in children older than age 7 years nor in those who have had pertussis.

Wound Management

- For patients with three or more previous tetanus toxoid doses, give Td (the adult form of DT) for clean, minor wounds if it has been more than 10 years since the last dose. For other wounds, give Td if it has been more than 5 years since the last dose.
- For patients with less than three or an unknown number of prior tetanus toxoid doses, give Td for clean, minor wounds and Td and tetanus immune globulin (TIG) for other wounds.

Haemophilus influenzae Type B

Haemophilus influenzae type B vaccine is not indicated in children older than age 5 years.

Polio

To eliminate the risk of vaccine–associated paralytic polio (VAPP), an all-IPV (inactivated poliovirus vaccine) schedule is now recommended for routine use in the United States. OPV may be used in the following special circumstances:

- Mass vaccination campaigns to control outbreaks of paralytic polio.
- Unvaccinated children who will be traveling in <4 weeks to areas where polio is endemic or epidemic.
- Children of parents who do not accept the recommended number of vaccine injections. These children may receive OPV only for the third or fourth dose or both. Risks of VAPP should be discussed with the parents.

Measles–Mumps–Rubella

- The MMR vaccine is not as effective if given before age 1 year because maternal antibodies interfere with the development of immunity.
- MMR suppresses tuberculin reactivity. A PPD skin test should either be given on the same day as the MMR or should be delayed 4 to 6 weeks.

Pneumococcal Vaccines

- The two pneumococcal vaccines available are the older pneumococcal polysaccharide vaccine (23PS; see Table 9-2 for recommendations) and the recently released heptavalent pneumococcal conjugate vaccine (PCV7).
- Children younger than age 5 years have a greater immune response to PCV7 than to 23PS; however, 23PS provides coverage against a broader range of pneumococcal serotypes. Thus, for high-risk children (see Table 9-2), the use of both vaccines is recommended.
- For healthy children, the schedule is listed in Table 9-1. A modified catch-up schedule is as follows: If the series is started at 7–11 months, only three doses are needed. If the series is started at 12–23 months, only two doses are needed. Low-to-moderate risk children older than 2 years do not need to be vaccinated.

HIV Disease

Epidemiology

The AIDS epidemic in the United States was first identified among homosexual men in the early 1980s. In addition to homosexual and bisexual men, IV drug users, heterosexual partners of high-risk individuals, and infants born of infected mothers are all at risk of becoming infected. African-Americans and Latinos are disproportionately represented in the epidemic (40% and 20% of those living with AIDS, respectively, vs. 12% and 13% of the population). Recipients of blood products after 1985 are at low risk because the United States blood supply is tested for HIV; however, a small risk still exists because of the possibility of an individual giving blood during the "window period" after infection but before seroconversion (Figure 9-1).

In Africa, the epidemic has very different characteristics, and the virus is spread primarily via heterosexual contact. Worldwide, 34.3 million people were living with HIV and AIDS at the end of 1999 and 18.8 million had died of the disease since the beginning of the epidemic.

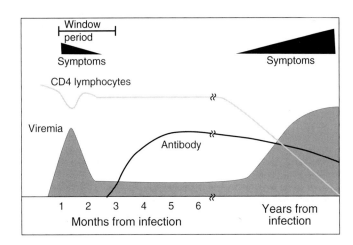

Figure 9-1. Natural history of human immunodeficiency virus infection. *Viremia* refers to the presence of detectable virus in the plasma.

IMMUNOLOGY

The Virus

HIV is an RNA retrovirus. After it infects a cell, it uses an enzyme, reverse transcriptase, to make a DNA copy of itself. The DNA version of the virus is then integrated into the cellular DNA. HIV infects T-helper cells, which are marked with a membrane glycoprotein called CD4. The progressive loss of these cells, which are integral in the immune system, and the quantity of virus in the blood (viral load) are the most significant prognosticators of HIV infection.

Acute Infection

HIV transmission requires contact with body fluids, including blood, semen, vaginal secretions, or breast milk. The presence of other sexually transmitted diseases makes viral transmission during intercourse more likely, presumably because of breaks in the mucosal tissue. The initial infection with HIV may be completely asymptomatic but is often accompanied by several weeks of a flu-like illness with symptoms including fever (96%), tender lymphadenopathy (74%), pharyngitis (70%), and a skin rash (70%). During this window period, viremia (and thus infectivity) is high, but antibody tests are still negative (see Figure 9-1).

Diagnosis

One to six months after the initial infection, antibodies to HIV can be detected in the blood. The standard test to detect antibodies is the enzyme-linked immunosorbent assay (ELISA). This test is 99% sensitive (i.e., anyone with anti-HIV antibodies will have a positive test) but not as specific (i.e., a few people without the infection will test positive as well). When an ELISA test is positive, the result should be confirmed with the more specific Western blot. Diagnosis by HIV PCR is not recommended for adults because it is slightly less sensitive than the antibody-based tests.

Post-exposure Care for Health Care Workers

Overall, the rate of HIV transmission due to occupational exposures from an HIV-infected source is about 1 in 300. Recommendations for post-exposure prophylaxis with antiretroviral medication are based on the severity of the exposure and the HIV status of the source patient. If indicated, prophylaxis with zidovudine (AZT) and lamivudine (3TC) should be started within an hour. Indinavir is added for very high-risk exposures. Prophylaxis beginning 2–3 days after exposure probably has no benefit. A baseline HIV antibody test should be drawn at the time of exposure and repeated at 6 weeks, 3 months, and 6 months.

Perinatal Care of the HIV-infected Patient

- All pregnant women should be offered HIV testing, regardless of risk factors.
- The rate of perinatal transmission of HIV correlates directly with the mother's viral load at the time of delivery. Transmission when the mother's viral load is less than 1000 is rare. Pregnant women should receive antiretroviral therapy according to the same guidelines as nonpregnant patients, although some authorities counsel against giving antiretroviral therapy during the first trimester of pregnancy. AZT should be given intravenously during labor and orally to the newborn for 6 weeks.
- Prolonged rupture of membranes (>4 hours) and fetal scalp electrodes should be avoided if possible.
- All infants of HIV+ mothers will have maternal HIV antibodies, so diagnosis must be made by detecting the HIV virus in the infant's blood. Only 30%–50% of infected infants test positive at birth, but virtually 100% test positive by 6 months of age.
- Breast-feeding is contraindicated for HIV positive mothers who have access to safe formula because of the 14%–30% increase in HIV transmission in breast-fed infants.

Natural History of HIV and Diagnosis of AIDS

Among untreated adults who contract HIV through sexual intercourse or IV drug use, approximately half become ill with AIDS within 10 years. Progression to disease occurs faster in patients with higher viral loads and can be greatly altered by antiretroviral therapy. A diagnosis of AIDS is made when the CD4 cell count falls below 200 cells/μL or when any of the conditions listed in Table 9-3 is diagnosed. Although many states do not require patients with positive HIV tests to be reported, all states have mandatory reporting laws for new diagnoses of AIDS.

Table 9-3. AIDS-defining conditions (partial list)

Candidiasis of esophagus, trachea, bronchi, or lungs

Cervical cancer, invasive[a]

Cryptococcosis, extrapulmonary

Histoplasmosis, extrapulmonary[a]

Kaposi's sarcoma

Mycobacterium avium, disseminated

Pneumocystis carinii pneumonia

Pneumonia, recurrent bacterial[a]

Toxoplasmosis (internal)

Tuberculosis[a]

[a]Requires positive HIV serology.

IMMUNOLOGY

Antiretroviral Therapy

There are currently three classes of antiretroviral medications:

- Nucleoside reverse-transcriptase inhibitors
- Non-nucleoside reverse-transcriptase inhibitors
- Protease inhibitors

Medications are used in combinations of three or more to prevent the virus from developing resistance to individual drugs. Therapy is recommended when viral load rises above 5,000–10,000 and when CD4 counts fall to less than 350–500. The goal of therapy is to lower the viral load so that it is undetectable in the serum (<50). Two common reasons for a rise in viral load are patient nonadherence and viral resistance. If viral resistance does develop, all three drugs must be changed at the same time. Resistance testing can help guide clinical choices.

Prevention in HIV Disease

Health Maintenance

On diagnosis, patients should have certain baseline laboratory tests checked. These include CD4 count, viral load, complete blood count, chemistry panel, lipid panel, toxoplasmosis serology, hepatitis serologies, VDRL or RPR for syphilis, PPD for tuberculosis, and a Pap test in women. The Pap test should be repeated at least yearly, and the PPD and VDRL or RPR should be checked yearly in high-risk patients.

Immunizations

The patient's adult vaccinations should be kept up-to-date. Influenza vaccine should be administered yearly. Vaccination against pneumococcus and hepatitis B should be given early in the course of the infection. As CD4 counts fall, the benefit of immunizations is less certain because the body is less able to mount an effective immune response.

Chemoprophylaxis

Taking prophylactic medication helps prevent illness from *Pneumocystis, Toxoplasma,* and *Mycobacterium avium* complex (MAC) when CD4 counts fall below certain levels. If a patient's immune system improves with antiretroviral medication and the CD4 counts are consistently above these levels for 3–6 months, prophylaxis can be stopped. Prophylaxis against TB should be given for 1 year regardless of CD4 levels. Recommendations are listed in Table 9-4.

AIDS-related Illnesses

Respiratory Diseases in HIV

- The most common lower respiratory tract infection in HIV disease is **community-acquired bacterial pneumonia,** typically caused by *Streptococcus pneumoniae* or *H. influenzae.* The pa-

Table 9-4. Recommended prophylactic medications

Disease	Indication	Preferred agent
Pneumocystis pneumonia	CD4 <200	Trimethoprim-sulfamethoxazole
Toxoplasmosis	CD4 <100 and positive serology (IgG)	Trimethoprim-sulfamethoxazole
MAC	CD4 <50	Daily clarithromycin or weekly azithromycin
Tuberculosis	PPD >5 mm induration Close contact of person with active TB	Daily INH for 12 mos

tient has a rapid onset of illness with cough productive of purulent sputum and high fevers. Gram's stain and culture of the sputum show bacteria, and chest x-ray often shows a lobar consolidation. Standard treatment is with a second-generation cephalosporin.

- *Pneumocystis carinii* **pneumonia** is common in patients with CD4 counts less than 200 and can occur despite adequate prophylaxis. Symptoms develop gradually and classically include nonproductive cough, dyspnea on exertion, and fever. Even in early or mild disease, exercise-induced oxygen desaturation is common. The classic x-ray finding is diffuse, bilateral interstitial infiltrates, but lobar, focal, or cystic disease may be seen. Lactate dehydrogenase (LDH) is usually elevated because of lung tissue damage. Diagnosis is based on visualizing the organism in an induced sputum or bronchoalveolar lavage specimen. Treatment of choice is trimethoprim-sulfamethoxazole (TMP-SMX, Septra, Bactrim). If the initial PaO_2 is less than 70, a tapering course of prednisone is added.
- **Tuberculosis** occurs more frequently in HIV-positive patients from certain high-risk groups, such as substance abusers, prison inmates, homeless, and people from endemic areas. Symptoms include cough, fever, night sweats, and weight loss. PPDs may or may not be positive, depending on the degree of immunocompromise. Chest x-ray may show the classic cavitary apical infiltrate or may show diffuse disease with hilar adenopathy. Diagnosis is based on acid-fast bacilli stains and cultures. Treatment of active disease requires multiple drug therapy.

Gastrointestinal Disease in HIV

- **Infectious esophagitis** can be due to *Candida,* cytomegalovirus (CMV), or herpes simplex virus (HSV) and usually occurs in patients with CD4 <100. Symptoms are pain and difficulty swallowing. Diagnosis is made using endoscopy with biopsy. *Candida* is treated with fluconazole, CMV with ganciclovir, and HSV with acyclovir.
- **Diarrhea** occurs in 30%–60% of HIV patients in the United States and can be bacterial (*Salmonella, Campylobacter, Clostridium difficile, Escherichia coli,* MAC, etc.), parasitic (*Cryptosporidia, Microsporidia, Giardia,* etc.), viral (CMV, enteric viruses), iatrogenic (medications), or idiopathic. A reasonable diagnostic approach is first to send stool for bacterial culture, ova and parasite evaluation, and *C. difficile* toxin. If these tests are negative, consider endoscopy with biopsy. Treatment depends on etiology.

Neurologic Disease in HIV

- *Cryptococcus neoformans* causes **cryptococcal meningitis.** Symptoms include headache, fever, and confusion. Neck stiffness may or may not be present. CT and MRI are normal. Lumbar puncture often reveals an elevated opening pressure. Diagnosis is made by finding the encapsulated, yeast-like organisms on India ink preparation of the CSF (75% sensitive), by getting a positive CSF cryptococcal antigen (CRAG; 90% sensitive), or by getting a positive serum CRAG (99% sensitive); thus, a negative serum CRAG effectively rules out disease. Treatment is with amphotericin B or fluconazole.

- Symptoms of **cerebral toxoplasmosis** include headache, confusion, and focal neurologic abnormalities. Serum *toxoplasma* IgG is present 85%–95% of the time. Multiple ring-enhancing lesions are identified on CT or MRI. Although brain biopsy is definitive, the diagnosis is commonly made by observing improvement with empiric therapy of pyrimethamine and sulfadiazine. Chronic maintenance therapy is necessary to prevent relapse.

- **CNS lymphoma** is another cause of mass lesions in the brain. Symptoms are similar to those of toxoplasmosis. Imaging studies are more likely to show a single lesion that enhances irregularly with contrast. Brain biopsy provides the definitive diagnosis but is usually only done if the patient fails to respond to an empiric trial of anti-toxoplasmosis medication. Steroids and radiation may be used for palliation, but survival is poor.

- The most common cause of visual loss in HIV is **CMV retinitis,** which usually occurs when the CD4 count falls below 50. Symptoms include floaters and areas of decreased vision. Advanced disease causes a characteristic "scrambled eggs and ketchup" appearance of the retina, with yellow infiltrates and hemorrhage. Treatment is with ganciclovir and must be ongoing to prevent relapse and worsening of vision.

Miscellaneous Disorders in HIV

- **Kaposi's sarcoma** is a common dermatologic neoplasm in HIV, although it also can occur in the GI tract and lungs. It is caused by human herpes virus 8. Patients have painless, purple subcutaneous nodules on the face, chest, or extremities. Diagnosis is based on biopsy, and local treatments, radiation, and chemotherapy are all used with moderate success.

- *M. avium* **complex** (MAC) is composed of two related, atypical mycobacteria that frequently cause disseminated disease in advanced AIDS. Symptoms include spiking fevers, night sweats, fatigue, weight loss, abdominal pain, and diarrhea. Adenopathy and hepatosplenomegaly may occur. Diagnosis is based on positive blood cultures. As in TB, treatment requires the use of multiple drugs to avoid resistance. Options include clarithromycin, azithromycin, rifampin, rifabutin, ethambutol, and ciprofloxacin.

Cell-mediated Immune Deficiencies

DiGeorge Syndrome (Thymic Aplasia)

DiGeorge syndrome involves a congenital defect of thymus and parathyroid glands. As a result, patients experience a severe lack of T cells and develop recurrent viral and fungal infections. Associated findings include congenital heart disease and craniofacial abnormalities. Within the first few days of life, these patients present with hypocalcemia and tetany due to lack of parathyroid function. Treatment is with calcium and vitamin D and surgery to correct the heart defects. Immunocompromise may resolve spontaneously or may require thymus grafting.

Chronic Mucocutaneous Candidiasis

Individuals with chronic mucocutaneous candidiasis have a T-cell deficiency that is specific to *Candida albicans.* As a result, these patients develop candidiasis on the scalp, skin, nails, and mucous membranes. Treatment is with antifungal medications.

Ataxia-telangiectasia

Ataxia-telangiectasia is an autosomal-recessive disorder that first presents in early childhood. It consists of worsening ataxia (gait abnormalities), telangiectasia (localized blood vessel dilatation on the skin), lymphopenia, and IgA deficiency. Recurrent infections and malignancies are common.

Wiskott-Aldrich Syndrome

Individuals with Wiskott-Aldrich syndrome, an X-linked disorder, are unable to mount antibody responses against polysaccharide-encapsulated bacteria such as pneumococci. Associated signs include bleeding (due to decreased platelets), eczema, and recurrent bacterial infections. Treatment consists of splenectomy (to alleviate platelet destruction), antibiotics, immunoglobulin, and bone marrow transplantation.

Chronic Granulomatous Disease

Chronic granulomatous disease is a disorder in which defective neutrophils ingest but cannot destroy bacteria. It can be autosomal recessive or X-linked. Patients experience recurrent bacterial and fungal infections, particularly of the skin and lymphoid tissue. Common organisms are *Staphylococcus aureus, Escherichia coli, Pseudomonas,* and *Aspergillus,* which form granulomas. Treatment is with prophylactic antibiotics.

Chédiak-Higashi Syndrome

Chédiak-Higashi syndrome is an autosomal-recessive disorder that results in ineffective neutrophilic enzymes, leading to recurrent streptococcal and staphylococcal infections. Other features of the disease include partial albinism due to melanocyte dysfunction and a mild bleeding disorder due to platelet dysfunction. Treatment is with antibiotics.

Severe Combined Immunodeficiency

Severe combined immunodeficiency is a group of X-linked and autosomal recessive disorders that involve deficits of both B- and T-cell function and is usually fatal within the first few years of life. Patients experience recurrent infections from bacteria, viruses, fungi, and protozoa. Laboratory results show lymphopenia and decreased serum antibodies. Immunoglobulin, antibiotics, and bone marrow transplantation may be helpful in some cases.

IMMUNOLOGY

Humoral Immune Deficiencies

Common Variable Immunodeficiency

Common variable immunodeficiency is a defect of B cell differentiation and antibody production. Onset typically occurs between the ages of 15 and 40 years, at which time patients experience recurrent sinus and respiratory tract infections. Diagnosis is made by finding low levels of IgG in the serum or by documenting a lack of antibody production after immunization. Regular IV immunoglobulin and antibiotics to treat infections are the mainstays of treatment.

X-linked Agammaglobulinemia (Bruton's Disease)

In X-linked agammaglobulinemia, B-cell precursors do not develop into B cells, resulting in low or absent B cells and antibody levels. Affected boys begin to experience recurrent bacterial infections after approximately 6 months of age (once maternal antibodies have been depleted). The patient's tonsils are small. Treatment consists of immunoglobulin infusions and antibiotics.

Immunoglobulin A Deficiency

Individuals with IgA deficiency may be asymptomatic or may experience recurrent infections, particularly of the respiratory and GI tract. Patients typically do not receive any treatment. The administration of immunoglobulin is contraindicated in these patients because they may develop antibodies against them, thereby depleting already low levels.

Hypersensitivity Reactions

Type I—IgE-Mediated (Immediate) Hypersensitivity. Allergen-specific IgE antibodies are attached to mast cells. When an allergen links two adjacent IgE molecules, the mast cell degranulates and releases histamines and other inflammatory response mediators. This causes symptoms of atopy (allergic rhinitis and asthma [see Chapter 3] and atopic dermatitis [see chapter 11]) and anaphylaxis (urticaria, angioedema, bronchospasm, and shock [see below]).

Type II—Antibody-Mediated (Cytotoxic) Hypersensitivity. Allergen-specific IgM and IgG circulate in the bloodstream. They bind antigens located on cells and initiate the complement cascade to destroy the cell. Examples include immune hemolytic anemia and Rh hemolytic disease of the newborn (see Chapter 8).

Type III—Immune Complex-Mediated Hypersensitivity. Circulating IgM and IgG form complexes with allergens. These complexes are deposited in tissues and initiate the complement cascade. Examples in-

IMMUNOLOGY

clude the Arthus reaction, in which immunization causes a localized inflammation, and serum sickness, a reaction to drugs or blood products characterized by fever, arthralgias, and dermatitis.

Type IV—T Cell-Mediated Hypersensitivity (Delayed Hypersensitivity). Antibodies are not involved in this type of reaction. Allergens are presented to T cells by macrophages. The T cells release lymphokines that, in turn, activate the macrophages to attack the allergen and surrounding tissue. The process takes 1–2 days. The most common manifestation of type IV hypersensitivity is allergic contact dermatitis (e.g., poison oak or ivy; see Chapter 11).

Anaphylaxis

Anaphylaxis occurs when a person who has been previously sensitized to an allergen is re-exposed. Medications (especially penicillin), bee stings, nuts, seafood, and latex are common causes of anaphylaxis.

SIGNS & SYMPTOMS

Anaphylactic reactions range from mild to fatal. The first sign is often warmth and tingling of the skin. Itching and urticaria (hives) then develop. Bronchospasm may cause cough, chest tightness, and wheezing. Angioedema of the pharynx or larynx causes throat tightness and difficulty swallowing and breathing. Increased vascular permeability and vasodilatation leads to light-headedness, tachycardia, and hypotension and can lead to arrhythmias and cardiac arrest.

DIAGNOSIS

The preceding symptoms provide the diagnosis. A history of exposure is helpful. Skin testing can help determine specific allergens.

TREATMENT

Epinephrine should be given immediately. If the airway is compromised, intubation may be necessary. Antihistamines block further histamine action. Blood pressure is maintained with Trendelenburg positioning, IV fluids, and vasopressors, if necessary. Bronchospasm is treated with inhaled β-agonists. Steroids take 4–6 hours to begin working but are useful to control a persistent reaction. Patients with severe reactions should be observed for 24–48 hours.

PREVENTION

Avoidance of the allergen is the best prevention. Susceptible patients should carry epinephrine auto-injection kits and antihistamine tablets. Desensitization therapy is occasionally warranted.

Transplantation

Organ transplants are generally limited to patients who will benefit significantly in both quality and quantity of life. The timing of transplantation varies depending on the organ being transplanted and in the underlying disorder. For example, cardiac transplantation is generally not performed until a patient has end-stage congestive heart failure. On the other hand, kidney transplants in diabetic patients are often performed when retinopathy begins because progression of the disease can be halted if kidney function improves. Many comorbid conditions are relative contraindications to transplantation. For example, transplants are virtually never performed in patients with acute infections, neoplasms, or HIV. Social resources, psychological stability, and ability to adhere to complex immunosuppressive regimens are also considered when determining transplant eligibility.

Rejection of transplanted tissue may occur by both cell-mediated and antibody-mediated responses to tissue antigens. The most important of these antigens are the HLA groups and the ABO blood group antigens. T cell-mediated rejection (host versus graft reaction) is the principal mechanism of acute transplant rejection, whereas later graft rejection generally occurs as a result of antibody-mediated damage. If the host has been presensitized against particular antigens (e.g., through a previous blood transfusion), hyperacute graft rejection occurs, in which the transplanted tissue is destroyed within minutes. A graft versus host reaction occurs when blood cells in the transplanted organ attack an immunocompromised host. Methods that are used to control transplant rejection include immunosuppressive drugs, antilymphocyte globulin, and irradiation of the graft and local recipient tissue.

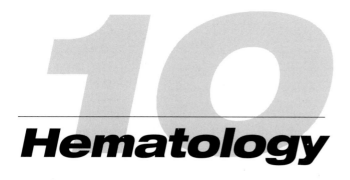

Hematology

Table 10-1. Common causes of anemia by mean corpuscular volume

Microcytic anemia (MCV <80 μL)	Normocytic anemia (MCV 80 to 100 μL)	Macrocytic anemia (MCV >100 μL)
Iron deficiency	Early iron deficiency	B$_{12}$ or folate deficiency
Thalassemia	Chronic disease	Liver disease
Lead poisoning	Hemolysis	Alcoholism
—	Bone marrow suppression (drugs, leukemia)	Hypothyroidism

MCV, mean corpuscular volume.

Anemia

Anemia is defined as any condition with less than normal amounts of hemoglobin, hematocrit, or number of red blood cells. It is typically classified according to whether red blood cells are microcytic [mean corpuscular volume (MCV) <80 μL], normocytic (MCV 80 to 100 μL), or macrocytic (MCV >100 μL) [Table 10-1]. Specific etiologies and diagnoses are described in the following sections.

Iron-deficiency Anemia

Iron-deficiency anemia (IDA) is the most common type of anemia. The reduction in heme production from lack of iron is usually due to blood loss through the GI system (e.g., ulcers, cancer, or chronic rectal bleeding) or menstruation. Dietary iron deficiency can contribute as well. Pregnancy is a common cause of IDA because of expanding maternal blood volume and high fetal iron requirements.

Fatigue, pallor, dizziness, and shortness of breath. In severe cases, angular cheilosis (irritation at the corners of the mouth and lips), koilonychia (spooning of the nails), and pica (the craving to eat unusual things such as dirt) may occur.

Hematocrit, hemoglobin, and RBC count are decreased. RBCs are usually microcytic but can be normocytic in early stages. Peripheral blood smear typically shows microcytic cells with increased central pallor (hypochromia; see Figure 10-1 in the color insert). Ghost and pencil cells may be present. Reticulocyte count may be low or normal, depending on the severity of the iron deficiency.

The single best test for diagnosing iron deficiency is measurement of the level of serum ferritin, an iron storage protein. Ferritin levels are proportional to iron stores and will therefore be low in IDA. Less reliable tests include low serum iron, high total iron-binding capacity (TIBC or transferrin), and low transferrin saturation (serum iron to TIBC ratio). Bone marrow biopsy reveals low or absent iron stores but is usually not indicated in simple IDA.

Oral iron supplements. IDA should be fully corrected in 6 to 8 weeks, but an additional 4 to 6 months of treatment are required to replenish iron stores. Common side effects of oral iron treatment are nausea and constipation.

HEMATOLOGY

Anemia of Chronic Disease

Anemia of chronic disease is the most common anemia in hospitalized patients. It is seen in patients with bacterial infections, malignancies, chronic inflammatory diseases, and diabetes. The anemia is caused by the production of lactoferrin, a storage protein with a greater affinity for iron than transferrin.

The classic symptoms of anemia are present, including fatigue, shortness of breath on exertion, and pallor.

Hematocrit levels are reduced but generally do not fall below 25%. MCV may be normal or low. RBC morphology and reticulocyte count are usually normal.

Laboratory analysis shows decreased serum iron and decreased transferrin. Ferritin levels are generally high because ferritin is an acute-phase reactant and these patients have some type of inflammatory condition. Bone marrow biopsy shows normal or increased iron stores.

Treat the primary disorder, if possible. Do not give these patients iron supplementation or transfusions; they may experience iron overload.

Megaloblastic Anemias

Megaloblastic anemia is most often due to folate or vitamin B_{12} deficiency, but it can also result from drugs that inhibit DNA synthesis. It is seen in liver disease, particularly in alcoholics. Features include macrocytosis, with macro-ovalocytes (large, elliptically shaped RBCs) and hypersegmented neutrophils (nuclei containing five or more lobes).

> **Folic acid** is used in DNA synthesis. It is found in green, leafy vegetables and citrus fruits and is absorbed throughout the small intestine. **Vitamin B_{12}** is important for DNA synthesis and myelin formation. It is found in meat, eggs, and milk. Once ingested, vitamin B_{12} binds to **intrinsic factor (IF),** which is produced in the gastric parietal cells, and the complex is absorbed in the terminal ileum.

Folate-deficiency Anemia

Folic acid deficiency is the most common cause of megaloblastic anemia, because folic acid stores last only 2 to 3 months. Inadequate dietary supply, from either decreased intake (seen

HEMATOLOGY

in alcoholics, elderly, and the poor) or increased demand (in pregnancy), is usually the cause. Some drugs, such as sulfasalazine and phenytoin, may reduce the availability of folic acid.

In addition to general symptoms of anemia, signs of impaired epithelial cell proliferation (e.g., sore, beefy tongue, and diarrhea) result from inadequate DNA synthesis. **In contrast to vitamin B$_{12}$ deficiency, no neurologic symptoms are seen.**

Hematocrit, hemoglobin, and RBC count are decreased and MCV is high. Peripheral blood smear reveals macro-ovalocytes and hypersegmented neutrophils. Bone marrow biopsy shows unusually large erythroblasts—hence the name *megaloblastic anemia*. Serum folate or RBC folate levels are low, and the vitamin B$_{12}$ level is normal. Serum folate levels correct quickly on a hospital diet, whereas the RBC folate level reflects long-term stores.

Daily oral folate supplement.

Vitamin B$_{12}$-deficiency Anemia

Vitamin B$_{12}$ (cobalamin) deficiency is usually caused by inadequate absorption because of pernicious anemia (lack of IF caused by autoimmune destruction of parietal cells), resection of the terminal ileum, intestinal overgrowth of bacteria, or presence of the fish tapeworm *Diphyllobothrium latum*. Vitamin B$_{12}$ deficiency due to diet is rare and seen only in strict vegans.

In addition to general signs and symptoms of anemia, vitamin B$_{12}$ deficiency can cause severe neurologic disturbances. These may occur with or without the presence of anemia and include symmetric paresthesias, loss of proprioception, and ataxia. Psychosis and irreversible dementia may develop.

The serum vitamin B$_{12}$ level is decreased, but serum folate measurements should be normal. Other findings are similar to those of folate deficiency.

The definitive diagnosis of pernicious anemia is made with the Schilling test, which involves administering an oral dose of radioactively labeled vitamin B$_{12}$ and measuring its urinary excretion. Decreased excretion indicates a lack of appropriate vitamin B$_{12}$ absorption. The test is repeated with the addition of IF. If absorption is normal with exogenous IF, the patient has pernicious anemia. If absorption is still low, an intestinal cause of vitamin B$_{12}$ malabsorption is likely.

Intramuscular injections of vitamin B$_{12}$ are given for as long as the need persists, which may be lifelong.

Aplastic Anemia

Aplastic anemia is pancytopenia (lack of all three blood cell lines: RBCs, WBCs, and platelets) resulting from bone marrow failure. It is associated with an almost complete lack of progenitor cells in the bone marrow. The most common cause of aplastic anemia is a drug reaction, frequently involving chloramphenicol, phenylbutazone, gold salts, sulfonamides, or phenytoin. Less common causes include chemotherapy, radiation therapy, and toxins.

SIGNS & SYMPTOMS

Symptoms result from the lack of blood cells and include anemia (fatigue, pallor), neutropenia (recurrent or persistent nonhealing infections), and thrombocytopenia (abnormal or uncontrolled bleeding).

DIAGNOSIS

The numbers of RBCs, WBCs, and platelets are decreased, and bone marrow biopsy shows hypocellularity.

TREATMENT

Potential causative agents should be stopped. Further treatment includes immunosuppressive drugs, transfusions, and bone marrow transplant.

Hemolytic Disease

Coombs' Test

There are two types of Coombs' tests used in the diagnosis of hemolytic disorders. Coombs' reagent consists of a rabbit IgM that is directed against human IgG and complement (anti-human globulin). The **direct Coombs' test** consists of mixing the Coombs' reagent with the patient's red blood cells; agglutination indicates that the patient's red blood cells are coated with IgG and complement. The **indirect Coombs' test** consists of first mixing the patient's serum with type O red blood cells; if the serum has anti-RBC antibodies, they will bind to the type O red blood cells. Then, the type O red blood cells are mixed with Coombs' reagent; agglutination occurs if the patient's serum contained anti-RBC antibodies.

Hemolytic Anemia

The average life span of an RBC is approximately 120 days. Hemolytic anemia occurs when the normal RBC life span is shortened and marrow production can no longer compensate for the increased destruction. Specific etiologies are generally grouped into three categories: defects external to the RBC (immune hemolysis, mechanical hemolysis, hemolytic disease of the newborn), defects of the RBC membrane (hereditary spherocytosis), and defects of the RBC interior [glucose 6-phosphate dehydrogenase (G6PD) deficiency]. These etiologies are described in greater detail in the following sections.

Mild cases are asymptomatic. Patients with severe cases have palpitations, dyspnea, pallor, hepatosplenomegaly, chills, fever, abdominal pain, back pain, and shock. Jaundice occurs when hemoglobin from destroyed RBCs cannot be converted to conjugated bilirubin fast enough to be excreted and unconjugated bilirubin builds up in the tissues. Hemoglobin may be excreted in the urine, causing brownish discoloration.

Reticulocyte count increases as the bone marrow tries to replenish the RBC supply. Unconjugated (indirect) bilirubin may be increased. Increased serum lactate dehydrogenase (LDH), released from RBCs, is also seen. Blood smear findings often reveal helmet cells, burr cells, RBC fragments, and a relative lack of platelets (see Figure 10-2 in the color insert).

Drug-induced Anemia

There are three mechanisms by which certain drugs provoke hemolytic anemia. First, some drugs can act as haptens, bind to the RBC membrane, and induce the synthesis of antidrug antibodies. One common drug in this category is penicillin. Hemolysis occurs approximately 7 to 10 days after starting the drug. The direct Coombs' test, which detects the presence of antibody or complement on the RBC, is positive with immunoglobulin G (IgG) reagent during hemolysis.

Some drugs form immune complexes with immunoglobulins and start fixing complement, which leads to hemolysis. Quinidine is one example. During hemolysis, the direct Coombs' test is positive with anticomplement reagents.

The third type of drug-induced anemia is induction of synthesis of anti-Rhesus (Rh) antibodies, which cause hemolysis. This may involve loss of suppressor cell activity. L-Dopa and alpha-methyldopa are examples of drugs that can cause this reaction, which may continue even after the drug is discontinued.

Immune Hemolysis

Immune hemolysis is usually caused by anti-RBC IgG antibodies that attach most effectively above 31°C (warm-reacting antibodies). Antibody-coated RBCs are removed from circulation by the spleen, resulting in anemia. Thirty percent of cases are idiopathic. An additional 30% are drug induced (penicillin, quinidine, methyldopa), and the rest are associated with underlying disease, including systemic lupus erythematosus (SLE), lymphoma, and chronic lymphocytic leukemia (CLL).

Peripheral blood smear shows spherocytes, which arise from partial consumption of RBCs by the reticuloendothelial system. The direct Coombs' test, which detects the presence of antibody or complement on the RBC, is positive.

In drug-induced disease, discontinue the offending drug immediately. Give corticosteroids to suppress the immune response. Splenectomy may be necessary to control hemolysis.

Cold-reacting antibodies form RBC complexes only below 31°C. These IgM antibodies can cause either hemolysis or agglutination of RBCs, leading to infarction of tissues in colder areas of the body (fingers and toes). This form of hemolytic anemia occurs in patients with certain infections (*Mycoplasma,* malaria, Epstein-Barr virus) and with lymphoproliferative diseases. Avoiding exposure to cold is the primary treatment.

Mechanical Hemolysis

Mechanical hemolysis occurs when RBCs are fragmented by shear forces or by turbulence. Injury to cells can arise in the heart (aortic stenosis, prosthetic heart valve), in the arterioles (malignant hypertension), or in other vessels [thrombotic thrombocytopenic purpura (TTP), disseminated intravascular coagulation (DIC)].

Peripheral blood smear shows odd-shaped RBCs, including schistocytes (helmet cells).

Directed at the underlying process.

Hereditary Spherocytosis

Hereditary spherocytosis is a dominantly inherited defect in RBC membrane proteins that results in spherical RBCs. Although functionally normal, these abnormally shaped cells are trapped in the spleen and destroyed.

Splenomegaly is the major finding. Hepatomegaly and cholelithiasis are also common. Aplastic crises can occur during infections.

Spherical RBCs and reticulocytosis are seen on peripheral blood smear. Coombs' test is negative, as no antibodies are involved.

HEMATOLOGY

Splenectomy will stop the hemolysis, although the underlying defect is unchanged.

Glucose 6-phosphate Dehydrogenase Deficiency

Glucose 6-phosphate dehydrogenase is an enzyme required by the RBCs to cope with oxidative damage. Its deficiency is an X-linked disease. Without G6PD, damaged hemoglobin accumulates in the RBCs as small densities called *Heinz bodies.* These cells are then taken out of circulation by the spleen. This sequence of oxidation and subsequent hemolysis occurs when a patient with G6PD deficiency ingests oxidative drugs (antimalarials, sulfa drugs, aspirin) or fava beans, as well as during febrile illnesses or acidosis. A mild form of the disease is found in 10% of African-American men, and a more severe form occurs in Mediterranean and Middle Eastern men.

Symptoms of acute hemolysis include palpitations, breathlessness, and dizziness, usually occurring 1 to 3 days after ingestion of an oxidant. Jaundice and splenomegaly are common.

Heinz bodies and "bite cells"—cells in which the Heinz body has been "bitten" out during a pass through the spleen—are visible on peripheral blood smear before the onset of hemolysis.

Assay of G6PD levels.

Discontinue the oxidative drug and counsel the patient to avoid future oxidants. Transfusion may be necessary.

White Blood Cell Disorders

Agranulocytosis (Neutropenia)

Agranulocytosis is a deficit of neutrophils. Because neutrophil half-life is only 6 to 7 hours, this disorder can develop rapidly. Causes include inadequate granulopoiesis, as seen in aplastic anemia and leukemia, or accelerated destruction of neutrophils, which is usually caused by drugs such as chloramphenicol, sulfonamides, chlorpromazine, thiouracil, and phenylbutazone.

HEMATOLOGY

Constitutional symptoms include fever, chills, weakness, and fatigue. Infections, including ulcerating and necrotizing surface lesions, are common.

CBC shows decreased neutrophils. Bone marrow biopsy is helpful in discerning the exact cause.

Granulocyte colony-stimulating factor (G-CSF) may be used to increase neutrophil counts. Antibiotics, steroids, and neutrophil transfusions may also be useful.

Eosinophilia

Eosinophilia is characteristic of allergic disorders, asthma, and parasitic diseases. The most common source of eosinophilia in hospitalized patients is an allergic drug reaction. It is also seen in Löffler's syndrome (endocardial fibrosis), pulmonary infiltrates with eosinophilia, and Addison's disease. (A mnemonic for the most common causes of eosinophilia is NAACP: **n**eoplasm, **a**llergy/asthma, **A**ddison's disease, **c**ollagen vascular disease, and **p**arasites.)

Asymptomatic, except as related to the underlying disorder.

Increased eosinophil count on CBC.

Remove any allergenic stimuli as soon as possible. Otherwise, treat the underlying disorder.

Hemoglobin Abnormalities

Thalassemia

In thalassemia, diminished or absent production of a particular globin chain causes unbalanced amounts of alpha and beta chains. Sufficient normal hemoglobin, comprised of two alpha and two beta chains, cannot be produced, resulting in microcytic anemia. Unpaired chains become tetramers and precipitate, damaging the RBC membrane and causing hemolysis.

Two types of thalassemia are commonly seen:

- α-**Thalassemia** refers to a group of structural deletions of the alpha chain of hemoglobin. It is seen more frequently in Asians. Depending on the number of deletions, patients may be asymptomatic, experience a mild anemia, or have more severe manifestations. In the most severe form, **hemoglobin H disease,** alpha-globin is completely absent. Infants with this disorder are often stillborn. Some may survive for a short time because of the presence of fetal hemoglobin, but they will have very severe anemia and splenomegaly.
- β-**Thalassemia** is characterized by defective expression of the beta chain of hemoglobin. It is generally seen in Mediterranean and African populations. Heterozygous patients have β-**thalassemia minor** and may be asymptomatic. Homozygotes have β-**thalassemia major,** with severe anemia, delayed growth and development, and shortened life expectancy.

MCV is severely decreased (typically out of proportion to the reduction in hematocrit), reticulocytes are increased, and peripheral blood smear shows abnormal RBC morphology. α-Thalassemia is characterized by target cells and acanthocytes (cells with rounded projections). Peripheral blood smear in β-thalassemia shows basophilic stippling, nucleated RBCs, anisocytosis (variations in size), and poikilocytosis (variations in shape).

Diagnosis may be made with hemoglobin electrophoresis. However, α-thalassemia often has normal electrophoresis results, and definitive diagnosis may require further molecular biology testing.

Transfusions are important for symptomatic disease, with iron chelation therapy to prevent iron overload. Supplemental iron should never be given to thalassemic patients. Bone marrow transplant has been used with some success, and genetic counseling is important to help prevent the most severe forms of both α- and β-thalassemia.

Mentzer's Index

Microcytic anemia is seen in both iron-deficiency anemia and thalassemia. One quick rule of thumb used to differentiate the two is calculation of the **Mentzer's index:**

$$\text{Mentzer's index} = \frac{\text{Mean corpuscular volume}}{\text{Red blood cell count}}$$

$$> 13 \Rightarrow \text{Iron deficiency}$$

$$< 13 \Rightarrow \text{Thalassemia}$$

If Mentzer's index is greater than 13, it is likely to be iron-deficiency anemia, while less than 13 indicates likely thalassemia.

Sickle Cell Anemia

Sickle cell anemia is a recessively inherited disease in which the beta-hemoglobin chain is altered, resulting in the production of hemoglobin S (HbS) instead of the normal hemoglobin A. When exposed to a low-oxygen environment, HbS molecules join together to form long crystalline structures that distort the RBC into the classic sickle shape. Acidosis and dehydration also promote sickling. The HbS gene is more common in African-American populations, and 1 in 400 births of African-American infants results in a child with sickle cell anemia (approximately 8% of African-Americans are carriers of the gene). Carriers are referred to as having **sickle cell trait,** and they are asymptomatic except under extreme conditions. These carriers have a beneficial increased resistance to malaria.

Patients are rarely symptomatic until 6 months of age because of the presence of fetal hemoglobin. Chronic anemia arises from constant destruction of sickled cells. Most other manifestations are due to vascular sludging and thrombosis, which result in damage to multiple organs as well as acute, painful crises. Common manifestations include stroke, osteonecrosis, pulmonary hypertension, and acute chest syndrome (characterized by fever, pain, dyspnea, and a pneumonia-like infiltrate on x-ray). Multiple infarcts of the spleen result in autosplenectomy, and patients are susceptible to *Streptococcus pneumoniae* sepsis and salmonella osteomyelitis. Aplastic crises may be triggered by infection of any kind.

Peripheral blood smear may not show sickled cells unless the blood sample is deoxygenated first (sickle cell preparation) [see Figure 10-3 in the color insert]. Hematocrit is low (20% to 30%), and the reticulocyte count is high (10% to 25%), except during an aplastic crisis. Neutrophilia is chronic but may become extreme during a painful crisis, even in the absence of infection.

Solubility tests (Sickledex) may be used, but hemoglobin electrophoresis showing HbS without HbA is the gold standard.

Hydroxyurea may decrease the number of sickle cell crises by increasing production of hemoglobin F and decreasing adherence of sickle cells to the vascular endothelium.

Preventive care includes avoidance of dehydration or low-oxygen environments. Prophylactic penicillin should be given to children to decrease risk of pneumococcal sepsis, and pneumococcal vaccine should be administered as soon as the child's system can respond to it (at 2 years of age). Treatment of crises includes oxygen, hydration, and narcotic analgesics. Blood transfusions may be required in aplastic crises, but iron overload is a concern.

Clotting Disorders

Hemophilia

Hemophilia A is an X-linked recessive disorder caused by reduced quantity or activity of factor VIII of the coagulation cascade (see Figure 10-4 in text). It is often asymptomatic

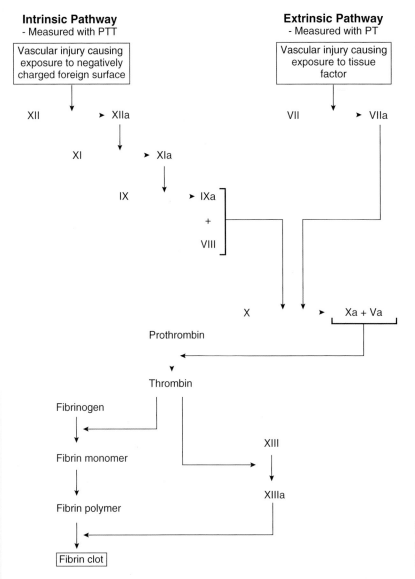

Figure 10-4. Coagulation cascade. PT, prothrombin time; PTT partial thromboplastin time.

but can become severe when factor VIII activity drops to less than 1% of normal. Incidence is approximately 1 in 10,000. **Hemophilia B** (Christmas disease) is also an X-linked recessive disease. It is similar to hemophilia A but is much less common, with an incidence of 1 in 100,000. Hemophilia B is due to factor IX deficiency.

Uncontrolled bleeding can arise spontaneously or after minor trauma. Bleeding occurs most often in the joints (hemarthroses) and soft tissues, but also in the GI tract, genitourinary tract, central nervous system, and elsewhere.

Laboratory evaluation shows a prolonged partial thromboplastin time (PTT). Definitive diagnosis is made with factor activity assays showing low activity of factor VIII (hemophilia A) or factor IX (hemophilia B).

Infusions of factor concentrates and fresh frozen plasma (FFP) may be useful. Desmopressin, an analogue of antidiuretic hormone, has been shown to raise factor VIII levels. Most adults with hemophilia are HIV positive if they received transfusions before widespread blood screening was available.

von Willebrand's Disease

von Willebrand's factor (vWF) functions both in adherence of platelets to the endothelium and in maintenance of normal plasma levels of factor VIII. von Willebrand's disease, an autosomal-dominant condition, involves deficiencies in both factor VIII and vWF, resulting in a disorder of both coagulation and platelet function.

Bleeding from the skin and mucous membranes, including epistaxis, menorrhagia, and bruising. Hemarthroses are rare, even though these patients have some factor VIII deficiency.

Prolonged PTT and bleeding time (time taken for bleeding to stop after a skin cut) are typical. Ristocetin cofactor assay or vWF immunologic assay shows specific deficiencies and provides the definitive diagnosis.

Cryoprecipitate and FFP.

Vitamin K Deficiency

Vitamin K is a cofactor in the liver's synthesis of clotting factors II, VII, IX, and X (mnemonic: "1972"). It is supplied by leafy green vegetables as well as by normal bacteria in the intestine. Thus, poor diet or prolonged antibiotic treatment may lead to a deficiency. The drug warfarin acts by interfering with vitamin K–mediated clotting factor synthesis and therefore patients using this drug appear to have a vitamin K deficiency.

The primary symptom is spontaneous bleeding or prolonged oozing.

Prothrombin time (PT) and PTT are prolonged, although the PT is generally more dramatically affected.

HEMATOLOGY

Platelet Disorders

Qualitative Platelet Disorders

Qualitative platelet disorders involve malfunctioning platelets. The hereditary forms are rare and include abnormalities of platelet membranes, attachment, and storage. Acquired platelet disorders occur with the use of aspirin, which irreversibly acetylates cyclo-oxygenase, resulting in deficits of platelet aggregation. The effect lasts for the life of the platelet (approximately 7 to 10 days) and is not dose dependent. Uremia can cause a platelet disorder that is associated with renal failure, although the mechanism by which this occurs is unknown. Symptoms of qualitative platelet disorders include easy bruising, epistaxis, prolonged oozing, and menorrhagia. Treatment with cryoprecipitate and renal dialysis may be helpful. Platelet transfusions are not beneficial.

Quantitative Platelet Disorders

Quantitative platelet disorders involve inadequate numbers of circulating platelets, which can result from a variety of etiologies. The following causes are most common:

- **Decreased production of platelets,** as a result of aplastic anemia, bone marrow damage (e.g., secondary to drugs, radiation), myelophthisis (reduction of cell-forming ability of the bone marrow), or ineffective thrombopoiesis (e.g., vitamin B_{12} and folate deficiency)
- **Increased destruction of platelets,** as a result of idiopathic thrombocytopenic purpura (ITP; see following section), underlying disease (e.g., SLE, CLL), drug-induced antibodies (e.g., quinine, quinidine, thiazide diuretics, sulfa drugs, heparin), or viral infections (e.g., CMV, EBV, HIV)
- **Increased consumption of platelets,** as a result of DIC (see following section), TTP (see following section), or hemolytic-uremic syndrome (HUS, see following section)

Common symptoms of quantitative platelet disorders include petechiae (small hemorrhages in the skin) and purpura (larger skin hemorrhages).

Diagnosis and treatment are discussed with the individual disorders.

Disseminated Intravascular Coagulation

Disseminated intravascular coagulation is caused by widespread activation of the coagulation sequence. Formation of microthrombi causes infarcts, and massive consumption of platelets, fibrin, and coagulation factors causes uncontrolled bleeding. Significant damage may occur in the kidneys, lungs, and brain. Common causes include obstetric complications (50%), malignancy (33%), infections, and massive tissue trauma.

Presentation varies widely. Physical manifestations include hemolytic anemia, respiratory difficulty, neurologic symptoms, acute renal failure, and shock.

SIGNS & SYMPTOMS

Decreased platelets, fragmentation of RBCs, prolonged PT and PTT, decreased fibrinogen, and increased fibrin degradation products. Slide review often shows hallmarks of hemolysis.

DIAGNOSIS

Coagulation factors can be replaced with FFP, and fibrinogen can be replaced with cryoprecipitate. Platelet transfusions may be necessary. In cases involving thrombosis, heparin may also be indicated. Heparin will not be effective if antithrombin III levels are low.

TREATMENT

Thrombotic Thrombocytopenic Purpura

Thrombotic thrombocytopenic purpura involves the reaction of platelets with endothelial cells, resulting in occlusion of vessels and platelet consumption. The cause of TTP is unknown but is not thought to be autoimmune. It is often seen in association with HIV disease. Patients are generally between the ages of 20 and 50 years.

TTP is characterized by the acute onset of thrombocytopenia, fever, anemia, jaundice, fluctuating neurologic deficits, and renal failure.

SIGNS & SYMPTOMS

Laboratory evaluation shows low platelet count, decreased hematocrit, and increased reticulocytes. Serum LDH levels and indirect bilirubin are usually elevated because of hemolysis of RBCs.

LABS

Diagnosis is established by the presence of hemolytic anemia, thrombocytopenia, fever, fluctuating neurologic signs, and renal failure.

DIAGNOSIS

Corticosteroids, platelet aggregation inhibitors (aspirin), and plasma exchange transfusions are generally effective. Splenectomy may be necessary. If untreated, TTP is usually fatal within 3 months.

TREATMENT

Idiopathic Thrombocytopenic Purpura

Idiopathic thrombocytopenic purpura is an autoimmune disease caused by the development of antibodies against the patient's own platelets. Massive phagocytosis of platelet-antibody immune complexes occurs in the spleen. ITP is more common in children and frequently follows a mild viral infection. The childhood form has a better prognosis than the adult form. ITP is also common in AIDS patients.

Patients are generally asymptomatic except for mucosal and skin bleeding that is due to lack of platelets. Purpura, petechiae, epistaxis, and menorrhagia are common.

Platelet counts are markedly low (less than 10,000/μL). Other blood cell counts are generally normal, and the peripheral blood smear is normal.

ITP is usually self-limited in children, but the condition may require treatment in adults. Medical treatment consists of corticosteroids. Splenectomy may be indicated if phagocytosis is severe and the disorder is unresponsive to steroids. If the bleeding is life-threatening, high-dosage IV immunoglobulin and plasmapheresis are indicated. Approximately 40% to 50% of ITP patients are cured within a short time, and the rest go on to have chronic ITP.

Hemolytic-Uremic Syndrome

In hemolytic-uremic syndrome, rapid destruction of RBCs causes acute renal failure, in part because of obstruction of small renal arteries. The associated thrombocytopenia (secondary to thrombi formation) can result in severe hemorrhage. This disorder is mainly seen in infants and children, but it can occur in adults, particularly pregnant women or patients with infectious diseases. Toxin-producing *Escherichia coli* (strain O157:H7) is associated with 75% of HUS cases.

Patients present with abdominal pain and diarrhea, usually following a flu-like prodrome. Manifestations are similar to TTP and include thrombocytopenia, anemia, and renal failure. Hypertension may be seen, but unlike TTP, CNS involvement is not common.

The hallmark finding is RBC fragments on peripheral blood smear in association with the preceding symptoms. Platelet counts are low, and serum LDH is usually markedly elevated.

Conservative management is generally sufficient. FFP and plasmapheresis are sometimes necessary.

HEMATOLOGY

Infection

The host response to infection is usually reflected in hematologic abnormalities. WBC differentials may indicate a specific class of etiology. For example, leukocytosis is common in bacterial infection, whereas eosinophilia is a hallmark of parasitic infection (as well as allergy). Immature WBCs can be found in the setting of excessive leukocytosis, a phenomenon known as a *leukemoid reaction*. Leukocytosis, thrombocytopenia, and DIC can occur in septic shock (see following sections).

Bacteremia and Septicemia

Bacteremia is the term used to describe bacteria in the bloodstream, regardless of whether the patient is symptomatic. **Septicemia** means that bacteria are in the bloodstream of a patient who has signs and symptoms of systemic infection.

SIGNS & SYMPTOMS

Fever, chills, and malaise are typical. Intermittent temperature spiking may occur. Nausea, vomiting, and other GI symptoms may also be present.

DIAGNOSIS

Possible sources of infections, such as surgical sites, wounds, IVs, urine, and drainage tubes, should be cultured. Serial blood cultures should ideally be drawn from two different sites while the patient's temperature is spiking. Chest x-ray and sputum culture are important if respiratory illness is suspected. Intravenous drug users often have *Staphylococcus* bacteremia that is due to introduction of bacteria through the skin.

TREATMENT

Broad-spectrum antibiotics should not be started until after the first blood cultures have been drawn. If no improvement is seen, consider occult abscesses that may serve as a source of infection.

Septic Shock

Septic shock is the circulatory collapse and multiple organ failure that occur as a result of infection. The release of bacterial toxins is thought to elicit the immune response cascade that results in circulatory failure. **High-output septic shock** refers to the early stages of shock, during which blood pressure drops and cardiac output is normal or increased. **Low-output septic shock** refers to the later stages, characterized by decreased cardiac output. Septic shock is seen primarily in immunocompromised people. Approximately 70% of infections are due to nosocomial gram-negative bacilli, and the remaining 30% are due to gram-positive cocci and fungal infections.

SIGNS & SYMPTOMS

The initial stages of septic shock involve fever, chills, and altered mental status. Low blood pressure is accompanied by paradoxically warm, dry skin and extremities. Increased heart and respiratory rates are common. Late-stage shock is characterized by cool, pale extremities, oliguria, adult respiratory distress syndrome, and DIC.

WBC counts, especially neutrophils, may be quite low at the onset of septic shock. Leukocytosis and significant thrombocytopenia or thrombocytosis can develop over a few hours. Increased BUN and creatinine are signs of impending renal failure. Increased lactic acid production can cause metabolic acidosis; this is partially compensated by a respiratory alkalosis as the patient hyperventilates and blows off CO_2.

The preceding symptoms combined with a likely infectious source should raise suspicion for septic shock. Blood cultures may confirm bacteremia, identify an infecting organism, and direct therapy.

Septic shock has a high fatality rate, so intensive care treatment is a must. Respiratory support, including intubation, is provided if necessary. Fluid status must be monitored and IV antibiotics given. Dopamine is often necessary to preserve renal perfusion and support blood pressure.

Malaria

Although uncommon in the United States, malaria is one of the most common infectious diseases worldwide. It is a parasitic disease involving infection of a human by the Anopheles mosquito vector with any of four species of *Plasmodium: P. vivax, P. falciparum, P. ovale,* and *P. malariae.* The cyclical rupture of RBCs as a result of parasite maturation causes the classic symptoms of recurrent fever and chills.

Periodic fever and chills occur at regular 2- to 3-day intervals. Anemia and splenomegaly are common. Severe parasitemia often is associated with hypoglycemia. *P. falciparum* infection can progress to coma (cerebral malaria), to pulmonary edema, and to hemoglobinuria (blackwater fever) with possible renal failure.

Giemsa-stained peripheral blood smears ("thick" and "thin" preparations) identifying the parasite are diagnostic. The specific *Plasmodium* species involved should be determined to direct therapy.

Antimalarials, such as chloroquine. In cases of chloroquine-resistant *P. falciparum,* mefloquine, quinidine, or quinine.

Chloroquine is recommended as chemoprophylaxis for areas not known to have chloroquine-resistant *P. falciparum.* Mefloquine is recommended for areas with chloroquine-resistant strains of *P. falciparum.* Doxycycline is appropriate in Southeast Asia, where mefloquine resistance is developing. Chemoprophylaxis should be taken during exposure and for 4 weeks after.

HEMATOLOGY

Mononucleosis

Infectious mononucleosis is caused by the Epstein-Barr virus (EBV) of the herpes family. EBV infects B lymphocytes and oropharyngeal epithelial cells, so it is transmitted by oropharyngeal contact or, less frequently, by blood transfusion. Infection is often subclinical. Because of its transmission by kissing, most people are exposed by early adulthood.

After an incubation period of 2 to 5 weeks, the patient typically presents with fatigue, pharyngitis, fever, malaise, and lymphadenopathy (typically bilateral). Splenomegaly and hepatitis are common.

Infected B lymphocytes secrete antibodies (heterophile antibodies) that cross-react with sheep and beef erythrocyte antigens. These antibodies are typically present after the first week of illness. EBV-specific serologic tests can be pursued in the absence of heterophile antibodies. Leukocytosis, with many atypical lymphocytes, is present.

Symptoms typically disappear over 2 to 6 weeks without therapy.

Neoplastic Disorders

Acute Lymphocytic Leukemia

Acute lymphocytic leukemia (ALL) is the malignant expansion of the lymphoid line of white cells (B and T cells) [see Figure 10-5 in text]. It comprises 80% of all childhood leukemias, with peak ages of incidence from 3 to 7 years. Eighty percent of ALL is of B-cell origin.

Symptoms are varied and result mainly from bone marrow infiltration. Pale skin and mucosa and fatigue result from anemia. Infections are common as a result of leukopenia. Purpura, petechiae, and bleeding occur as a result of thrombocytopenia. Splenomegaly, hepatomegaly, lymphadenopathy, and bone tenderness may also be present.

Blasts are usually abundant, although they may be absent in some cases. Total WBC count may vary from low to high. Decreased RBC and platelet count occur because the bone marrow has been taken over by lymphocytic cells. Hyperuricemia may be noted.

Bone marrow biopsy reveals many lymphoblasts and few other cells. Hyperdiploidy (>50 chromosomes) in the nuclei of B cells is associated with a good prognosis. The **Philadelphia chromosome,** a translocation of chromosomes 9 and 22 that is found in approximately 15% of adult ALL, is associated with a poorer prognosis.

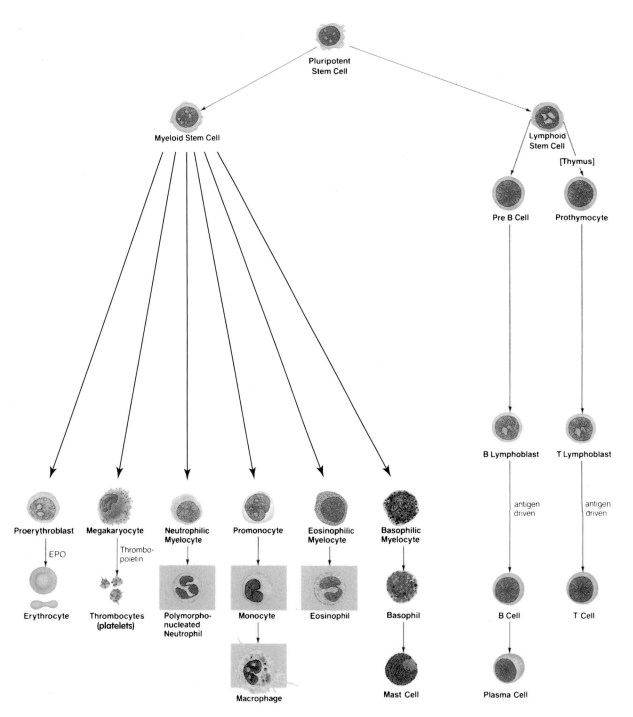

Figure 10-5. Development of lymphoid and myeloid cell lines. EPO, erythropoietin. (Adapted with permission from Turgeon M: *Clinical Hematology: Theory and Procedures,* 2nd ed. Boston, Little, Brown, 1993.)

ALL must be differentiated from a **leukemoid reaction,** in which patients with infections or severe inflammatory diseases have increased numbers of WBCs and blasts.

Chemotherapy alone achieves a cure rate of 60% in children and 40% in adults. Typical choices for induction chemotherapy include vincristine, doxorubicin, prednisone, and 1-asparaginase. Maintenance chemotherapy consists of methotrexate or 6-mercaptopurine. Those who are not cured may be candidates for bone marrow transplant.

Acute Myelocytic Leukemia

Acute myelocytic leukemia (AML) affects the myeloid cells (neutrophils, basophils, eosinophils, erythrocytes, and megakaryocytes) [see Figure 10-5 in text]. In contrast to ALL, AML is more common in adults.

Symptoms are similar to those of ALL and include infections and bleeding. DIC may be seen with AML. Neutropenic patients are at risk for a number of infections with gram-negative bacteria and fungi, such as *Candida* and *Aspergillus.*

An increased number of cells from one cell line may be seen. Examination of the cells may show the presence of **Auer rods,** red-staining intracellular inclusions that are pathognomonic for AML. Bone marrow histochemistry reveals staining with myeloperoxidase or *para*-aminosalicylic acid.

The majority of patients go into remission with chemotherapy (such as cytarabine or daunorubicin), but they tend to relapse within 12 to 18 months. Bone marrow transplant may be beneficial to those who relapse. Long-term (5-year) survival is generally only 10% to 15%.

Chronic Myelocytic Leukemia

Chronic myelocytic leukemia (CML) describes a group of disorders of myeloid cells. Unlike AML, the tumor cells are more mature myeloid forms rather than blasts, and they retain the ability to differentiate. The disease may remain stable for several years before progressing to an acute leukemia. It is usually diagnosed in middle age. Genetically, CML is characterized by the **Philadelphia chromosome,** an acquired translocation of chromosomes 9 and 22.

Fatigue, night sweats, chronic low-grade fevers, and splenomegaly.

Leukocytosis is often an incidental finding, with WBC counts greater than 150,000/μL. Other laboratory abnormalities include increased uric acid and increased serum vitamin B_{12} because the vitamin B_{12} carrier protein is produced by WBCs. Leukocyte alkaline phosphatase may be low or absent. RBCs are normal in appearance and number.

Treatment with chemotherapy (busulfan, hydroxyurea) and alpha-interferon is palliative, not curative. As the disease progresses, patients eventually experience a "blast crisis," which signifies rapid worsening of the disease. Survival is typically approximately 4 years after onset. Bone marrow transplant increases survival time but is rarely curative.

Chronic Lymphocytic Leukemia

Chronic lymphocytic leukemia (CLL) is a neoplastic disorder of mature B cells (T-cell types are rare). Typically, these B cells do not differentiate into plasma cells. Some B cells may create autoantibodies to RBCs and platelets, resulting in hemolytic anemia and thrombocytopenia. CLL strikes men more often than women. Patients are generally older than age 50 years, with 65 years the median age at diagnosis.

Patients with CLL are often asymptomatic or experience nonspecific symptoms such as fatigue and anorexia. Generalized lymphadenopathy, splenomegaly, and hepatomegaly may be noted on physical examination. Because of a relative lack of plasma cells, many patients have hypogammaglobulinemia and experience frequent infections as a result.

WBC count is elevated, with an isolated increase in lymphocytes. Peripheral blood smear shows numerous small, mature-appearing lymphocytes. Small amounts of IgM paraprotein may be detected in the patient's serum.

Treatment is primarily symptomatic, with benefit in some patients from chemotherapy, such as chlorambucil and cyclophosphamide. Prognosis varies, but median survival is 6 years. Unlike CML, there is no "blast crisis" transformation to acute leukemia, signaling a poorer prognosis. Radiation therapy, splenectomy, and leukapheresis are also used in treatment.

Hairy Cell Leukemia

This neoplastic transformation of B cells involves tumor cells with fine, hair-like projections. It is predominantly a disease of middle-aged men.

Symptoms are nonspecific, often including generalized fatigue. Unlike CLL, there is usually no lymphadenopathy, and virtually all patients have splenomegaly. Recurrent infections, especially of mycobacteria, are common.

Laboratory evaluation is notable for pancytopenia, with leukocytosis in only 25% of patients. Peripheral blood smear reveals the "hairy cells." Bone marrow may be inaspirable but may show infiltration. Infiltration of the red pulp of the spleen is also present (as opposed to white pulp infiltration, which is common in lymphomas).

Chemotherapy achieves complete remission in more than 80% of patients. The course of the disease is indolent, with survival of 10 years or more.

Hodgkin's Lymphoma

Hodgkin's lymphoma, a cancer of macrophage origin, has a bimodal distribution, with peak ages of presentation in patients in their 20s or later in their 50s.

HEMATOLOGY

Patients present with painless lymphadenopathy, especially in the neck, and generalized symptoms, such as fever, weight loss, night sweats, and pruritus.

Lymph node biopsy shows Reed-Sternberg cells. These large, multinucleated, reticular cells are pathognomonic of Hodgkin's disease (see Figure 10-6 in color insert).

Radiation therapy and chemotherapy. Currently, patients with Hodgkin's disease have a good prognosis, and cure rates approach 80% even for stage III disease.

Non-Hodgkin's Lymphoma

Non-Hodgkin's lymphoma (NHL), a large group of neoplasms of the lymphocytes, has a wide range of severity and prognoses. In general, however, prognosis is poorer for NHL than for Hodgkin's disease.

As in Hodgkin's disease, patients usually present with localized or generalized painless lymphadenopathy, as well as with nonspecific symptoms of fever, night sweats, and weight loss.

Laboratory evaluation is often normal, although one-third of patients have anemia that is due to bone marrow infiltration. Peripheral blood smear may be normal or reflect the overgrowth of a particular white cell line. At this point, it is often difficult to distinguish NHL from other types of leukemia. Serum LDH is increased if the disease has spread.

Definitive diagnosis is made by lymph node biopsy. The disease is often disseminated by the time of diagnosis, and bone marrow is frequently involved. Bone marrow biopsy shows lymphoid aggregates around the bone trabeculae.

Treatment is primarily palliative, although radiation therapy and chemotherapy are used with variable effectiveness. Survival ranges from months to several years depending on the aggressiveness of the disease.

One form of NHL is **Burkitt's lymphoma,** which affects B cells. It is endemic in parts of Africa, and it is more common in children and young adults. In the United States, symptoms include abdominal pain and fullness because of a predilection of the disease for the abdomen, whereas jaw involvement is common in Africa. Burkitt's lymphoma has been associated with chromosomal translocation (8;14), and the African form is related to EBV.

Multiple Myeloma

Multiple myeloma is a neoplastic proliferation of plasma cells and monoclonal immunoglobulin. The disorder strikes men and women equally, and peak incidence occurs between 50 and 60 years of age. Monoclonal IgG is more commonly produced than IgA. Some plasma cell tumors secrete only monoclonal kappa or lambda light chains, known as *Bence Jones protein.*

Replacement of the bone marrow with plasma cells results in anemia, bone pain, and pathologic fractures. Immunoglobulin deposition contributes to nephrosis. Plasma cell infiltration of the liver, lungs, and nodes also occurs. Because of leukopenia, infections may be frequent, especially with encapsulated organisms such as *S. pneumoniae.*

Diagnosis is made by finding "paraproteins" (abnormal plasma immunoglobulins) in the blood via serum protein electrophoresis (SPEP). X-rays may show osteolytic bone lesions.

Chemotherapy and radiation therapy may be effective, depending on the stage of the disease. Bone marrow transplant has also been used with the potential for cure. Palliative care includes treatment of infections and the hypercalcemia that results from bone degradation. Survival is generally 1 to 3 years from diagnosis.

Waldenström's Macroglobulinemia

Waldenström's macroglobulinemia is characterized by malignant transformation of a single B-lymphocyte cell line, resulting in monoclonal IgM overproduction. Peak incidence is in the sixth decade.

Constitutional symptoms of weakness, fatigue, and weight loss are seen initially. Hyperviscosity may occur, along with bleeding, visual, and neurologic problems. Cellular proliferation in the liver and spleen causes hepatomegaly and splenomegaly.

Decreased hematocrit, usually with normal WBC and platelet counts. Peripheral blood smear reveals RBCs in a *rouleau formation,* in which several RBCs pile on one another, forming a cylinder. Bone marrow biopsy shows increased plasma cells, but no osteolytic lesions are seen on x-ray.

Definitive diagnosis is made by the presence of a monoclonal IgM spike on SPEP.

Plasmapheresis to reduce hyperviscosity and chemotherapy to slow lymphocyte production are commonly used. Survival is approximately 3 to 5 years from diagnosis.

HEMATOLOGY

Mycosis Fungoides

Mycosis fungoides is a neoplastic tumor involving clonal proliferation of CD4 T cells. It usually infiltrates the dermis and epidermis but may involve lymph nodes and viscera.

Skin lesions may initially be confused with eczema, psoriasis, or contact dermatitis. They later thicken and become nodular, with an area of central clearing.

Skin biopsy.

Topical medications and phototherapy may be used for early lesions. Further progression of the disease requires systemic chemotherapy such as methotrexate and cyclophosphamide. Cure is usually possible in early stages, and median survival is usually 8 to 9 years.

Polycythemia Vera

Polycythemia vera is a common, acquired disorder of the bone marrow stem cells that results in overproduction of all three blood cell lines, but predominantly RBCs. RBC counts can exceed $1,000,000/\mu L$ and hematocrit can rise above 60%. Polycythemia vera is seen in both men and women, with peak incidence around age 60 years. The disease can last for decades but may progress to leukemia.

Symptoms are due to increased blood viscosity. Headache, dizziness, blurred vision, and fatigue are common. Some patients may experience generalized pruritus, especially after a hot bath, which is attributed to the increased number of basophils. Splenomegaly and hepatomegaly may be present. Major morbidity and mortality are primarily related to thrombotic events, particularly strokes and deep venous thrombosis.

Hematocrit and RBC count are increased. Bone marrow biopsy shows hypercellular marrow with absent iron stores. Biopsy differentiates polycythemia vera from increased hematocrit as a response to decreased oxygenation (e.g., high altitude) or resulting from dehydration.

Phlebotomy is used to maintain hematocrit below 45%. Allopurinol may be given for hyperuricemia, antihistamines for itching, and aspirin to prevent thrombotic events. Iron should not be given despite low or absent iron stores, as it may exacerbate the overproduction.

Basic Principles of Blood Loss and Replacement

Blood Loss

Blood loss may occur as a result of injury, bleeding disorders, ulcers, complications of pregnancy, complications of surgery, and many other conditions. Hemorrhage can occur externally or internally, as large amounts of blood can collect in the abdomen, pelvis, or pleural space. Fractures of the pelvis and long bones generally result in significant blood loss. Rapid hemorrhage can be fatal in minutes.

SIGNS & SYMPTOMS

Although many hemorrhages are visible and obvious, internal blood loss is not always evident. Signs of hypovolemia include rapid heart rate and low blood pressure, especially orthostatic hypotension. Abdominal bleeding is suggested by bluish discoloration in the flank or abdomen and by peritoneal signs, such as guarding and rebound tenderness. Hemothorax causes difficulty breathing, dullness to percussion, and decreased breath sounds. Retroperitoneal bleeds may be virtually asymptomatic.

DIAGNOSIS

Presentation and vital signs are usually diagnostic of blood loss. Heart rate typically increases before blood pressure drops. Hemoglobin and hematocrit are not good indicators of acute blood loss because these measures remain normal for several hours before equilibration occurs. CT scan is useful for the diagnosis of intra-abdominal and retroperitoneal bleeding, and diagnostic peritoneal lavage is also used to assess intra-abdominal bleeds.

TREATMENT

If the source of blood loss can be identified, it should be addressed immediately. For stabilization, patients are given crystalloid infusion through a large-bore IV needle while blood is sent for chemistries, clotting parameters, counts, and crossmatch. O-negative blood may be given in an emergency if the patient's blood type is unknown. Transfusions are required for a patient in clinical shock or for patients whose vital signs do not stabilize after crystalloid infusion. The final stabilized hematocrit should be at least 20% in otherwise healthy patients.

Red Blood Cell Transfusions

Transfusions are generally given to raise hematocrit or blood volume in patients with inadequate blood volume or severe anemia. There are four major replacement products used:

- **Fresh whole blood** has RBCs, plasma, and platelets. It is used in cases of massive hemorrhage when clotting factors and platelets are needed in addition to RBCs.
- **Packed RBCs** will raise the hematocrit approximately 3% per unit given. If need is anticipated—for example, before surgery—the patient may opt to store his or her own blood for autologous transfusion.
- **Leuko-poor blood** is the name given to packed RBCs from which leukocytes have been removed. It is given if patients have histories of severe leukoagglutinin reactions (described later in this chapter).
- **Frozen blood** can be stored for 3 years. The process is very expensive, so its use is lim-

HEMATOLOGY

ited to transfusion of individuals with rare blood types. Frozen blood has no WBCs or plasma.

Blood for transfusions is currently screened by antigen or antibody testing for a number of viruses, including hepatitis B, hepatitis C, and HIV. The risk of getting blood contaminated with HIV in the United States is now 1 in 400,000 units. There is a higher risk of getting the hepatitis C virus, which currently infects about 0.01% of blood supplies.

Compatibility testing of the donor blood is crucial. If the incorrect blood is given, patients can experience severe intravascular hemolysis and death. The most important factor to match is the ABO blood type (Table 10-2). The Rh type should then be considered. Care should be taken with female patients who may later bear children to ensure that they do not receive Rh-positive blood if they are Rh-negative. However, in an emergency, type-specific Rh-positive blood is not life-threatening. If possible, the patient should have an antibody screen and crossmatch performed to assure that cross-reactions will be minimized. In an emergency, when type is not known, give type O-negative packed cells.

The threshold hematocrit at which patients should receive blood transfusions is controversial and varies from institution to institution. Typically, however, patients' hematocrits should be kept above 20, with levels above 25 in patients with cardiac problems.

Transfusion Reactions

Transfusion reactions are usually due to clerical errors, so it is vital that all identification labels are checked and confirmed. Immediate reactions to incorrect blood transfusion occur within the first 2 hours, and symptoms include fever, chills, back pain, chest pain, headache, pulmonary edema, urticaria, and hematuria. If a reaction is suspected, the transfusion must be discontinued immediately, and antihistamines and epinephrine should be administered. Delayed reactions can also occur over days to weeks after the transfusion and include hemolysis, thrombocytopenia, rash, fever, and GI symptoms.

Leukoagglutinin Reactions

Leukoagglutinin reactions occur when the patient reacts to antigens on the donor WBCs or platelets. These reactions are usually seen in patients who have had previous transfusions that sensitized them to these antigens. Presentation includes fever and chills, shortness of breath, and pulmonary edema, which can become life-threatening. Treatment includes antihistamines, acetaminophen, and steroids. The patient may require leuko-poor blood for future transfusions.

Table 10-2. ABO blood type frequencies

Blood type	Percentage of the white population	Antibodies present
O	45	Anti-A, anti-B
A	42	Anti-B
B	10	Anti-A
AB	3	—

Platelet Transfusions

Platelet transfusions are given to patients with thrombocytopenia, as platelet levels below 20,000/μL can result in spontaneous bleeding. One unit of platelets elevates platelet count by approximately 10,000/μL. Platelet transfusions are not useful if the thrombocytopenia is caused by autoimmune destruction because the transfused platelets will quickly be destroyed as well. Transfused platelets may also have poor survival if human leukocyte antigen (HLA) types are very dissimilar. Platelet concentrate is also available; it contains 6 units of platelets and will raise the platelet level approximately 60,000/μL.

Coagulation Factor Transfusions

Fresh frozen plasma is given to patients with coagulation factor deficiencies. It is also given to patients with TTP and DIC. FFP contains normal levels of the coagulation factors found in blood.

Cryoprecipitate contains fibrinogen, factor VIII, and vWF. It is given to patients with factor VIII deficiency, von Willebrand's disease, fibrinogen deficiency, and DIC.

HEMATOLOGY

11

Dermatology

Skin Disorders Secondary to Sun Exposure

Sunburn is an acute reaction to sun overexposure. It may range in severity from mild erythema to severe pain, swelling, and blisters, with constitutional symptoms of fever and even shock.

Effects of chronic sun exposure include wrinkling and precancerous lesions known as *actinic keratoses* (described later in this chapter). The incidence of squamous and basal cell carcinoma increases in proportion to the amount of previous sun exposure. Melanoma incidence may also increase with sun exposure. Darker-skinned individuals have more melanin, which protects against all types of sun damage, including cancer.

Prevention of these effects through the use of sunscreen is simple and effective. Sunscreens containing para-aminobenzoic acid (PABA) or opaque creams with zinc oxide protect the skin well. Sunscreens are rated on the U.S. Food and Drug Administration's sun protection factor scale, with a rating of 15 considered adequate protection.

Drug Reactions

Any medication can cause an allergic reaction with cutaneous manifestations. Antibiotics, nonsteroidal anti-inflammatory drugs, and anticonvulsants are common offenders, but all medications, including nonprescription medicines, must be considered in a careful history. Skin eruptions can vary in severity from a mild maculopapular rash to the potentially lethal **toxic epidermal necrolysis,** in which large areas of epidermis become loosened and detached. The edematous wheals of urticaria ("hives") are common, especially with penicillin allergies.

Dermatitis

Contact Dermatitis

There are two types of contact dermatitis. **Primary irritant contact dermatitis** is caused by direct injury to the skin, affects all individuals who contact the irritant, and occurs at the first exposure to the irritant. **Allergic contact dermatitis** (ACD) is a type IV delayed hypersensitivity reaction. It never occurs at first exposure because susceptible individuals must first be sensitized to the agent. Common substances causing ACD are poison oak, poison ivy, ragweed, nickel, latex, and topical medications, such as neomycin.

Occupational dermatitis is most often an irritant contact dermatitis, resulting from detergents, solvents, and other caustic chemicals. Occupational dermatitis can also be of the allergic type. This is seen commonly in agricultural and forestry operations.

Effects range from redness to severe swelling and blistering. Itching is common. Distribution of the reaction depends on the area of contact; the extremities and face are commonly affected (see Figure 11-1 in color insert).

If the history is not diagnostic, patch testing may be useful.

DERMATOLOGY

Compresses are useful if the lesion is weeping. An antihistamine for itching and topical—or, in severe cases of ACD, systemic—corticosteroids may be used. Remove or avoid the offending substance.

Seborrheic Dermatitis

Seborrheic dermatitis is a chronic, inflammatory hyperproliferation of the epidermis. It occurs in teens and adults and is generally worse in winter and in times of stress. Mild scalp involvement is called dandruff or, in infants, "cradle cap." Eyelid involvement is called **seborrheic blepharitis.**

Involved skin is erythematous. Greasy yellow scales are typically noted on the scalp, forehead, nasolabial folds, ears, umbilicus, and body folds (see Figure 11-2, A & B, in color insert).

Selenium, tar, or ketoconazole shampoo reduces the severity of the symptoms. A mild corticosteroid cream may be used on the face intermittently, but chronic, regular use should be avoided. Baby shampoo is usually sufficient to treat cradle cap. Recurrence is likely.

Psoriasis

Psoriasis, a condition of increased proliferation of epidermal tissue, can be acute or chronic and is often familial. **Psoriatic arthritis** is a condition found in 20% of patients with psoriasis. It is associated with HLA-B27 and a family history of psoriasis. Its symptoms are similar to those of rheumatoid arthritis, but patients are rheumatoid factor negative.

Sharply demarcated, salmon-colored papules or plaques covered by silvery scales are typical. Most common locations are the scalp, knees and elbows, intergluteal cleft, and back. Pinpoint bleeding results if scales are removed. Nails are frequently pitted or thickened (see Figure 11-3 in color insert).

Topical corticosteroids, topical tar, and topical retinoids may be used to decrease epidermal proliferation. Ultraviolet light is effective and indicated in diffuse disease. Methotrexate and azathioprine may be used to control symptoms of psoriatic arthritis.

Atopic Dermatitis

Atopic dermatitis (eczema) is a common, chronic, and recurrent skin condition characterized by pruritus and a range of skin manifestations. It is more common in patients with asthma or allergic rhinitis or with a family history of them. Together, atopic dermatitis, asthma, and allergic rhinitis form the atopic triad. While the adult form of atopic der-

DERMATOLOGY

matitis is often relapsing and remitting, the infantile form often disappears or significantly improves after the age of 3 to 4 years.

SIGNS & SYMPTOMS

In adolescents and adults, lesions are pruritic and show marked dryness, thickening, and excoriation. They typically occur on the antecubital and popliteal folds (flexor surfaces), on the dorsal surfaces of hands and feet, and on the face, neck, and upper truck (see Figure 11-4 in color insert). In infants, lesions tend to show blistering, oozing, crusting, and excoriation and are often found on the face, scalp, and extremities.

DIAGNOSIS

Clinical presentation is diagnostic. Blinded food challenges and skin tests may identify causes of allergy.

TREATMENT

Drying soaps, lanolin preparations, and wool should be avoided, and emollients should be used regularly. Topical corticosteroids and tar preparations are useful, but systemic corticosteroid therapy may be indicated in severe or extensive cases. Antihistamines will relieve severe pruritus.

Acne Vulgaris

Acne vulgaris, or simple acne, is an inflammation of hair follicles and sebaceous glands. Although pathogenesis is unclear, it is thought that the bacterium *Propionibacterium acnes* causes the degradation of lipids into irritating fatty acids, resulting in inflammation. A contributing factor in the development of acne is the presence of sex hormones, especially androgens. Males are more often affected than females, and adolescents are frequently affected because of the presence of increased sex hormone production. The role of diet and genetic influences is controversial.

SIGNS & SYMPTOMS

Erythematous pustules and cysts are found predominantly on the face and trunk. Chronic inflammation may lead to scarring.

DIAGNOSIS

Clinical inspection of the lesions.

TREATMENT

Topical drying agents, such as benzoyl peroxide, allow drainage of the sebum from the follicles, preventing obstruction and subsequent pustule development. Topical or oral antibiotics (e.g., tetracycline) are thought to be effective as a result of inhibition of *P. acnes* growth. Vitamin A analogs, topical retinoic acid, and oral isotretinoin (Accutane) decrease sebaceous gland size and sebum production. However, isotretinoin therapy causes birth defects and must be used with extreme care in women of childbearing age.

DERMATOLOGY

Decubitus Ulcer

Decubitus ulcers, also called *pressure sores,* result from ischemic damage when tissues are exposed to continuous pressure. They are most commonly seen in patients who do not sense pain and pressure or cannot move to alleviate this pressure (e.g., paralyzed, bedridden, or comatose patients). They may also occur under casts and on the legs of diabetic patients with poor circulation and sensation. Sores are most frequent over bony prominences, including the sacrum, trochanter, ankles, and heels.

The first sign of pressure sores is redness of the skin. The ulcer that then develops may ultimately extend through fat and muscle to bone.

Relieve pressure and keep wounds clean and dry. Severe sores may require surgical debridement and closure. Deep infections are treated with systemic antibiotics.

Change patient's position at least every hour. Keep skin clean and dry. Water beds, "egg-crate" mattresses, and protective padding at susceptible sites may help. Avoid oversedation and encourage activity. Diabetic patients should be taught how to examine and care for their feet.

Infections

Herpes Simplex

Herpes simplex virus (HSV) HSV-1 and HSV-2 generally cause oral and genital herpes lesions, respectively, although there is considerable overlap and any inoculated site can develop infection. Transmission usually occurs via oral or genital secretions from active and, occasionally, inactive cases. The virus infects its new host, and the viral DNA remains in the neurons of the sensory ganglia, becoming periodically reactivated by sunlight, illness, or stress and causing recrudescent lesions in the distribution of that sensory nerve. (See Chapter 6 for a discussion of genital herpes.)

The most common site of oral herpes lesions is the lower lip. Recurrences are often preceded by a prodrome of local itching or burning. Small, painful vesicles on an erythematous base are characteristic. After a few days, the vesicles crust over and heal (see Figure 11-5 in color insert). Ocular involvement most often presents as keratitis.

Microscopic examination of the vesicular fluid using a Tzanck preparation reveals multinucleated giant cells. Viral culture of the fluid is diagnostic, as is polymerase chain reaction (PCR). In ocular HSV, dendritic corneal ulcers that stain with fluorescein are characteristic.

DERMATOLOGY

Acyclovir shortens the duration and severity of the recurrence and may be taken prophylactically in an attempt to prevent recurrence.

Chickenpox

Chickenpox is a highly contagious, acute viral illness caused by the varicella-zoster virus. The virus is spread by infectious respiratory droplets and direct contact with skin lesions. Symptoms develop in 2 to 3 weeks, but communicability begins only 10 days after exposure and continues until skin lesions have crusted over. Epidemics tend to occur in winter.

A prodrome, which becomes more severe with age, includes headache, malaise, and fever and is usually present for 24 to 36 hours before pruritic skin lesions appear. The typical skin lesion progresses from macule to papule to vesicle ("dew drops on a rose petal") before it crusts over. New lesions, which appear in crops as old lesions are crusting over, may continue to appear for 5 to 6 days. Skin lesions may become secondarily infected. Pneumonia is a complication seen more frequently in adults and immunocompromised patients.

Clinical inspection of the lesions is generally all that is necessary. Tzanck preparation shows multinucleated giant cells on microscopic examination.

In mild cases, symptomatic treatment to control itching is helpful to prevent later scarring. In severe cases or in immunocompromised patients, IV acyclovir may be given. Acetaminophen is preferred over aspirin due to the risk of Reye's syndrome.

For exposed newborns and immunocompromised patients, intramuscular varicella-zoster immunoglobulin given within 4 days of exposure may prevent or lessen the severity of disease.

Varicella vaccination is now recommended for all children at 12 to 18 months. Unvaccinated older children with no history of chickenpox should be vaccinated at age 12. Other susceptible persons older than age 12 should receive two doses of vaccine given 1 month apart.

Herpes Zoster

Also known as *shingles,* herpes zoster is caused by the varicella-zoster virus, which can remain dormant in the sensory nerve root ganglia for years after the patient has chickenpox. Reactivation of the virus characteristically affects only one dermatome. Unlike herpes simplex infections, recurrence is rare. Zoster occurs frequently in the elderly and immunocompromised.

After a 3-day prodrome of fever and malaise, pain followed by crops of vesicles on an erythematous base appear along one dermatome (see Figure 11-6 in color insert). Vesicles begin to scab over after 4 to 5 days, but the lesions and pain remain for approximately 2 to 6 weeks. The most common site of eruption is the thorax; however, herpes zoster ophthalmicus, which results from involvement of the ophthalmic branch of the trigeminal nerve, can have the most serious consequences. Vesicles on the tip of the nose may portend involvement of the cornea and risk to vision. Elderly patients are particularly susceptible to **postherpetic neuralgia,** which is pain at the site that may last for months or years.

Vesicles in a characteristic dermatomal distribution are usually diagnostic. Viral culture of the lesion may be obtained; Tzanck preparation shows multinucleated giant cells for rapid diagnosis. Newer laboratory techniques, such as ELISA and PCR, are also becoming available.

Pain medication. Corticosteroids may reduce subsequent postherpetic neuralgia. Acyclovir is used in immunocompromised patients and in involvement of the ophthalmic division of the fifth cranial nerve (V_1).

Cellulitis

Cellulitis is an acute, spreading infection of the skin and subcutaneous tissues most often caused by streptococci, although *Staphylococcus aureus* and gram-negative rods are also common culprits. Polymicrobial infections are seen in IV drug abusers and after animal bites.

Typically, infection begins on the lower extremities at the site of a break in the skin, although this break may not be evident. The area is erythematous, hot, tender, and edematous. Regional lymphadenopathy may be present. Systemic symptoms, such as fever and chills, tachycardia, and hypotension, may precede cutaneous findings by a few hours.

Leukocytosis.

Diagnosis is based on clinical findings because culturing the organism is often difficult.

Penicillinase-resistant penicillins (e.g., nafcillin, dicloxacillin) can be used in uncomplicated cases.

Necrotizing Fasciitis

Severe necrotizing fasciitis is caused by group A β-hemolytic streptococcus. It is initially difficult to distinguish from cellulitis on a clinical basis. One diagnostic clue is the presence of anesthesia on the involved skin that is due to destruction of nerves in the fascial planes.

As the disease progresses, the skin may turn purple, crepitus may be appreciated, and bullae and dermal gangrene develop. Systemic toxicity can be severe. Necrotizing fasciitis requires broad-spectrum antibiotics and extensive wound debridement. Mortality is 30%.

Carbuncle

A carbuncle is an abscess of the skin and subcutaneous tissue that is created when several follicular infections (called *furuncles* or *boils*) coalesce. Carbuncles are most common on the back or nape of the neck. Multiple drainage sites may develop and the patient may be febrile. *S. aureus* is frequently the cause, although gram-negative bacteria may be involved. Treatment is with drainage, culture, and antibiotics. Usually, a penicillinase-resistant penicillin or cephalosporin is used.

Abscess

An abscess is a collection of pus, usually from a bacterial infection. Cutaneous abscesses result from implantation of bacteria through breaks in the skin. The most common causative organisms are *S. aureus* and *S. epidermidis.* Perineal abscesses are frequently caused by anaerobic bacteria (e.g., *Peptococcus, Bacteroides*). Examination reveals fluctuant soft-tissue swelling surrounded by erythema. Treatment involves incision and drainage, followed by gauze packing. Antibiotics are only necessary if the patient has signs of systemic infection or is immunocompromised or if the abscess is in an area of the face drained by the cavernous sinus. If not properly treated, orbital or central facial abscesses can lead to **cavernous sinus thrombosis** (see Chapter 13).

Gangrene

Gangrene is tissue necrosis resulting from lack of circulation. The skin is blackened and wrinkled in "dry" gangrene. When bacterial superinfection occurs, "wet" gangrene results, and the tissue oozes fluid.

Gas gangrene results from a wound contaminated with gas-producing anaerobes, usually of the *Clostridium* species. Infection develops hours to days after a severe crushing or penetrating injury. The patient has severe pain, fever, and shock. Crepitus (a crackling sound or sensation) is noted in the subcutaneous tissues, and the wound may have a foul-smelling discharge. X-ray will show gas in the fascial planes. Treatment requires immediate wound debridement and antibiotics.

Dermatophytoses

Dermatophytes are fungi that cause dermatophytoses, also known as *tinea* or *ringworm.* These fungi invade dead tissue, including the epidermis, nails, and hair. Common causative organisms include *Microsporum, Trichophyton,* and *Epidermophyton.* Certain types of fungal infections are more common in warm weather and in warm, moist areas of the body, such as between toes and in skin folds. Scalp infections are contagious and primarily affect children.

Tinea corporis (ringworm of the body) and **tinea cruris** ("jock itch") have characteristic round lesions with raised borders that expand peripherally and clear centrally (see Figure 11-7 in color insert). **Tinea pedis** ("athlete's foot") occurs between the toes and on the sole of the foot. The skin may be scaly or macerated (soft and pulpy). **Tinea unguium** (onychomycosis) involves infection of toenails or, rarely, fingernails, which become thickened and discolored. **Tinea capitis** (ringworm of the scalp) causes patchy hair loss, with or without scalp inflammation.

Clinical presentation is often sufficient. KOH preparation showing hyphae and fungal culture are diagnostic.

Topical antifungals (miconazole, clotrimazole) or oral antifungals (griseofulvin) may be used.

Pilonidal Cyst

In pilonidal cysts, a congenital tract exists in the skin of the sacrococcygeal area. This tract is lined with hair and forms a cavity. Infection of the cavity results in a tender, erythematous pilonidal cyst. Treatment is by incision and drainage, followed by excision of the tract.

Viral Warts

There are 35 different types of human papillomavirus (HPV), all of which can cause epithelial tumors, or viral warts. Some HPV types are associated with malignancies, such as cervical cancer. Warts are contagious and frequently occur at a site of local irritation or trauma. Common warts (**verrucae vulgaris**) are sharply demarcated, rough tumors as large as 1 cm in diameter (see Figure 11-8 in color insert). Color may vary. Plantar warts are common warts on the sole of the foot. They are flat, surrounded by cornified epithelium, and frequently tender. Warts occasionally disappear spontaneously, but chemical or cryotherapy may be used to destroy them. Moist warts, condyloma acuminata, are discussed in Chapter 6 (Gynecology).

Neoplasms

Actinic Keratosis

Actinic keratosis is a precancerous lesion that develops on sun-exposed skin and may lead to squamous cell carcinoma. Atypical keratinocytes grow to form a firm, well-marginated, reddish papule with rough, yellow-brown scales (see Figure 11-9 in color insert). Diagnosis is made by biopsy. Cryotherapy and topical 5-fluorouracil are used to destroy the lesion.

DERMATOLOGY

Squamous Cell Carcinoma

A squamous cell carcinoma may arise from normal tissue or from a pre-existing actinic keratosis. It occurs on sun-exposed areas of the body and is more common in outdoor workers and frequent sunbathers. Light-skinned individuals are more susceptible.

SIGNS & SYMPTOMS

The tumor is initially a red papule with a crusted surface but later can become nodular, ulcerate, and invade the underlying tissue (see Figure 11-10 in color insert). Metastasis occurs infrequently.

DIAGNOSIS

Biopsy.

TREATMENT

Excision.

Basal Cell Carcinoma

Basal cell carcinoma is the most common cancer found in humans. Similar to squamous cell carcinoma, it is found in light-skinned patients on sun-exposed areas.

SIGNS & SYMPTOMS

The typical lesion is a pearly papule with dilated blood vessels (telangiectasia) and a central depression or ulceration (see Figure 11-11 in color insert). Lesions grow but rarely metastasize.

DIAGNOSIS

Biopsy.

TREATMENT

Treatment is usually with excision, but radiation, electrocautery, or cryotherapy may also be used. Excision permits assessment of margins, which, if positive, necessitate further excision.

Nevi

Pigmented nevi (benign moles) vary widely in size, color, and texture, but they are generally uniform in appearance. Most appear on sun-exposed areas in childhood or adolescence. Half of malignant melanomas arise from melanocytes in moles, so a biopsy should

DERMATOLOGY

be performed on any mole that enlarges suddenly, changes color, ulcerates, bleeds, or begins to itch or hurt.

Dysplastic nevi are generally larger (5 to 12 mm in diameter) and more irregular than simple moles. They occur more frequently on unexposed areas of the body and continue to appear into adulthood. The syndrome of **multiple dysplastic nevi** runs in families and is associated with a high risk of melanoma. Dysplastic nevi should be carefully monitored, and the threshold for biopsy should be low. People with dysplastic nevi should avoid sun exposure, as they are at risk for melanoma.

Melanoma

Melanoma is a malignant tumor of melanocytes that may occur in the skin, mucous membranes, eye, or central nervous system. Although four types have been described, the superficial spreading type accounts for 70% of cases. Lesions may arise from pre-existing nevi or from normal skin in sun-exposed areas. The prognosis is much worse than for other skin cancers and is correlated with the amount of vertical extension of the tumor. Metastasis occurs to the skin or internal organs with increasing frequency as the lesion invades deeper than 0.76 mm.

SIGNS & SYMPTOMS

The patient may report that a mole has increased in size. The lesion has irregular borders and color. Initially brown or black, later stages may show spots of red, white, or blue. Plaques and nodules may itch, ulcerate, and bleed (see Figure 11-12 in color insert).

DIAGNOSIS

Biopsy, preferably excisional.

TREATMENT

Wide excision is the treatment for local disease. Chemotherapy is added if metastasis has occurred.

Hemangioma

Hemangiomas are benign tumors of hyperplastic blood vessels and are present in one-third of newborns. They are either congenital or occur shortly after birth. There are three types of hemangiomas. A **nevus flammeus** (port wine stain—think Mikhail Gorbachev) is a flat purple lesion that usually does not fade with time. Laser treatment is used with some success. **Capillary hemangiomas** (strawberry marks) are raised, bright red lesions that usually regress spontaneously by age 5 years. Treatment with prednisone is indicated only when the lesion is obstructing the eye, urethra, or anus. **Cavernous hemangiomas** are raised red or purple lesions created by enlarged vascular spaces. Prednisone or surgical excision is a treatment option, but lesions usually regress by age 4 years.

DERMATOLOGY

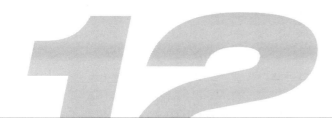

Musculoskeletal and Connective Tissue Disorders

Degenerative Disorders

Degenerative Joint Disease

Degenerative joint disease, or osteoarthritis (OA), affects all of us lucky enough to reach age 70 years. Joint cartilage wears away with age and exposes subchondral bone, which then proliferates to form bone spurs, or osteophytes. There is no associated inflammation.

SIGNS & SYMPTOMS

OA manifests with the gradual onset of pain in the affected joints made worse with activity and relieved by rest. Morning stiffness is common and is usually transient. Distal and proximal interphalangeal joints are commonly affected, as are hips, knees, and joints of the cervical and lumbar spine. Deformities of the distal interphalangeal (DIP) joints (**Heberden nodes**) and proximal interphalangeal (PIP) joints (**Bouchard nodes**) are caused by bony protuberances at the joint. Degenerative joint disease can also arise at any joint following joint injury.

DIAGNOSIS

X-rays show osteophytes, irregular narrowing of the joint space, and increased radiologic density of subchondral bone (Figure 12-1).

TREATMENT

Joint rest, local heat, and analgesics. Weight reduction may be helpful. In severe cases, joint replacement may be indicated.

Degenerative Disk Disease

The intervertebral disk consists of the nucleus pulposus surrounded by the anulus fibrosus (Figure 12-2). Degenerative changes allow the nucleus to herniate posteriorly or postero-

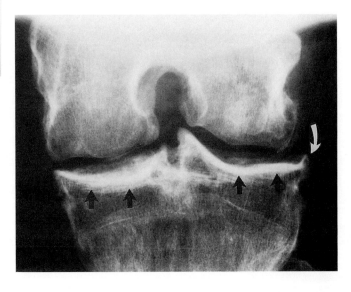

Fig. 12-1. Osteoarthritis of the knee. There is subchondral sclerosis (*straight arrow*) and a large marginal osteophyte (*curved arrow*) laterally. (Reprinted with permission from Daffner R: *Clinical Radiology: The Essentials,* 2nd ed. Baltimore, Williams & Wilkins, 1999, p 473.)

MUSCULOSKELETAL

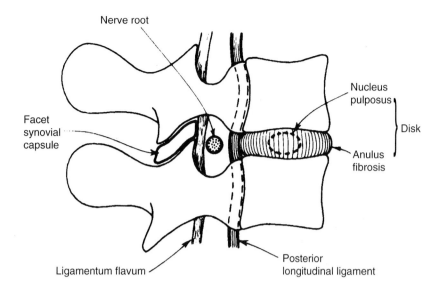

Fig. 12-2. Intervertebral disk and surrounding structures. (Reprinted with permission from Samuels M: *Manual of Neurologic Therapeutics,* 5th ed. Boston, Little, Brown, 1995.)

laterally through the anulus fibrosus and impinge on the spinal cord or roots. This occurs most commonly in the lumbosacral region, but it may occur in the cervical region as well. Thoracic herniations are rare.

Pain is felt both locally and along the distribution of the affected nerve root. In lumbosacral herniations the L4–5 or L5-S1 disks are most often involved, and sciatica (pain down the leg in the L5–S1 distribution) is characteristic (Figure 12-3). Pain is aggravated by movement and by the Valsalva maneuver, in which increased pressure of the subarachnoid space is transmitted to the herniated disk during coughing or straining. Passive straight leg lifts elicit pain that extends below the knee in lumbosacral herniations. There may be muscle weakness and depressed reflexes at the affected nerve level (Table 12-1). The **cauda equina syndrome** is caused by a large midline posterior herniation that compresses the cauda equina. Urinary and bowel incontinence and bilateral leg weakness are classic symptoms.

In L5 radiculopathy, dorsiflexion of the foot and toes is weak. In S1 radiculopathy, plantar flexion is weak and the ankle jerk reflex is reduced. CT or MRI is useful in demonstrating the disk protrusion and ruling out spinal tumors (primary or metastatic) in the cauda equina syndrome. Electromyography (EMG) will help assess nerve damage.

Conservative approaches include bed rest, local heat, NSAIDs, and physical therapy. Symptoms frequently resolve in 4 to 6 weeks. Surgery may be necessary for unrelenting pain, progressive neurologic impairment, or the cauda equina syndrome.

Spinal Stenosis

Spinal stenosis, or narrowing of the spinal canal, occurs most commonly as a result of osteoarthritis of the cervical or lumbar spine. Patients with congenitally narrow spinal canals may be predisposed to stenosis. Patients are usually middle-aged and may have no other evidence of osteoarthritis.

MUSCULOSKELETAL

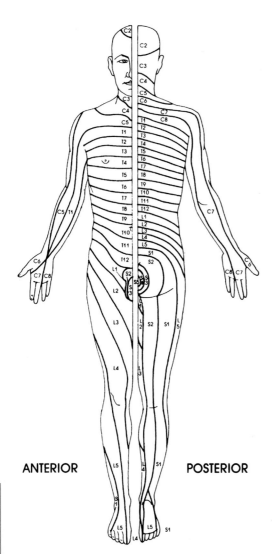

ANTERIOR   **POSTERIOR**

Fig. 12-3. Sensory dermatomes. (Reprinted with permission from Guberman A: *An Introduction to Clinical Neurology.* Boston, Little, Brown, 1994.)

SIGNS & SYMPTOMS

Patients present with pain and weakness in the distribution served by the compressed cord or root, which is often elicited by walking (pseudoclaudication). Unlike true claudication, pain also occurs with standing and extension of the spine. Symptoms improve with rest and flexion of the stenotic area.

DIAGNOSIS

CT or MRI. EMG may help to localize the lesion.

TREATMENT

Conservative treatment includes anti-inflammatory medications, corsets, and abdominal muscle strengthening to decrease stress on the lumbar spine. Surgical decompression is necessary in more severe cases.

Table 12-1. Signs and symptoms of nerve root compression

Nerve root	Location of pain	Muscle weakness	Diminished reflex	Sensory deficit
C5	Shoulder, outer aspect of upper arm	Deltoid	Biceps	Shoulder
C6	Shoulder, scapula, inner aspect of upper arm	Biceps, wrist extension	Brachioradialis	Lateral forearm
C7	Shoulder, scapula, back of upper arm, forearm	Triceps, wrist flexor	Triceps	Middle finger (inconsistent)
C8	Scapula, back of entire arm, medial forearm	Finger flexion	—	Medial forearm, ring and little finger
L4	Hip, front of thigh, knee	Quadriceps, foot inversion	Knee jerk	Medial leg and foot
L5	Outer thigh and leg, dorsal foot	Extension of great toe (patient cannot heel-walk), dorsiflexion of foot	—	Lateral leg and dorsum of foot
S1	Back of thigh and leg, heel	Plantar flexion and eversion of foot, gastrocnemius, gluteus maximus	Ankle jerk	Lateral and plantar surface of foot

Metabolic and Nutritional Disorders

Osteoporosis

Osteoporosis is a progressive decrease in the mass of otherwise normal bone. This condition is most common in postmenopausal white and Asian women. Smoking, excessive alcohol intake, sedentary lifestyle, and low estrogen or androgen levels all predispose to disease. Secondary causes of osteoporosis include long-term corticosteroid therapy, Cushing syndrome, hyperparathyroidism, and hyperthyroidism. It is estimated that hundreds of thousands of fractures in the United States each year are due to osteoporosis.

SIGNS & SYMPTOMS

The disease is usually asymptomatic until a fracture occurs. Hip (neck of the femur) and wrist [distal radius (Colles)] fractures are common. Vertebral compression fractures cause back pain, loss of height, and kyphosis.

DIAGNOSIS

Quantitative CT, densitometry, and dual energy x-ray absorptiometry studies show decreased bone density, particularly in the spine and pelvis. Serum calcium, phosphorus, and parathyroid hormone (PTH) are normal.

Sufficient dietary calcium and vitamin D, weightbearing exercise, and estrogen (or testosterone) all help slow bone loss. Bisphosphonates (etidronate, alendronate) inhibit osteoclast activity, increase bone density, and decrease risk of fracture. Calcitonin and estrogen analogues (raloxifene) are also useful.

Bone density is built up until roughly age 35 years. Thereafter, bone is lost with age. Prevention of osteoporosis involves maximizing total bone density and slowing bone loss. These goals are achieved with high dietary calcium, weightbearing exercise, and, if necessary, exogenous estrogen.

Gout

Gout is a peripheral arthritis that results from the deposition of sodium urate crystals in the joints. Primary gout is usually idiopathic, although patients with renal disease are predisposed because of decreased urate clearance. The majority of patients are middle-aged men, and there is often a familial component.

The typical presentation is the sudden nocturnal onset of excruciating pain and swelling in a single joint, most commonly the metatarsophalangeal joint of the big toe (**podagra**), but also other foot joints, the ankle, or the knee. The joint is exquisitely tender, and the overlying skin is tense and dark red or purple. The patient may also have fever, chills, or malaise. Initial attacks resolve spontaneously, but later attacks may last for weeks and involve multiple joints. Half of patients with untreated gout will develop chronic tophaceous gout, in which urate crystals are deposited in the joints, ear cartilage, or other tissues, and can be appreciated as nodular tophi. Permanent deformity results.

The diagnosis is suspected in a patient with the typical presentation and a high serum uric acid level, although uric acid level may be normal at times during an attack. If necessary, the diagnosis is confirmed by analyzing the synovial fluid and finding negatively birefringent needle-shaped crystals within leukocytes. X-rays show tophi as "punched out" radiolucent areas.

NSAIDs (such as indomethacin), colchicine, or steroids are used to treat and terminate an acute attack. Preventive measures include limiting alcohol and foods high in purines (e.g., liver, sardines, anchovies), avoiding thiazide and loop diuretics, and adequate hydration. Chronic low dose colchicine is often employed prophylactically.

Xanthine oxidase inhibitors, such as allopurinol, inhibit the formation of uric acid and are used in conditions of high nucleic acid turnover, such as leukemia or psoriasis. Uricosuric drugs, such as probenecid, inhibit uric acid resorption by the kidney and may be used for chronic gout. These drugs and low-dose aspirin are not recommended during an acute attack because they may transiently raise serum uric acid concentration.

Pseudogout

Pseudogout, a calcium pyrophosphate dihydrate deposition disease (CPPD), is a condition caused by inflammation due to calcium pyrophosphate dihydrate crystals in the synovial fluid. It is often familial and frequently associated with endocrine diseases, such as

MUSCULOSKELETAL

diabetes mellitus (DM) and hyperparathyroidism. Although the overall presentation is similar to that of gout, the knee and wrist are most commonly affected, and positively birefringent rhomboid crystals of calcium pyrophosphate are found in the synovial fluid. (Remember, *p*seudogout has *positively* birefringent crystals.) NSAIDs are useful for acute attacks, and colchicine can be used for prevention.

Rickets and Osteomalacia

Rickets is a disease of bone mineralization in children that results most often from vitamin D deficiency but can also occur with calcium or phosphorous deficiency. In vitamin D deficiency, lack of exposure to sunlight and poor dietary intake are necessary for clinical disease to develop in otherwise normal patients. Defects in vitamin D metabolism may also predispose to disease. Clinical disease results when the epiphyseal cartilage of growing bones becomes hypertrophic without calcification. Decreased bone mineralization in adults causes **osteomalacia.** Osteomalacia differs clinically from rickets because of the different effects of defective mineralization on growing bone compared to the mature skeleton.

In young children with rickets, walking is delayed, and bowlegs and kyphoscoliosis may occur. In older children and teenagers, walking causes pain, and bowlegs may develop in extreme cases. In osteomalacia, adults tend to develop proximal muscle weakness, bone pain and tenderness, and fractures with minimal trauma.

Very low levels of the vitamin D metabolites 25-hydroxyvitamin D_3 (calcifediol) and 1,25-dihydroxy cholecalciferol (calcitriol) are detected in the serum. Parathyroid hormone is elevated, serum phosphorus is low, and calcium may be low or normal. In osteomalacia, alkaline phosphatase is elevated. X-rays will identify skeletal abnormalities.

Vitamin D, calcium, and phosphorus supplementation.

Infections

Septic Arthritis

Septic arthritis, an infectious monoarthritis, is usually caused by hematogenous spread of microorganisms. *Staphylococcus aureus* is the most common causative organism, except in sexually active young people, in whom *Neisseria gonorrhoeae* is more frequent. Gram-negative rods account for only 10% of cases and usually occur in patients with diabetes, cancer, or other underlying illnesses. Joints with pre-existing arthritis (often rheumatoid) are particularly susceptible to infection. IV drug use and endocarditis from any cause are also major risk factors.

Patients present with sudden onset of arthritis in one joint, most often the knee. The affected joint is warm, red, tender, and swollen. Movement causes intense pain. Fever is common, but the patient may or may not appear acutely ill.

Synovial fluid has markedly elevated leukocyte counts, decreased glucose, and positive cultures. Blood cultures and Gram's stains of synovial fluid often reveal the organism but cannot be relied on.

A penicillinase-resistant penicillin (e.g., nafcillin) should be used. An aminoglycoside should be added if the patient is susceptible to gram-negative infections. Local aspiration relieves symptoms caused by the effusion itself and can be repeated for recurrence of the effusion. If patients do not improve over 2 to 4 days, surgical drainage is indicated. Delay of treatment can result in articular destruction.

Gonococcal Arthritis

Approximately 1% of all *N. gonorrhoeae* infections are complicated by joint involvement that is due to disseminated gonococcal disease, making this the most common septic arthritis of young adults. The typical patient is a young woman who is pregnant or menstruating. Instead of arthritis, some patients develop **tenosynovitis,** in which the synovial tunnel surrounding tendons becomes inflamed, resulting in pain on muscle movement.

A few days of migrating polyarthralgias involving the hands, wrists, elbows, knees, and ankles tend to precede onset of either tenosynovitis or a septic monoarthritis (usually of the knee). The affected joints are red, hot, swollen, and tender. Most patients have associated skin lesions, such as petechiae, pustules, or necrosis, which are located on the extremities, palms, and soles and indicate disseminated gonococcal infection. Half of patients are afebrile and most patients deny genitourinary complaints.

Synovial fluid has elevated WBC count, although not as markedly as in other types of septic arthritis (less than 100,000/µL). Gram's stain and synovial fluid culture are positive in less than 50% of patients, whereas blood cultures are positive in 25% of patients. Urethral, throat, and rectal cultures may be positive even without local symptoms.

Ceftriaxone is given in any cases of suspected gonococcal arthritis.

Use of condoms during intercourse prevents the spread of gonorrhea. Prompt treatment of persons with symptoms of genital tract infection and their partners prevents the development of disseminated disease.

MUSCULOSKELETAL

Osteomyelitis

Osteomyelitis is an infection of the bone that may develop locally, by extension from a nearby infection site, or via hematogenous spread. Local spread is usually initiated by a fracture, surgery, bite, or other trauma. Hematogenously spread osteomyelitis generally occurs in bones with rich blood supplies, such as long bones and vertebral bodies. Before puberty, infection usually occurs in the metaphysis (shaft) of long bones because the epiphysis is protected by the epiphyseal plate. Common infecting organisms are *S. aureus* and *Pseudomonas.* In patients with sickle cell anemia, salmonella osteomyelitis can be seen.

Pain, tenderness, redness, and swelling are present over the involved bone. Fever and chills may be present in acute presentations. Subacute and chronic osteomyelitis are subtle and may escape detection until a sinus draining to the skin develops.

Leukocytosis and elevated erythrocyte sedimentation rate (ESR).

X-rays are not helpful in diagnosing early disease because lesions are not visible until 10 to 14 days after clinical onset. Radionuclide bone scans will show the lesion within 72 hours. Blood cultures or needle biopsy with Gram's stain and culture are necessary to select appropriate antibiotics.

Drainage of pus and debridement of dead tissue are required, followed by a long course (4 to 6 weeks) of organism-specific intravenous antibiotics. Urgent surgical decompression is indicated for vertebral body osteomyelitis.

Lyme Disease

Named after the town in Connecticut where it was first described, Lyme disease is caused by the spirochete *Borrelia burgdorferi,* which is transmitted to humans by the *Ixodes* tick. The disease has a variety of presentations and may affect the joints, heart, or nervous system.

Within a month of being bitten, the patient develops an expanding, erythematous rash with central clearing (**erythema chronicum migrans**). Accompanying symptoms include fever, chills, fatigue, arthralgias, and headache. Weeks to months later, cardiac and neurologic sequelae may develop. Cardiac complications include myocarditis, arrhythmias, and heart block. Neurologic involvement includes Bell's palsy, sensory or motor neuropathies, aseptic meningitis, and meningoencephalitis. Months to years later, the patient may develop chronic synovitis or mono-oligoarticular arthritis, usually in the larger joints, particularly the knees. Late neurologic sequelae include subacute encephalopathy and axonal polyneuropathy.

MUSCULOSKELETAL

In early stages, diagnosis relies on clinical presentation, including history of exposure and rash. Later, evidence of late manifestations of disease is supported with immunologic assays, such as the enzyme-linked immunosorbent assay, which detects antispirochete antibodies, and Western blot, which detects IgM and IgG. Synovial fluid culture is not helpful in diagnosis.

Choice and duration of antibiotic depends on clinical presentation, but doxycycline is typically used, with amoxicillin a useful alternative, for example in children and pregnancy. IV antibiotics are reserved for central nervous system and advanced cardiac involvement.

Prevention centers around avoidance of tick bites (e.g., insect repellent and long sleeves) and early detection of tick bites (e.g., inspection of arms and legs after walking in areas of potential exposure).

Inflammatory and Immunologic Disorders

Polymyalgia Rheumatica

Polymyalgia rheumatica is an inflammatory connective tissue disorder that primarily affects older patients, particularly women. There is a strong association with giant cell (temporal) arteritis.

Symmetric pain in the neck, shoulder, or pelvic girdle muscles, often with fever, malaise, and weight loss. Morning stiffness is so extreme that patients may have difficulty getting out of bed. Swelling may occur in only one or two joints, unlike rheumatoid arthritis. There is no muscle weakness, unlike polymyositis. If temporal arteritis is present, the patient may have headaches, blurred vision, jaw claudication, or blindness (see Giant Cell Arteritis in Chapter 2).

Anemia is common.

A very elevated ESR is characteristic. Rheumatoid factor (RF) is negative. The pattern of illness, including morning stiffness and prompt response to corticosteroids, confirms the diagnosis. If temporal arteritis is present, biopsy will show giant cells and inflammation.

If temporal arteritis is suspected, high-dose corticosteroids must be started immediately to avoid blindness, and ophthalmologic consultation is necessary. Lower dose steroids may be used in polymyalgia rheumatica. Improvement is seen within 3 days. Most patients may be tapered off steroids gradually, but some continue to take small doses for years.

MUSCULOSKELETAL

Systemic Lupus Erythematosus

Systemic lupus erythematosus (SLE) is a multisystem, autoimmune disorder associated with a variety of autoantibodies. Most manifestations occur because antigen-antibody complexes trigger inflammatory responses in various locations of the body. This disease occurs predominantly in young women and is more common in blacks. The most common causes of death in lupus are infection, nephritis, and central nervous system disease.

Certain drugs, including procainamide, hydralazine, isoniazid, methyldopa, quinidine, and chlorpromazine, can cause lupus-like syndromes, which are reversible after discontinuing the medication.

Presentation varies widely and may involve all body systems. Most patients have constitutional symptoms and cutaneous and musculoskeletal manifestations (Figure 12–4). Other common clinical effects are listed in Table 12-2.

If renal disease is present, there may be proteinuria and elevated BUN and creatinine. If anemia is present, check for hemolytic anemia with a Coombs' test. Several antiphospholipid antibodies are important in lupus. Lupus anticoagulant is a risk factor for miscarriage and thrombosis. Anticardiolipin antibody increases the risk of fetal death, and a third antiphospholipid antibody causes a false-positive syphilis test.

Clinical presentation and serum antibody tests. Antinuclear antibodies (ANA) are found in more than 95% of lupus patients, but they may be found in other autoimmune diseases as well, including rheumatoid arthritis and autoimmune hepatitis (i.e., the test is sensitive, but not specific to lupus). Anti-dsDNA (double-stranded DNA) antibodies are found in only 60% of cases, but they are not found in other disorders (i.e., the test is not as sensitive, but it is very specific to lupus). Anti-Sm (smooth muscle) antibodies are also very specific but are less frequently observed.

Avoidance of sunlight reduces cutaneous effects. Control joint pain with NSAIDs or hydroxychloroquine, an antimalarial medication. Corticosteroids should be used to control systemic manifestations. Other immunosuppressants, such as cyclophosphamide, are given in steroid-unresponsive cases. Anticoagulation is indicated for patients with arterial or venous thrombosis.

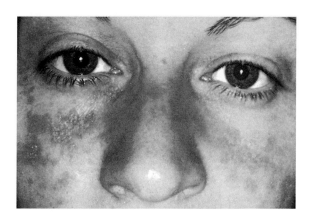

Fig. 12-4. Systemic lupus erythematosus. Showing classic "butterfly" eruption. (Reprinted with permission from Hall J: *Sauer's Manual of Skin Diseases,* 8th ed. Philadelphia, Lippincott Williams & Wilkins, 2000, p 248.)

MUSCULOSKELETAL

Table 12-2. Clinical manifestations of systemic lupus erythematosus

Organ system	Manifestations
Constitutional	Fever, malaise, anorexia, weight loss
Mucocutaneous	"Butterfly rash" (erythematous rash on bridge of nose and cheeks; Figure 12-4), discoid rash (erythematous patches), cutaneous vasculitis, photosensitivity, Raynaud's phenomenon, alopecia, oral ulcers
Musculoskeletal	Arthritis (distribution similar to RA, including symmetric involvement of PIP, MCP, wrists, knees, and feet), morning stiffness, myalgias
Renal	Immune-complex glomerulonephritis (mesangial, membranous, focal proliferative, diffuse proliferative), interstitial nephritis
Neurologic	Psychosis, seizures, strokes, aseptic meningitis, neuropathies
Cardiovascular	Pericarditis, myocarditis, arrhythmias, verrucous (Libman-Sacks) endocarditis
Pulmonary	Pleuritis, pneumonitis, pleural effusion
Gastrointestinal	Abdominal pain, vomiting
Ocular	Conjunctivitis, episcleritis, episodic or permanent monocular blindness
Hematologic	Anemia of chronic disease, autoimmune hemolytic anemia, leukopenia, thrombocytopenia, venous and arterial thrombosis

MCP, metacarpophalangeal (joint); PIP, proximal interphalangeal (joint); RA, rheumatoid arthritis.

Polymyositis and Dermatomyositis

Polymyositis and dermatomyositis are diseases involving inflammation of skeletal muscle. In dermatomyositis, patients also have cutaneous involvement. Women are more likely than men to get either disease, as are African-Americans. A coexisting occult malignancy is present in 25% of cases of dermatomyositis.

Symmetric, progressive, proximal muscle weakness develops. Hips and legs are typically affected first, and the typical first symptom is difficulty climbing stairs. Muscle pain or tenderness may also be present, and atrophy can develop in advanced disease. Patients with dermatomyositis have a red, scaly rash of the face, neck, shoulders, upper back, and/or chest and may have a violet discoloration of their upper eyelids. This **heliotrope** rash is pathognomonic of the disease. They may also have characteristic scaly patches over the joints of the hand.

Elevation of serum muscle enzymes [creatine phosphokinase, aldolase, serum glutamic-oxaloacetic transaminase (SGOT), serum glutamate pyruvate transaminase (SGPT), lactate dehydrogenase]. Positive ANA is common. Anti-Jo-1 antibodies are found in patients with associated interstitial lung disease.

EMG shows spontaneous fibrillations, but this is nonspecific. Muscle biopsy is diagnostic but can be insensitive. In polymyositis, biopsy shows lymphoid inflammatory infiltrates in the muscle and muscle necrosis. In dermatomyositis, the inflammatory cells are perivascular and surround muscle fascicles.

MUSCULOSKELETAL

TREATMENT

Treatment is with high-dose corticosteroids or other immunosuppressants, if necessary, which can be tapered over many months. Monitor improvement by measuring muscle enzymes. Search for occult malignancy.

Rheumatoid Arthritis

Rheumatoid arthritis (RA) is a chronic inflammatory disorder in which the synovial joints are infiltrated by inflammatory cells, resulting in progressive destruction of the cartilage and bone and eventually in severe disability. Middle-aged women are most often affected.

SIGNS & SYMPTOMS

RA is a symmetric polyarthritis. Systemic symptoms of malaise, weight loss, and low-grade fever often precede development of diffuse joint pain, tenderness, and swelling. Morning stiffness is common. Any synovial joint may be affected, but the PIP and metacarpophalangeal (MCP) joints of the hands and the metatarsophalangeal joints of the feet are often the first to be involved. The DIP joints are seldom affected. Advanced cases will show a typical **swan neck** deformity (flexed DIP and hyperextended PIP) and the **boutonnière** deformity (flexed PIP). Extra-articular manifestations include subcutaneous nodules (common over bony prominences), pleuritis, pericarditis, scleritis, and chorea.

LABS

RF (antibodies against the Fc portion of IgG) is present in at least 75% of patients. ANA is found in less than half of patients. Elevated ESR, IgG and IgM, and normocytic, hypochromic anemia are common. X-rays may show soft-tissue swelling or periarticular osteoporosis, joint space narrowing, marginal erosions, and possibly subluxation (Figure 12-5). Synovial fluid analysis shows 30,000–50,000 WBCs with a polymorphonuclear (PMN) predominance, without purulence or crystals.

DIAGNOSIS

A number of the above laboratory findings in the appropriate clinical setting must be met for the diagnosis to be made formally.

TREATMENT

Supportive treatment, physical therapy, and splints can reduce pain, decrease joint use, and prevent contracture. The first-line drug is an NSAID. Methotrexate should be used for treatment failure with NSAIDs. Gold salts, antimalarials, and tumor necrosis factor inhibitors offer another tier of treatment options for methotrexate failure. Immunosuppressive agents are third-line drugs. Corticosteroids may be used to control flare-ups and can be injected intra-articularly, but they should not be used on a chronic basis.

Overlap (Mixed) Connective Tissue Disease

Overlap connective tissue disease, also known as mixed connective tissue disease (MCTD), is a clinical entity characterized by overlapping features of SLE, scleroderma, and polymyositis. Over time, however, the clinical picture refines itself, and many patients proceed to develop SLE, scleroderma, or polymyositis. Early presentation may include Raynaud's phenomenon, polyarthralgia and arthritis, swollen hands with "sausage" fingers, proximal muscle

MUSCULOSKELETAL

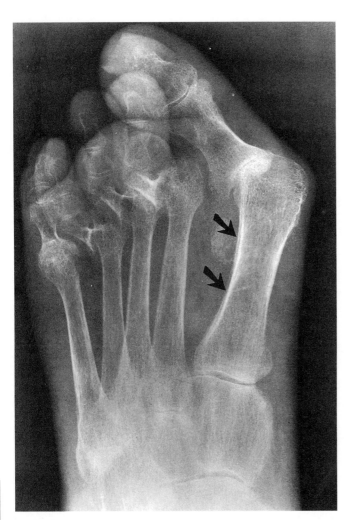

Fig. 12-5. Rheumatoid arthritis of the foot with lateral subluxation of the metatarsophalangeal (MTP) joint. There are erosive changes in the second through fifth MTP joints, as well as periosteal reaction (*arrows*) along the shaft of the first metatarsal. (Reprinted with permission from Daffner R: *Clinical Radiology: The Essentials,* 2nd ed. Baltimore, Williams & Wilkins, 1999, p 473.)

weakness, esophageal hypomotility, and pulmonary abnormalities. Lupus-like and heliotrope rashes are common. ANAs directed against ribonucleic protein (anti-RNP) are present in high titers but are also found in SLE. Corticosteroids are often useful. However, scleroderma-like manifestations are generally not responsive to corticosteroids, permitting only supportive measures.

Ankylosing Spondylitis

Ankylosing spondylitis (AS) is a seronegative spondyloarthropathy often associated with HLA-B27. It is a chronic inflammatory disease of the axial skeleton and large peripheral joints in which involvement of the sacroiliac joint is considered diagnostic. The disease is frequently mild, but it can result in permanent, extreme kyphosis and spinal fusion. AS is most common in white, young adult men.

SIGNS & SYMPTOMS

Insidious onset of back pain, often nocturnal, with progressive spinal stiffness, restricted range of motion, and restricted chest expansion is the typical presentation. Patients unconsciously ease back pain by bending over slightly, so some absence of normal lordosis is seen. Transient or permanent arthritis of the hips, shoulders, and knees in an asymmetric distribution affects less than half of patients. Some patients have self-limited episodes of anterior uveitis, an inflammation of the iris and ciliary body.

Elevated ESR. Absence of both RF and ANA. HLA-B27 is present in 90% of patients but is not specific.

Presence of sacroiliitis on x-ray with erosion and sclerosis of the sacroiliac joints. The classic "bamboo spine"—with vertebral squaring, bony outgrowths, and paraspinal ligament calcification—is a late finding.

Indomethacin or another NSAID controls pain and allows the patient to do maintenance exercises. Strengthening and breathing exercises and diligent attention to posture may help prevent permanent deformity.

Bursitis

A bursa is a fluid-filled sac located at sites of friction between tendons, muscles, or bones. Bursitis is the chronic or acute inflammation of the bursa. Bursitis of the shoulder (subdeltoid or subacromial) is most common, although any bursa may be involved. Trauma, infection, gout, RA, or osteoarthritis may be the cause. In the case of semimembranous-gastrocnemius bursitis (Baker's cyst), rupture can cause calf pain and swelling and can be clinically difficult to distinguish from thrombophlebitis.

Pain and limitation of movement are common and can be abrupt in onset. Swelling and redness are seen if the bursa is superficial or if a bacterial infection is present, and aspiration is necessary in this setting. The WBC count is often >50,000 in septic bursitis. Ultrasound can differentiate thrombophlebitis from a ruptured Baker's cyst.

Local heat, immobilization, and NSAIDs. If due to trauma, local corticosteroid injections are useful. Use antibiotics if infection is present. Repeated aspiration of the bursa will help relieve symptoms. Exercises to improve range of motion and strength can be started when symptoms subside. Ruptured Baker's cysts are treated with leg rest, elevation, and corticosteroid injection into the knee.

Tendonitis

Tendonitis is inflammation of the tendon or tendon sheath (**tenosynovitis**). Trauma, strain, or excessive exercise are the most common causes. Incidence is higher in older patients, presumably because of decreased blood flow in the tendons, which makes the tendons more susceptible to microtrauma. In young adults, disseminated gonococcal infection may cause gonococcal tenosynovitis or gonococcal arthritis.

MUSCULOSKELETAL

Pain with movement and tenderness along the tendon. The tendon sheath may be visibly swollen because of fluid accumulation. If it is dry, friction rubs may be felt or heard with a stethoscope.

Immobilization, hot or cold compresses (whichever the patient prefers), and NSAIDs relieve discomfort. Injection of corticosteroids into the tendon sheath may also help. Increase exercise as tolerated. Gonococcal infection must be treated with appropriate antibiotics.

Fibromyalgia

Fibromyalgia is a common syndrome of unknown etiology that causes chronic pain in muscles and tendons, with increased involvement of the neck, shoulders, back, and hips. No objective abnormality has yet been identified. The disorder is most commonly seen in middle-aged women. Hypothyroidism, RA, and sleep apnea may predispose.

Diffuse, achy muscle pain, poor sleep, fatigue, headache, and irritable bowel syndrome are common. "Trigger points" are present, which, when palpated, reproduce the pain.

Once other systemic diseases have been ruled out, diagnosis is made on the basis of the clinical presentation.

Stretching exercises, tricyclic antidepressants, and SSRIs may be beneficial. Trigger points may be injected with local anesthetics.

Neoplasms

Osteosarcoma

Osteosarcoma is the most common primary bone cancer. It is most common in rapidly growing teenage boys. Although it can occur in many bones, the most frequent sites are the distal femur and proximal tibia. Metastases occur in the lung. Patients usually present with bone pain and swelling, at times associated with limitation of movement of an associated joint, often the knee. Pathologic, spontaneous fracture can also occur. X-ray shows bone destruction and a soft-tissue mass, usually in the metaphysis, often with periosteal elevation. Biopsy is necessary for diagnosis. Treatment involves aggressive chemotherapy and surgery, which can be "limb-sparing" or involve amputation.

MUSCULOSKELETAL

Bone Metastases

The most common cancers that metastasize to bone are carcinomas of the breast, lung, prostate, kidney, and thyroid. Symptoms of bony metastases (pain or pathologic fracture) may occur before a primary tumor is suspected. Although advanced lesions will be visible on x-ray, early bony metastases may be identified only by using whole-body bone scans with radioisotopes. Bone biopsy may help identify the primary tumor, and treatment will depend on this identification.

Pulmonary Osteoarthropathy

Pulmonary osteoarthropathy is a paraneoplastic disorder (i.e., a syndrome caused by the indirect effects of a malignancy) that presents with polyarthritis and can resemble RA clinically. This disorder involves inflammation of the periosteum of the long bones of the extremities and digits, with subperiosteal formation of new bone and frequently associated synovitis. The distal long bones of the arms and legs are most commonly involved, and the sites may be tender and swollen. Clubbing of the fingers is also frequently present. Pulmonary osteoarthropathy occurs in patients with lung and thorax cancers (except small cell carcinoma) as well as in patients without malignancies who have cyanotic heart disease, cirrhosis, or lung abscess. Surgical treatment of the malignancy improves the joint pain. If unresectable, NSAIDs are often useful, and surgical vagotomy is sometimes effective.

Miscellaneous Disorders

Shoulder-Hand Syndrome

Shoulder-hand syndrome is a variant of **reflex sympathetic dystrophy,** a rare disorder thought to be caused by unchecked sympathetic nerve hyperactivity and vasomotor instability. The shoulder-hand syndrome is characterized by reduced shoulder range of motion, along with burning pain, diffuse swelling, and skin atrophy or excess sweating in the ipsilateral hand. It can develop weeks to months after a myocardial infarction or neck or shoulder injury but can also occur following direct hand trauma. Treatment is with physical therapy and analgesics. Corticosteroids are used in resistant cases. Prognosis is best with early treatment.

Dupuytren's Contracture

Thickening and contracture of the palmar fascia result in limitation of finger extension in Dupuytren's contracture. This condition typically occurs in middle-aged and older men and is more common in alcoholics and patients with epilepsy, tuberculosis, diabetes, and liver disease. Diagnosis is by inspection and palpation of the palm. Surgery is required in severe cases. Nodules, if present, can be injected with corticosteroids.

Carpal Tunnel Syndrome

Neuropathy in carpal tunnel syndrome is caused by compression of the median nerve as it passes through the carpal tunnel. More common in women and in occupations that require repetitive hand movements, this syndrome is also associated with pregnancy, RA, acromegaly, myxedema, DM, hyperparathyroidism, and hypocalcemia.

Numbness, tingling, and/or pain occur in the first three digits of the hand (in the distribution of the median nerve), and aching pain often radiates into the forearm. Pain is often worse with activity and worse at night. Gentle percussion of the palmaris longus tendon of the wrist causes tingling (Tinel sign). Placing the dorsal surface of the hands together with wrists flexed at 90 degrees for 60 seconds exacerbates symptoms (Phalen test).

History and physical, as described in preceding paragraphs. Decreases in nerve conduction can be measured.

Initial treatment is with nightly use of wrist splints. Elevation of the extremity can be helpful, and corticosteroid injection into the carpal tunnel is effective in some patients. Surgery to divide the volar carpal ligament may be necessary.

Paget's Disease of Bone

Paget's disease (osteitis deformans) is a skeletal disorder seen in adults. Overactive osteoclasts produce osteolytic lesions, and overactive osteoblasts fill these lesions with improperly formed, disorganized bone. Because the bone lesions are highly vascular, high-output cardiac failure may develop. Deafness and frequent fractures can occur. Osteosarcoma occurs in rare instances.

The disease is most often asymptomatic. Symptoms may include bone pain, headaches, hearing loss, increased skull size ("Doc, my hats don't fit anymore!"), and fractures with minimal trauma. The patient may have a visibly enlarged skull with rounded forehead (frontal bossing), bowed thighs, and a shortened, kyphotic spine because of vertebral flattening, giving the appearance of long arms.

Serum alkaline phosphatase is elevated. Calcium and phosphorus levels are normal. Urine hydroxyproline is elevated.

The disease is often diagnosed incidentally on x-ray. Early in the course of the disease, x-rays show osteolytic lesions. Later, bone is expanded and dense, and chaotic architecture may be seen. The skull may have a characteristic "cotton wool" appearance. Fractures may be evident.

No treatment is needed for asymptomatic cases. Bisphosphonates are the treatment of choice, but calcitonin can also be useful. Orthopaedic appliances or surgery may be needed to improve gait disturbances.

MUSCULOSKELETAL

13

Neurology and Special Senses

(continued)

Headache

Migraine

Migraine headaches are recurrent headaches with characteristic symptoms in each patient. They affect twice as many women as men, usually begin between the ages of 10 and 30 years, and often disappear spontaneously by age 50 years. Patients may have a family history of migraine. Precipitating factors include stress, fatigue, fasting, oral contraceptives, menstruation, and foods containing tyramine (cheeses), monosodium glutamate, and nitrites (hot dogs).

Presentations vary widely, but patients with classic migraines experience an aura before the onset of the headache. The aura often involves visual disturbances such as scintillating scotomas (small areas of vision loss that may enlarge and spread peripherally). The headache is dull, throbbing, and frequently unilateral. Nausea and vomiting, sensitivity to noise, and photophobia are common. Without medical intervention, migraines can last for hours or days.

The clinical presentation is diagnostic in the absence of abnormal neurologic findings.

Prophylaxis is useful for patients with frequent or severe migraine headaches. Prophylactic medications include amitriptyline, propranolol, valproic acid, calcium channel blockers, ergots, and NSAIDs. Treatment of an acute migraine attack includes NSAIDs, ergots, and sumatriptan.

Cluster Headache

Cluster headaches primarily affect men 20 to 50 years of age. Precipitating factors include alcohol and vasodilators.

Cluster headaches are severe, brief, nonthrobbing, periorbital, unilateral headaches that recur or "cluster" around the same time each day for weeks or months at a time. **Horner's syndrome** (ptosis, miosis, anhidrosis) and ipsilateral nasal congestion, rhinorrhea, and tearing are often associated. Remissions can last months or years.

Diagnosis is by presentation and exclusion of other disorders.

Treatment for an acute attack includes oxygen, ergots, and sumatriptan. Prophylactic therapies against recurrent symptoms include antimigraine agents, prednisone, and lithium.

Tension Headache

Chronic headaches that do not resemble migraine or cluster headaches may be "tension headaches." Despite its name, the cause of tension headaches is unknown. Tension headaches are by far the most common type of headache seen in adults, and they afflict more women than men. Precipitants include stress, fatigue, and glare.

Patients report a bilateral, occipital, constant head pain.

Tension headache is a diagnosis of exclusion and requires that no focal neurologic symptoms be present.

Relaxation techniques, massage, and biofeedback may be useful. If simple analgesics are not effective, antimigraine agents may be tried.

Giant Cell Arteritis

Also known as *temporal arteritis,* giant cell arteritis is a chronic inflammatory disease of large blood vessels, primarily the carotid and cranial arteries, and is discussed in more detail in Chapter 2. Patients typically present with a bilateral temporal or occipital headache and jaw claudication. Temporal artery tenderness may be present. Without treatment with steroids, patients are at risk for blindness.

Trigeminal Neuralgia

Also known as **tic douloureux,** trigeminal neuralgia is typically seen in older adults. Although its etiology is unknown, some theories suggest microvascular compression as a possible cause.

Excruciating, lightening bolt–like bouts of facial pain in the V_2 and V_3 distribution of the trigeminal nerve are characteristic. Stimulation of trigger zones (e.g., touching face, eating, or brushing teeth) can precipitate the neuralgia.

NEUROLOGY

The preceding symptoms in the absence of other neurologic abnormalities are diagnostic.

Medical approaches include carbamazepine, phenytoin, baclofen, and gabapentin. Patients unresponsive to medical therapy may benefit from surgical decompression of fifth cranial nerve fibers.

Tumor-associated Headache

Tumor-associated headaches typically present as intermittent, progressively increasing, dull, nonthrobbing headaches. They are frequently exacerbated by postural changes and exertion, tend to be maximal on waking, and often disrupt sleep. These headaches are often associated with nausea and vomiting. CT scan or MRI is required for definitive diagnosis.

Increased Intracranial Pressure

Increased intracranial pressure (ICP) can be caused by increased dural venous sinus pressure. This results from obstruction (e.g., sagittal sinus thrombosis, tumors), resistance to CSF outflow (e.g., meningitis or subarachnoid hemorrhage plugging the arachnoid villi, tumor obstructing CSF flow), or increased CSF production (e.g., choroid plexus papilloma, benign intracranial hypertension).

Headache, nausea and vomiting, and lethargy are common symptoms. Headache is worst in the morning because of peaks in ICP. Bilateral papilledema, bradycardia, and elevated systolic blood pressure may be seen on examination. Focal neurologic signs forecast impending herniation.

CT or MRI may reveal the diagnosis if increased ICP is suspected on examination. Lumbar puncture (LP) is contraindicated except in cases of benign intracranial hypertension because of the risk of transtentorial herniation.

Hyperventilation will immediately reduce ICP by reducing cerebral blood flow. Mannitol causes water to shift from the brain into the intravascular space by osmosis. Steroids may decrease edema. Ventricular puncture is used as a last resort to prevent herniation.

Epilepsy and Seizure Disorders

Seizures result from a synchronized discharge of neurons in the CNS and can have a variety of causes (Table 13-1). In idiopathic epilepsy, recurrent seizures arise from a focus of epileptic tissue within the brain. Electrical discharge of this focus may spread to other brain regions. Other

Table 13-1. Causes of seizures among different age groups

Children	Adults	Elderly
Fever	Idiopathic epilepsy	Neoplasms
CNS infections	Alcohol withdrawal	Stroke
Metabolic defects	Drug withdrawal	Trauma
Idiopathic epilepsy	Metabolic abnormality	
	Trauma	
	Eclampsia	

causes of seizures include CNS infections, fever, metabolic defects, tumor, congenital abnormality, or head trauma. Epilepsy is more likely following head trauma associated with a depressed skull fracture, a penetrating injury, or a subdural or intraparenchymal hemorrhage.

Partial Seizures

Partial seizures arise from a specific focus in the brain and generally begin with localized symptoms.

SIGNS & SYMPTOMS

Simple partial seizures involve a focal symptom, whether sensory (e.g., visual hallucinations), motor (e.g., lip smacking), or psychomotor (e.g., purposeless pattern of movement). There is no loss of consciousness. The seizure may spread to involve adjacent cortical regions. For instance, in **jacksonian seizures,** focal muscle twitches spread progressively from their initial source across the patient's body as adjacent motor cortex becomes involved. **Secondary generalization** refers to simple seizures that evolve into grand mal seizures. In these cases, consciousness is lost.

Complex partial seizures involve stereotyped, psychomotor symptoms that are due to an epileptic focus in the temporal or medial frontal lobes. Seizing patients may show automatisms (i.e., coordinated motor activity) and may experience olfactory hallucinations, fear, or déjà vu. In contrast with simple partial seizures, patients with complex partial seizures lose contact with their environment during the seizure and experience postictal confusion afterward.

DIAGNOSIS

Electroencephalogram (EEG) during or immediately after the episode shows distinctive changes. MRI may locate a focal abnormality.

TREATMENT

Control of seizures may be achieved with phenytoin, carbamazepine, or valproate. Surgery may be an option.

Generalized Seizures

Generalized seizures involve the entire cerebral cortex, but they may produce only minor symptoms. These seizures are frequently genetic and usually present during childhood.

Absence seizures, also known as *petit mal,* involve very brief and frequent losses of consciousness without loss of muscle tone. Rapid eye blinking is common during the seizure. Patients experience no aura or postictal confusion. Symptoms may resolve as the patient ages.

Tonic-clonic seizures, also called *grand mal seizures,* may be preceded by an aura of epigastric discomfort or mood change. In the tonic phase, which lasts up to 30 seconds, the patient falls unconscious to the ground in tonic contraction with an arched back. A 1-minute clonic phase follows, during which the patient undergoes rapid alternation of muscle contraction and relaxation. As long as 30 minutes may pass before the patient regains consciousness. Postictal confusion and headache can last another 10 to 30 minutes. Todd's paralysis refers to a focal neurologic deficit that is first observed in the postictal period and resolves within approximately 2 days. If present, it indicates an underlying brain lesion.

Symptoms and EEG are diagnostic in most cases. The EEG finding in absence seizures is a characteristic 3-cycle-per-second spike-and-wave pattern. In tonic-clonic seizures, laboratory and imaging studies may suggest an etiology.

Ethosuximide is the primary drug used for absence seizures, but valproate is also effective. Phenytoin, carbamazepine, or valproate is effective for control of tonic-clonic seizures. Surgery may be an option.

Status Epilepticus

In status epilepticus, seizure activity is not separated by any periods of regained consciousness. It is typically defined as active seizure for more than 20 minutes or more than 2 episodes of seizure without periods of regained consciousness. Status epilepticus may develop from any type of seizure disorder or from the rapid withdrawal of anticonvulsant medications.

Uninterrupted seizures may last hours or even days. If untreated, the patient may experience hypoxia, aspiration, hyperthermia, circulatory collapse, rhabdomyolysis, and brain damage.

The clinical presentation is generally diagnostic. However, nonconvulsive status can be a difficult clinical diagnosis and requires EEG. Laboratory studies—including blood glucose, electrolytes, and toxicology—and imaging studies may suggest an etiology.

Diazepam is typically given initially to abort the seizure over approximately 20 minutes, while airway, breathing, and circulation are maintained. Phenytoin, phenobarbital, or pentobarbital is then used in turn until the seizures are controlled, after which time diazepam is given. Glucose, thiamine, and naloxone may be given intravenously to treat potential causes. Fever is managed with cooling blankets and curare, if necessary.

NEUROLOGY

Cerebrovascular Disease

Ischemic Disorders

Ischemia of brain tissue occurs when the local blood supply becomes inadequate. Decreased blood flow to the brain can be due to atherosclerosis affecting the carotid or vertebral arteries, intracranial atherosclerosis and thrombosis, vascular inflammation, cerebral embolism arising from an atherosclerotic intra- or extracranial vessel or from a cardiac thrombus, a hypercoagulable state, or generalized hypoperfusion. If ischemic conditions persist, infarction of brain tissue results.

Transient Ischemic Attack

Transient ischemic attacks (TIAs) are sudden-onset, focal neurologic deficits that last less than 24 hours (typically lasting 1–2 hours). They are caused by sudden, brief episodes of impaired blood flow to the brain, generally due to emboli or arterial stenosis. Predisposing conditions for TIAs include hypertension, diabetes, hypercoagulable states, heart disease, smoking, hyperlipidemia, and stimulant abuse. TIAs are frequently recurrent and most commonly seen in elderly or middle-aged patients.

SIGNS & SYMPTOMS

Focal neurologic abnormalities begin suddenly and usually disappear within an hour but may last up to 24 hours. Consciousness is not impaired. Longer-lasting symptoms define **stroke** and suggest brain infarction. Carotid artery involvement (Figure 13-1) produces unilateral anterior circulation symptoms, including contralateral heaviness, weakness, tingling, or numbness of the face, arm, and/or leg, and aphasia if the dominant hemisphere is involved (Figure 13-2). **Amaurosis fugax** is brief, ipsilateral blindness caused by occlusion of the ophthalmic artery. Vertebrobasilar system involvement produces posterior circulation symptoms of brainstem, cerebellar, and visual cortex dysfunction, including vertigo, ataxia, dysarthria, dysconjugate gaze, diplopia, blindness, weakness, and/or paresthesias of the extremities or hemiface.

DIAGNOSIS

The clinical presentation and its duration suggests the diagnosis and the location of the impairment. Carotid bruits or thrills suggest carotid atherosclerosis and stenosis, which can be documented with carotid duplex ultrasonography. Magnetic resonance angiography or neuroangiography can identify stenosed intracranial arteries.

TREATMENT

Patients with carotid TIAs and marked (>70%) stenosis of the carotid arteries frequently benefit from surgical endarterectomy. Aspirin is recommended in patients with milder obstruction. Patients in atrial fibrillation benefit from anticoagulants. Risk factors should be minimized as much as possible.

Stroke

A stroke is a sudden-onset focal neurologic deficit that lasts more than 24 hours. It is caused by prolonged ischemia of the brain, resulting in infarction. Insufficient perfusion (ischemic stroke) and hemorrhage are the two etiologies of stroke.

NEUROLOGY

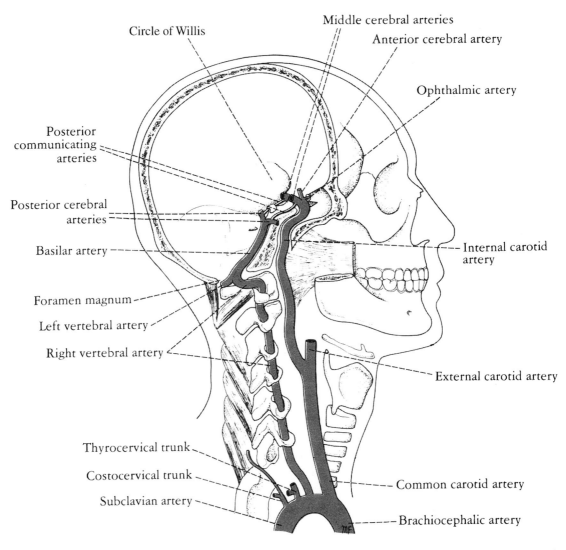

Fig. 13-1. Arteries of the head and neck. The anterior and middle cerebral arteries, fed by the internal carotid arteries, are the major vessels of the anterior circulation. The posterior cerebral arteries, along with the vertebral arteries and basilar artery, which perfuse the cerebellum and brainstem, comprise the major vessels of the posterior circulation. (Reprinted with permission from Snell R: *Clinical Neuroanatomy for Medical Students,* Boston, Little, Brown, 1980, p 450.)

Ischemic stroke results most often from embolic events, typically from the heart, carotids, aortic arch, or intracranial vessels. Thrombotic ischemic stroke occurs with the occlusion of an intra- or extracranial vessel with underlying atherosclerosis. Major risk factors for ischemic stroke include hypertension, diabetes, heart disease, hyperlipidemia, hypercoagulable states, and smoking.

Hemorrhagic stroke is characterized by the location of the bleed and can be epidural, subdural, intracerebral, or subarachnoid (Figure 13-3). Trauma is the major cause of hemorrhagic stroke, but rupture of berry aneurysms is an additional important cause of subarachnoid hemorrhage; and hypertension, stimulant abuse, and rupture of vascular malformations are important causes of intracerebral hemorrhage. Intracerebral and subarachnoid hemorrhages are discussed elsewhere in this chapter.

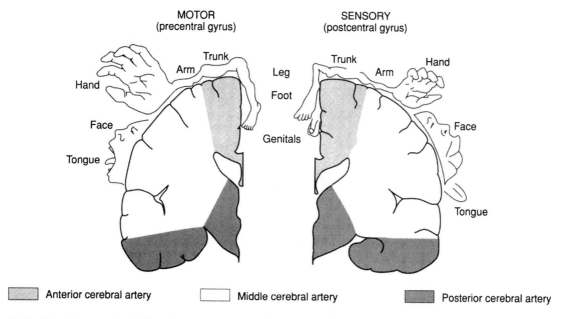

MOTOR
(precentral gyrus)

SENSORY
(postcentral gyrus)

Anterior cerebral artery   Middle cerebral artery   Posterior cerebral artery

Fig. 13-2. Arterial supply of the primary motor and sensory cortex, coronal view. The drawing indicates where different parts of the body are represented in the cortex and, thus, which areas of the body are affected by an occlusion of each artery. (Reprinted with permission from Greenberg D, Aminoff M, Simon R: *Clinical Neurology,* 2nd ed. Norwalk, Appleton & Lange, 1993, p 262.)

SIGNS & SYMPTOMS

Neurologic symptoms depend on the site of the infarct (see Figures 13-1 and 13-2), which can be broadly localized to the anterior or posterior circulation. The carotid arteries provide the major blood supply to the anterior circulation through the anterior cerebral artery and the middle cerebral artery. The vertebral arteries via the basilar artery are the major supply to the posterior circulation, including the posterior cerebral artery and vessels supplying the brainstem and cerebellum.

- The anterior circulation is more commonly affected in ischemic stroke, and the distribution of the **middle cerebral artery** is most often involved. Contralateral face and limb weakness (arm > leg), sensory loss, and homonymous hemianopsia (loss of half the visual field in both eyes) are com-

NEUROLOGY

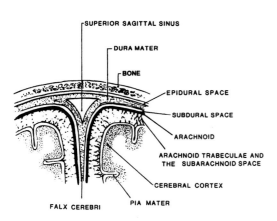

SUPERIOR SAGITTAL SINUS
DURA MATER
BONE
EPIDURAL SPACE
SUBDURAL SPACE
ARACHNOID
ARACHNOID TRABECULAE AND THE SUBARACHNOID SPACE
CEREBRAL CORTEX
FALX CEREBRI
PIA MATER

Fig. 13-3. Meninges and meningeal spaces, coronal view. (Reprinted with permission from Westmoreland B, Benarroch E, Daube J, et al: *Neurosciences: An Approach to Anatomy, Pathology and Physiology by Systems and Levels,* 3rd ed. Boston, Little, Brown, 1994, p 33.)

mon symptoms. Involvement of the dominant hemisphere leads to aphasia, whereas involvement of the nondominant hemisphere results in sensory neglect and apraxia (inability to perform learned actions—e.g., dressing). In addition, ipsilateral ocular defects may be present with internal carotid artery involvement, due to emboli to the ophthalmic artery.

- Occlusion of the **anterior cerebral artery** causes contralateral leg weakness.
- Occlusion of the **posterior cerebral artery** causes contralateral homonymous hemianopsia, and extraocular movement abnormalities may be present. Bilateral posterior cerebral artery occlusion can cause cortical blindness.
- **Vertebrobasilar artery** involvement is frequently fatal. Unilateral occlusion in the vertebrobasilar system compromises brainstem function, producing ipsilateral cranial nerve abnormalities and contralateral body weakness and sensory deficits. Cerebellar perfusion can also be compromised. Vertigo, ataxia, dysconjugate gaze, and dysarthria may all be observed. Complete occlusion of the basilar artery can cause ophthalmoplegia, defects of pupillary constriction, bilateral weakness or paralysis of the extremities, and, usually, coma (although consciousness can rarely be spared).

Lacunar infarcts, small infarcts in the distribution of arterioles, often occur in the brainstem, basal ganglia, cerebellum, internal capsule, and deep white matter. Their associated clinical syndromes include pure motor or sensory deficits, ataxia, and dysarthria with hand clumsiness. A completed stroke presents with stable neurologic deficits and most often develops within a few minutes. A stroke in evolution presents with a progressive, stepwise increase in neurologic abnormalities that can occur over 1 to 2 days. Severe brainstem signs, impaired consciousness, mental deterioration, and aphasia indicate a poor prognosis.

DIAGNOSIS

The clinical presentation is indicative of stroke and localizes the lesion. CT or MRI differentiates ischemic stroke from hemorrhage and rules out other possible causes, such as tumor. Shortly after an ischemic stroke, CT and MRI scans are usually negative, although a CT will identify a hemorrhagic stroke. New MRI techniques such as diffusion-weighted imaging permit early diagnosis of ischemic strokes.

TREATMENT

Heparin is not indicated in completed ischemic strokes but does help to stabilize evolving ischemic strokes and may also prevent additional cardiac emboli, if this is the source of the stroke. It is contraindicated in cases of hemorrhagic stroke. Hypertension should not be treated in the acute phase of a stroke to avoid further reduction of blood flow to ischemic areas. Intravenous thrombolytic therapy with recombinant tissue plasminogen factor (rt-PA) is beneficial in ischemic stroke within 3 hours of onset. Contraindications include evidence of hemorrhage on CT, recent hemorrhage, recent surgery, use of anticoagulants, systolic blood pressure above 185 mm Hg, diastolic blood pressure above 110 mm Hg, and puncture of an artery at a noncompressible site. Intra-arterial thrombolytic therapy under angiographic guidance appears to be effective within 6 hours of onset and is available at some tertiary care centers. The prognosis for recovery is better in younger patients and in patients with limited motor or sensory defects, intact mental function, and a strong support network. The prognosis for recovery from lacunar strokes is excellent. Physical, occupational, and speech therapy facilitate recovery.

Aneurysm

Aneurysms—localized dilations of blood vessels—are a common cause of hemorrhage in the subarachnoid space (Figure 13-4). Congenital berry aneurysms, occurring at arterial bi-

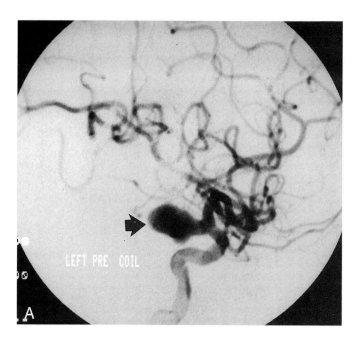

Fig. 13-4. Aneurysm of the intracranial portion of the internal carotid artery. (Reprinted with permission from Daffner R: *Clinical Radiology: The Essentials,* 2nd ed. Baltimore, Williams & Wilkins, 1999, p 527.)

furcations—often around the circle of Willis—are common and are often multiple. They can be associated with polycystic kidney disease and aortic coarctation.

The most dangerous feature of an intracranial aneurysm is its risk of rupture, which results in subarachnoid or intracerebral hemorrhage. Typically, aneurysms are asymptomatic until hemorrhage occurs. Headache, optic abnormalities, syncope, vomiting, and altered level of consciousness are common symptoms of hemorrhage. CT and lumbar puncture indicate hemorrhage, and angiography identifies the ruptured aneurysm and any other aneurysms. Treatment of ruptured or large unruptured aneurysms involves surgical clipping or endovascular coil embolization. Nimodipine decreases the incidence of arterial spasm.

Intracerebral Hemorrhage

Bleeding into the tissue of the brain usually results from hypertension. Stimulant abuse and rupture of vascular malformations are important causes. Intracerebral hemorrhages often extend into the subarachnoid space. Hypertensive hemorrhages are often large and frequently fatal.

As the vessel bleeds, pressure from the forming hematoma compresses and displaces adjacent brain regions. A supratentorial hematoma can cause transtentorial herniation, with brainstem compression and midbrain bleeding. Cerebellar hematomas can produce acute hydrocephalus by blocking CSF flow and can also cause brainstem compression.

SIGNS & SYMPTOMS

The acute onset of headache, nausea, and vomiting with progressive neurologic abnormalities is typical. Loss of consciousness, coma, focal or generalized seizures, and delirium are all common. Neurologic abnormalities frequently extend beyond vascular boundaries.

Symptoms may begin during exercise. Small cerebral hemorrhages cause focal neurologic deficits. Early supratentorial hemorrhages may produce hemiparesis, whereas subtentorial hemorrhages and supratentorial hemorrhages with transtentorial herniation produce brainstem or cerebellar defects.

NEUROLOGY

NEUROLOGY

CT is used to localize and quantify bleeding, assess compression, and rule out ischemic stroke (Figure 13-5).

Supportive care is the mainstay of treatment with particular attention to controlling intracranial pressure. Surgery may be life saving for large cerebellar hemorrhages and for decompression of supratentorial hemorrhages that are causing herniation. Many patients with large hemorrhages die within days of onset of the hemorrhage. Recovery is most dramatic with prompt decompression of cerebellar hemorrhages.

Subarachnoid Hemorrhage

Subarachnoid hemorrhage refers to bleeding between the pia and arachnoid layers of the meninges. It usually arises from rupture of a cerebral artery (berry) aneurysm or an arteriovenous malformation (AVM) or from trauma.

A sudden-onset, explosive headache is typically characterized as "the worst headache" of the patient's life. Patients may have loss of or a decreased level of consciousness, nuchal rigidity, and nausea and vomiting. Irritability and even combativeness are often observed.

CT scan shows subarachnoid blood. If negative, LP is mandatory to exclude CSF blood or xanthochromia. Once the patient is stabilized, neuroangiography can identify aneurysms and AVMs. Magnetic resonance angiography (MRA) can also be informative.

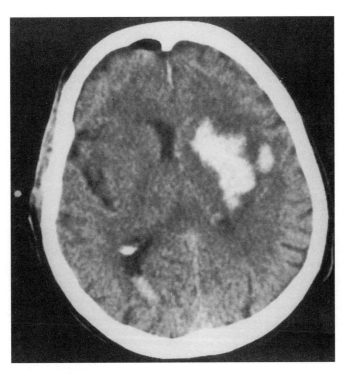

Fig. 13-5. Spontaneous intracerebral hemorrhage in a hypertensive patient, in a left periventricular distribution. (Reprinted with permission from Daffner R: *Clinical Radiology: The Essentials,* 2nd ed. Baltimore, Williams & Wilkins, 1999, p 526.)

Management of increased intracranial pressure includes intubation and hyperventilation, osmotic agents (e.g., mannitol), and elevation of the patient's head. Exertion, anticoagulants, and straining are contraindicated. Phenytoin prevents seizures. Nimodipine decreases the incidence of arterial spasm. Surgical clipping or endovascular embolization of an aneurysm or an AVM reduces both the long-term mortality and the probability of a recurrence.

Cavernous Sinus Thrombosis

Cavernous sinus thrombosis is a dangerous condition involving the presence of a thrombus in the cavernous sinus. Predisposing conditions include maxillofacial infections, hypercoagulable states, and dehydration. Chronic bacterial sinusitis may spread from the sphenoid or ethmoid air sinuses to form a septic thrombus.

The patient presents with cranial nerve palsies, as well as exophthalmos, papilledema, headache, decreased consciousness, and, occasionally, seizures. Fever is common in septic thrombosis.

CT scan of the cavernous sinus and the air sinuses confirms the diagnosis. Blood and nasal discharges are cultured to identify the infecting organism.

Intravenous antibiotics should be administered immediately. Surgical drainage of the air sinuses may be useful, especially if the patient does not respond to antibiotics. Hypercoagulable states should be treated if identified.

Toxic Neurologic Disorders

Toxic Vestibulopathies

Many drugs can interact with the peripheral nervous system, resulting in vestibular disorders.

- **Alcohol** can cause positional vertigo within 2 hours of ingestion, and symptoms may last as long as 12 hours. The patient experiences vertigo and nystagmus, especially while lying down and with closed eyes.
- **Aminoglycosides** are ototoxic agents that can produce symptoms of both vestibular and auditory dysfunction. Patients present with vertigo, nausea, vomiting, and ataxia. Romberg's sign may be present. These symptoms last 1 to 2 weeks and then gradually improve. Extended or repeated therapy can produce progressive vestibular dysfunction.
- **Salicylates** used chronically or in high doses can cause reversible vertigo, tinnitus, and sensorineural hearing loss. Headache, nausea, vomiting, tachypnea, and thirst may also be present. Arterial blood gas shows metabolic acidosis and compensatory respiratory alkalosis.

Toxic Neuropathies

Many chemical exposures may result in neurologic effects.

- **Lead** can produce a multiple motor mononeuropathy. It can also cause an acute encephalopathy in children.
- **Organophosphates** can cause delayed motor neuropathies, in addition to cholinergic crisis.
- **Alcohol** frequently causes a bilateral, distal sensorimotor neuropathy. Chronic use is also associated with Wernicke's encephalopathy and Korsakoff's amnestic syndrome.
- **Isoniazid,** used in the treatment of TB, produces a reversible sensory polyneuropathy that is prevented by concurrent pyridoxine (vitamin B_6) administration.

Carbon Monoxide Poisoning

Fetal hemoglobin's increased affinity for carbon monoxide makes fetuses especially susceptible. Hyperbaric oxygen has no proven benefit but is often employed in patients with seizures or coma and in pregnant women.

Metabolic Encephalopathy

Metabolic abnormalities can cause lethargy, confusion, and coma. In comatose states, pupillary reactivity is characteristically preserved, even though other brainstem functions are lost. Focal neurologic deficits, if any, cannot be explained by any one neurologic lesion. Asterixis is common. Laboratory tests may reveal uremia, hepatic failure, hypoglycemia, hypercalcemia, or hyponatremia. Drug overdoses may also cause metabolic encephalopathy. Imaging studies are normal, but EEG shows bilateral slowing. Infection should be ruled out with an LP. Treatment targets the underlying abnormality.

Infections

Bacterial Meningitis

Bacterial meningitis, an infection of the meninges of the spinal cord or brain, is most common in the first month of life. Group B streptococci and *Escherichia coli* predominate at this time. *Neisseria meningitidis* and *Streptococcus pneumoniae* are responsible for most meningitis in children older than 1 month, and *S. pneumoniae* causes the majority of cases in adults. *N. meningitidis,* harbored in the nasopharynx of 5% of the population, causes disease in people of all ages.

Bacteria reach the meninges from the blood, from nearby infected structures (such as the sinuses), and from contamination of the CSF. The bacteria then attract neutrophils. The resulting exudate may cause hydrocephalus, ischemia, and cranial nerve damage.

A sore throat may precede symptoms of fever, confusion, headache, vomiting, and neck stiffness. Stupor or coma may be present, in addition to cranial neuropathies and seizures. A petechial rash is found in more than half of patients with meningitis caused by *N. meningitides,* called meningococcemia. Brain infarction or systemic complications can cause death within hours. Signs of meningeal irritation include a positive Brudzinski's sign, in which neck flexion in the supine patient causes involuntary hip and knee flexion, and a positive Kernig's sign, in which extension of the knee in a patient with a flexed hip is painful.

CSF analysis confirms that meningitis is present. A low glucose level, a high neutrophil count, and a high protein concentration suggest bacterial meningitis (Table 13-2). CSF, Gram's stain, and culture may also be positive.

Administration of antibiotics should begin immediately after CSF has been taken for culture. Empiric therapy typically includes a third-generation cephalosporin in adults and in children older than 3 months and ampicillin and cefotaxime in infants and neonates. Once the culture results are available, an antibiotic specific to the infecting organism should be used.

People in close contact with patients with meningococcal meningitis should receive prophylaxis with rifampin. Children are now routinely immunized against *Haemophilus influenzae.*

Aseptic Meningitis

Aseptic meningitis is nonbacterial meningeal inflammation. Viruses are usually responsible and may be associated with community epidemics. Coxsackie viruses, echoviruses, and mumps virus are common.

Aseptic meningitis has the same clinical presentation as bacterial meningitis, including fever, headache, vomiting, neck stiffness, and an altered level of consciousness. The symptoms may be milder than with bacterial infection.

Table 13-2. Cerebrospinal fluid findings in different neurologic conditions

Condition	Pressure	Glucose	Protein	White blood cell count
Normal	70–180	15–85	15–45	0–5 WBCs
Bacterial meningitis	High	Low	High	High neutrophils (200–20,000)
Aseptic meningitis	Normal	Normal	Normal	High lymphocytes (25–2000)
Fungal or TB meningitis	High	Low	High	High lymphocytes (100–1000)
Guillain-Barré syndrome	Normal	Normal	High	Normal

TB, tuberculous; WBC, white blood cell count.

NEUROLOGY

CSF analysis shows high lymphocytes, normal glucose, normal or slightly increased protein, and a negative Gram's stain and bacterial culture.

Supportive treatment is usually sufficient, and the patients generally recover fully.

Subacute and Chronic Meningitis

Subacute and chronic meningitis involve the slow but progressive onset of meningeal infection. Subacute meningitis develops over 2 weeks in the absence of treatment. Chronic meningitis lasts longer than 1 month without antibiotic intervention.

Subacute or chronic meningitis can develop in patients with HIV, AIDS, cytomegalovirus, Lyme disease, syphilis, TB, sarcoidosis, or neoplasms. Immunosuppressive therapy and AIDS have increased the frequency of fungal meningitis, particularly *Cryptococcus.*

Symptoms of meningitis appear slowly over a period of several weeks.

CSF analysis confirms meningeal inflammation, showing a high lymphocyte count, low glucose (normal in syphilis), and sometimes high protein. Fungi may be seen in the CSF. TB can often be identified by acid-fast stain of the CSF; blood or CSF rapid-plasma reagin (RPR) is positive in syphilis. Because of the many treatment possibilities, the causative agent must be identified.

Treatment varies with etiology. Amphotericin B is used in fungal infections, and four-drug therapy is indicated in TB meningitis.

Encephalitis

Encephalitis, acute inflammation of the brain tissue, may be caused by direct viral invasion or by host hypersensitivity to a virus. Primary encephalitis may be sporadic, caused by endemic viruses, such as varicella-zoster virus, herpes simplex virus, and mumps, or it may be epidemic, caused by Coxsackie, polio-, echo-, or arboviruses. St. Louis and California encephalitis cause most arbovirus encephalitis in the United States. Secondary encephalitis arises from an immunologic response to viral infection, most commonly chickenpox, measles, and rubella.

Signs of cerebral dysfunction include seizures, paresis, cranial nerve defects, and altered level of consciousness. Symptoms and signs of meningitis may be present.

A viral etiology is suggested by CSF lymphocytosis, normal glucose, and a negative bacterial culture.

Supportive measures include reducing intracranial pressure. In cases of herpes encephalitis, acyclovir is started immediately and continued for 14–21 days. Permanent cerebral damage is more common in infants than in adults.

Reye's Syndrome

Reye's syndrome is a rare complication of a viral infection and involves acute hepatic failure and encephalopathy. It is seen primarily in children with influenza or chickenpox infection who are given aspirin products. For this reason, salicylates are contraindicated in children.

Symptoms of a viral infection (typically an upper respiratory tract infection) are followed by severe nausea, vomiting, and an acute change in mental status. Hepatic dysfunction is demonstrated by altered liver function tests and increased prothrombin time. Hypoglycemia may be present. Seizures, loss of muscle tone, fixed and dilated pupils, coma, respiratory arrest, and death may all result.

The sudden onset of encephalopathy, severe vomiting, and liver dysfunction in the appropriate clinical context suggests Reye's syndrome. CSF pressure is increased. Liver biopsy showing fatty infiltration provides the definitive diagnosis.

No treatment is available, but early and intensive supportive care is useful and includes management of cerebral edema.

Brain Abscess

A brain abscess is a collection of pus in the brain usually resulting from bacterial infection. It may be caused by extension from cranial infections (mastoiditis, sinusitis), by direct inoculation after a head wound, or by hematogenous spread from a bacterial source elsewhere in the body. Streptococci, staphylococci, or anaerobes are usually responsible.

NEUROLOGY

After an infection or injury, patients develop progressive headache, nausea, vomiting, lethargy, papilledema, and focal neurologic abnormalities. Seizures and personality changes may be present. Brain abscesses are fatal if left untreated.

CT or MRI is diagnostic and typically shows a ring-enhancing lesion. Because of the risk of herniation, LP is contraindicated.

High-dose, broad-spectrum antibiotics should be used if the organism is unknown. Steroids may reduce cerebral edema. The patient's response to medication may be evaluated by serial CT scans. Surgical drainage is indicated for large abscesses to reduce the mass effect and eliminate infection.

Neurosyphilis

Late or tertiary syphilis can cause CNS infection and symptoms. Symptomatic neurosyphilis develops in only 5% of patients with untreated syphilis infection.

Patients with meningovascular neurosyphilis present with headache, dizziness, decreased concentration, cranial nerve palsies, and neck stiffness. Rarely, stroke is the presentation. Patients may also develop **tabes dorsalis**, caused by bilateral lesions of the posterior columns. It is characterized by irregular, intense, stabbing leg pain; impairment of proprioception and vibration sense; a wide-based gait; and loss of tendon reflexes. A characteristic sign is the **Argyll-Robertson pupil**, an irregular, small pupil that reacts to accommodation but not to light. In general paresis, diffuse cortical involvement causes dementia, memory loss, personality change, irritability, dysarthria, and facial tremor. Psychiatric disorders, such as delusions of grandeur or psychosis, may develop.

Serum VDRL is positive and the CSF shows elevated WBCs, increased protein, and a positive RPR. With tabes dorsalis, however, the RPR may be negative.

High-dose aqueous penicillin G is given intravenously for 10 days and may be followed by 3 additional weeks of IM benzathine penicillin. Analgesics may be used to control pain from tabes dorsalis, but this manifestation may progress despite appropriate therapy. The CSF should be examined every 3 to 6 months until it has been normal for 2 years.

Poliomyelitis

Poliovirus is transmitted through fecal-oral contact and may spread to the brain and motor neurons. There is also a small risk of developing vaccine-associated poliomyelitis after immunization with the oral polio vaccine (OPV).

NEUROLOGY

Most polio infections, especially in infants and young children, are subclinical, do not involve the CNS, and have no sequelae. If the illness progresses, it usually presents with signs of aseptic meningitis, including headache, fever, stiff neck, sore throat, vomiting, and muscle weakness. Focal or extensive paralysis then occurs. Sensation is not compromised.

Asymmetric paralysis during a febrile illness suggests polio. CSF lymphocytes are usually increased. For diagnosis, the virus must be isolated from the throat or stools, or an increase in polio-specific antibody must be shown.

Therapy is palliative. Artificial respiration is necessary in cases of respiratory failure. More than half of patients with paralytic poliomyelitis recover completely, but bulbar involvement is a bad prognostic sign.

Immunization with OPV has almost completely eliminated polio from the United States. The inactivated polio vaccine (IPV) is not associated with vaccine-induced polio and is currently recommended for routine immunizations of children.

Botulism

Botulism is a syndrome of neuromuscular deficits produced by the *Clostridium botulinum* toxin. In **food-borne botulism,** the toxin is ingested. Home-canned foods are a frequent culprit. Exposure to high heat for 30 minutes kills the spores, and the toxins are easily destroyed by heat. **Infant botulism** results from ingestion of spores, which then colonize the GI tract and produce toxin in vivo. Honey may contain these spores and should not be given to infants younger than 1 year of age. **Wound botulism** occurs when spores present in the environment contaminate the wound site and produce toxin.

Food-borne botulism has an abrupt onset 12 to 36 hours after toxin ingestion, and cranial nerve palsies, particularly of the extraocular muscles; fixed, dilated pupils; and diplopia are characteristic signs. Dry mouth is common, and dysphagia may cause aspiration. Nausea and vomiting may be present. The muscles of respiration weaken, leading to respiratory failure. Patients remain afebrile. Wound botulism results in neurologic symptoms without GI involvement, and patients have evidence of an injury or puncture wound. In infant botulism, constipation is usually the first sign, followed by cranial nerve symptoms and neuromuscular paralysis.

The toxin is found in serum, feces, or the suspected food.

Induced vomiting and gastric lavage help eliminate any unabsorbed toxin. Hospitalization is mandatory because supportive respiratory treatment may be needed. An antitoxin is available to halt progression of the disease.

Neoplasms

Primary Neoplasms

Primary brain tumors present most commonly in young and middle-aged adults. Local growth causes most of the symptoms and complications. Increased intracranial pressure is common and can occur with mass effect, cerebral edema, hydrocephalus, obstructed venous sinuses, or obstructed CSF resorption. **Glioblastoma multiforme,** a malignant glioma, is the most common primary malignant brain tumor in adults, and it has a very high mortality rate. **Meningioma** is the most common benign tumor of adults. Meningiomas may grow very large before they create symptoms. The most common primary childhood tumors include **cerebellar astrocytomas** and **medulloblastomas.**

Headache, classically postural and worst on waking, and vomiting are prominent early symptoms. Patients may also present with lethargy, stupor, personality changes, and mental deterioration. Convulsive seizures are more frequent with lesions of the cerebrum, particularly meningiomas and slow-growing astrocytomas. Focal manifestations that are due to local mass effects are also commonly seen. An important syndrome is uncal herniation, in which the temporal lobe uncus compresses the third cranial nerve followed by the midbrain, resulting in ipsilateral fixed papillary dilation (blown pupil) followed by coma and then death.

CT, MRI, and biopsy are used in diagnosis.

Treatment involves resection when possible and debulking when necessary, as well as radiation and chemotherapy. Steroids reduce cerebral edema, and anticonvulsants prevent seizures. Prognosis varies depending on the tumor type and location.

Metastatic Neoplasms

Metastatic brain tumors are the most common brain tumors in adults and most frequently originate from bronchogenic carcinoma, breast adenocarcinoma, and malignant melanoma. They are uncommon in children. Presenting signs and symptoms are indistinuishable from those of a primary neoplasm. CT or MRI may show single or multiple lesions. Resection and irradiation can be used to treat single metastasis but are often not attempted for multiple metastases. The underlying cancer should be treated as much as possible. Prognosis is typically poor.

Neurofibromatosis

Neurofibromatosis is a neurocutaneous disease that can be sporadic or familial, with autosomal-dominant inheritance. Type 1 (von Recklinghausen's disease) is much more common than type 2 and presents with multiple cutaneous and noncutaneous neurofibromas, unilateral acoustic neuroma (a neurofibroma of the 8th cranial nerve), iris hamartomas, optic gliomas, bone lesions, café-au-lait-pigmented macules, and axillary freckles. Type 2 typically presents with bilateral acoustic neuromas in addition to multiple peripheral or central nervous system tumors, including neurofibromas, gliomas, schwannomas, and meningiomas. Surgical excision is indicated for symptomatic tumors. Plastic surgery is useful for cutaneous neuromas. Genetics counseling for the patient and the family is valuable.

Degenerative Disorders

Alzheimer's Disease

Alzheimer's disease is a slowly progressive dementia of unknown cause. It is the most common cause of dementia, affecting the elderly (typical onset after age 80 years), those with trisomy 21, and those with the autosomal-dominant familial Alzheimer's disease (typical onset after age 60 years). While normal aging can be associated with a mild reduction in short-term memory, the decline is more gradual and less severe, and intellectual function remains unimpaired. While advanced Alzheimer's disease can cause psychosis, dementia continues to be prominent, permitting distinction from other causes of psychosis.

SIGNS & SYMPTOMS

Progressive short-term memory loss is the first symptom, followed by disorientation, depression, agitation, apraxias, and anomia. Frontal release signs may be present. Later stages tend to show psychiatric abnormalities, such as personality changes, paranoia, delusions, and psychosis. Eventually, the patient becomes bedridden and incontinent. Death occurs within 5 to 10 years of onset of symptoms, usually secondary to aspiration.

DIAGNOSIS

No definitive premortem diagnostic test exists, so the diagnosis is made primarily on clinical grounds after ruling out other causes of dementia (e.g., syphilis, hypothyroid, HIV, vitamin B_{12} deficiency, multi-infarct dementia). CT shows cortical atrophy.

TREATMENT

No effective treatment exists, although cholinergic stimulants (e.g., tacrine, donepezil, and ginkgo biloba) may provide slight benefits in some patients. Well-established routines, tools for orientation, and supportive care are useful, and support for caregivers is essential.

Multi-infarct Dementia

Multi-infarct dementia, also known as vascular dementia, is a common cause of dementia. It is believed that the accumulation of multiple cortical infarcts, many subclinical, is responsible. Patients tend to have stroke risk factors—for example, chronic hypertension—and develop a stepwise progression of neurologic deficits.

SIGNS & SYMPTOMS

At the time of presentation, focal upper motor neuron and sensory deficits, ataxia, and gait apraxia may be present. Pseudobulbar palsy, with dysarthria, dysphagia, and uninhibited laughter or crying, also may be evident. The dementia proceeds with stepwise loss of impulse control, decreases in short-term memory, and disorientation. Personality changes may develop. On exam, frontal release signs may be present.

NEUROLOGY

MRI shows multiple small cortical and subcortical lesions. Etiologies of stroke, including embolic sources and meningovascular syphilis, should be sought.

No effective treatment exists. Hypertension and other stroke risk factors should be addressed.

Huntington's Disease

Huntington's disease is a progressive, hereditary disorder involving abnormalities in movement and mental function. It is transmitted in an autosomal-dominant pattern with complete penetrance but does not become symptomatic until patients are between the ages of 30 and 50 years.

Patients initially show subtle features of dementia, including irritability and antisocial behavior. Initial movement disturbances may also be subtle, but they eventually develop into chorea (rapid, irregular involuntary movements of the digits and extremities). The chorea and dementia progress slowly, leading to death approximately 15 years after onset.

A positive family history is very useful in diagnosis. CT or MRI shows atrophy of the caudate nucleus and cerebral cortex. Genetic screening is available for asymptomatic family members but should only be undertaken after extensive counseling.

No treatment exists for the disease itself. Chorea can be partially controlled with a dopamine antagonist, such as haloperidol. Genetic counseling for the patient and family is important.

Parkinsonism

Parkinsonism is a syndrome characterized by a resting tremor, decreased movement, muscular rigidity, and postural instability. Idiopathic Parkinson's disease involves the loss of dopaminergic cells in the substantia nigra, leading to an imbalance of cholinergic input into the striatum. Other etiologies include therapeutic drugs, such as phenothiazines, and MPTP, a by-product of the manufacture of illicit home-made recreational drugs.

Most patients develop a resting tremor that is initially confined to one limb (a "pill-rolling" tremor) but may eventually generalize. Voluntary movement and automatic movement decrease, and the patient develops mask-like facies, infrequent blinking, and a lack of arm-swinging while walking. The characteristic rigidity of the parkinsonian patient is caused by increased tone affecting both agonist and antagonist muscles, and cogwheel rigidity is common. Patients have difficulty initiating movement. They

NEUROLOGY

walk with small, shuffling steps, in some cases with increasing speed (festinating gait), and they often have difficulty stopping. Dementia occurs in some cases.

Clinical presentation.

Dopaminergic agonists and cholinergic antagonists are useful in the treatment of Parkinson's disease. Frequently used dopaminergic agents include levodopa (a dopamine precursor), pergolide, and bromocriptine. Amantadine is also beneficial. Levodopa is administered with carbidopa, which inhibits the breakdown of levodopa outside of the brain. Benztropine is a common anticholinergic agent. Pallidotomy or thalamotomy may be beneficial in patients with severe disease refractory to medical treatment. Chronic deep brain electrical stimulation of the subthalamic nucleus or globus pallidus appears to be an effective alternative and is being performed at some tertiary care centers.

Amyotrophic Lateral Sclerosis

Amyotrophic lateral sclerosis (ALS), also known as *Lou Gehrig disease,* is a disease of upper and lower motor neurons, involving a progressive loss of anterior horn cells and their afferents. Bulbar musculature may also be involved. Most cases of ALS are idiopathic, but 5% have a genetic, autosomal-dominant transmission. Middle-aged men are most commonly affected. Half of ALS patients die within 3 years of onset, and only a small minority live more than 10 years.

Upper or lower extremity weakness and atrophy reflect lower motor neuron dysfunction and are present in an asymmetric distribution. Muscle spasticity with increased deep tendon reflexes may be present and reflects upper motor neuron involvement. Dysarthria and dysphagia and other evidence of bulbar involvement may also be present. There are no sensory abnormalities.

Clinical diagnosis requires upper and lower motor neuron signs in three extremities or in two extremities and the bulbar region. Electromyography (EMG) and nerve conduction studies demonstrate upper and lower motor neuron abnormalities in at least three regions.

No effective treatment is known. Riluzole may slow progression of disease.

Demyelinating Disorders

Multiple Sclerosis

Multiple sclerosis (MS) is a progressive demyelinating disease that affects the brain, spinal cord, and optic nerve. The cause is unknown, but immune-mediated and viral etiologies are both popular theories. Women are more commonly affected than men, with peak ages of onset between 20 and 40 years.

Initial presentations are diverse, including unilateral optic neuritis, diplopia, focal paresthesias, focal weakness or unsteadiness, and bladder dysfunction. The disease progresses slowly and unpredictably, with periods of remissions and exacerbations. Infection, trauma, or childbirth may trigger relapses. Eventually, the patient may develop optic atrophy, nystagmus, dysarthria, upper motor neuron deficits, cerebellar dysfunction, and sensory abnormalities. Approximately half of patients are significantly disabled 10 years after symptoms begin.

Gradual onset of varied CNS deficits suggests MS. MRI shows multiple white matter lesions. CSF is abnormal in most patients, with mildly increased protein, mild lymphocytosis, and oligoclonal bands.

No treatment prevents progression of the disease, but avoiding stress and fatigue seems to help. In this regard, counseling, therapy, and rest may be useful. Corticosteroids may hasten the recovery from acute exacerbations. Interferon-γ and copolymer 1 decrease the frequency of exacerbations. At least partial recovery from an acute exacerbation is likely, but residual deficits are likely to accumulate with serial exacerbations.

Guillain-Barré Syndrome

Guillain-Barré syndrome, also known as acute idiopathic polyneuropathy, is a polyneuropathy of unknown cause that can follow minor viral infections, inoculations, or surgeries. It is presumed to be immune-mediated.

Patients present with progressive, bilateral weakness in the legs. Weakness is typically proximal and can extend to the upper extremities and face. Sensory deficits may be associated, and deep tendon reflexes are absent. Autonomic dysfunction may occur, including instability of temperature, blood pressure, heart rate, and sphincter control. Involvement of the respiratory muscles or the pharynx can be lethal. The disease generally stabilizes within 1 month of onset. Most patients recover completely, but some retain neurologic defects.

Diagnosis is largely clinical. CSF shows increased protein, with normal pressure, glucose, and cell number. Electrophysiologic studies show multiple, varied abnormalities.

Plasmapheresis accelerates recovery. Intravenous immunoglobulin (IVIG) is also beneficial. Corticosteroids are contraindicated, as they may exacerbate symptoms and delay recovery. Because of the risks of respiratory and vascular collapse, patients should be closely monitored.

NEUROLOGY

Neuromuscular Disorders

Myasthenia Gravis

Myasthenia gravis is an autoimmune disorder of neurotransmission and is slowly progressive. Antibodies against the acetylcholine receptor at the neuromuscular junction impair normal neuromuscular transmission. Myasthenia gravis is more common in women and occurs with greatest frequency between the ages of 20 and 40 years. Thymoma is frequently present.

SIGNS & SYMPTOMS

Episodic weakness and easy muscle fatigability may involve all muscles, particularly those innervated by the cranial nerves. The most common presentations involve ptosis, diplopia, difficulty swallowing, and limb weakness. Weakness is worsened by activity, improved by rest, and tends to fluctuate diurnally. Respiratory compromise may cause death.

DIAGNOSIS

Most patients have acetylcholine-receptor antibodies present in their serum. Chest x-ray or CT may show a thymoma. Diagnosis is confirmed when administration of an exogenous anticholinesterase, such as edrophonium or neostigmine, leads to increased levels of acetylcholine at the neuromuscular junction and provides transient relief of symptoms.

TREATMENT

Anticholinesterase drugs, such as neostigmine, provide symptomatic benefit. Thymectomy in patients younger than 60 years usually leads to improvement. Corticosteroids or azathioprine are used in patients unresponsive to other treatments, and plasmapheresis and IVIG provide additional alternatives.

Lambert-Eaton Syndrome

Lambert-Eaton syndrome, also known as myasthenic syndrome, is another autoimmune disorder of neuromuscular transmission. Often associated with an underlying malignancy, such as small-cell carcinoma, it involves the production of antibodies that cross-react with the voltage-gated calcium channels of the presynaptic terminal of the neuromuscular junction, inhibiting neuromuscular transmission.

SIGNS & SYMPTOMS

Patients present with proximal muscle weakness, but the extraocular muscles are typically spared. Autonomic impairment may also occur. In contrast to myasthenia gravis, weakness improves with sustained activity.

DIAGNOSIS

Demonstration of antibodies against the P/Q subtype of voltage-gated calcium channels is definitive. Electrophysiological studies show improved muscle response with repetitive activity.

TREATMENT

Corticosteroids, azathioprine, and plasmapheresis are all effective. An underlying malignancy should be treated, if present. Guanidine may be helpful in severe cases. Anticholinesterase drugs are of variable value.

NEUROLOGY

Miscellaneous Conditions

Peripheral Neuropathy

Dysfunction of the peripheral nerves may involve motor, sensory, or autonomic fibers. **Mononeuropathy** refers to involvement of a single nerve. Mononeuropathies are most commonly caused by trauma, particularly when entrapment or compression is involved. Leprosy can also cause a form of mononeuropathy. **Multiple mononeuropathy** (mononeuritis multiplex) refers to involvement of more than one nerve asymmetrically and in separate areas. Multiple mononeuropathies arise in collagen vascular disorders, such as systemic lupus erythematosus, rheumatoid arthritis, and vasculitis; in metabolic diseases, such as diabetes mellitus; and in infectious diseases, such as HIV, leprosy, or Lyme disease.

   Polyneuropathy is the involvement of many nerves simultaneously and in the same region. It usually develops slowly, affecting the distal lower extremities first. The disorder most often arises in the setting of metabolic disorders, such as diabetes or uremia, or nutritional deficiencies, such as deficiency of vitamin B_1 or B_{12}, but it may also arise with Guillain-Barré syndrome, hereditary conditions, malignancy, paraproteinemias, and toxins, such as alcohol, phenytoin, heavy metals, and industrial solvents.

SIGNS & SYMPTOMS

Clinical manifestations typically include muscle weakness and atrophy, decreased deep tendon reflexes, and/or sensory impairment.

DIAGNOSIS

EMG and nerve conduction velocity studies are useful in confirming neuropathy and distinguishing axonal from paranodal and segmental demyelination. General workup for etiology includes a complete blood count, renal function tests, glucose, erythrocyte sedimentation rate (ESR), serum protein electrophoresis, VDRL, rheumatoid factor, urine heavy metal levels, and thyroid function tests, as well as a thorough history and examination. Biopsy can diagnose infiltrative diseases and vasculitis.

TREATMENT

Treatment of the systemic disorders occasionally permits a slow recovery. Apposition of transected nerves is important in cases of trauma. Surgical decompression or corticosteroids can be useful in entrapment neuropathies.

Ataxia

Ataxia involves a lack of coordination caused by cerebellar, vestibular, or sensory dysfunction. It may present with abnormalities of gait, speech, or eye movement. **Cerebellar ataxia** presents with irregular voluntary movement. These patients have decreased muscle tone, decreased coordination, intention tremor, nystagmus, gaze paresis, and abnormal smooth pursuit and saccades.

   Vestibular ataxia presents as a lack of limb coordination that resolves while the patient is lying down. These patients may have a unilateral nystagmus and may report vertigo. **Sen-**

NEUROLOGY

sory ataxia is caused by lesions of the proprioceptive pathway. Lesions of the posterior columns and polyneuropathies tend to affect the legs symmetrically. Joint position and vibration sense are impaired.

Gait Abnormality

Normal gait requires intact coordination of the motor, vestibular, and proprioceptive pathways. Lesions at any level will produce characteristic abnormalities. A few examples follow:

- **Cerebellar lesions** cause a truncal ataxia, with a broad-based, unsteady, and irregular gait. Turning is impaired.
- In **corticospinal disorders** such as hemiparesis, the affected leg circumducts as it steps forward and may also drag somewhat, leading to asymmetric shoe wear. A scissors-like gait is typical of bilateral involvement.
- **Extrapyramidal lesions,** such as those seen in Parkinson's disease, cause a characteristic festinating gait. Patients assume a flexed posture and walk in small but rapid steps, without arm swinging.
- **Motor system lesions** (lesions of anterior horn cells, peripheral motor nerves, and skeletal muscle) cause footdrop if the anterior tibial muscle is involved. Calf muscle involvement prevents patients from being able to walk on their toes. Pelvic muscle involvement may cause a waddling gait.
- Patients with **sensory deficits** walk with their feet markedly raised in a steppage gait. They also have difficulty walking with closed eyes.

Syncope

Syncope (fainting) is an acute onset and transient loss of consciousness. It is frequently preceded by light-headedness, nausea, or weakness. Orthostatic hypotension, vasovagal, and cardiogenic syncope are the most common causes. Cardiac etiologies may lead to syncope if reduced cardiac output causes insufficient cerebral blood flow. In these patients, syncope is frequently related to exertion. Cardiovascular causes include arrhythmia, aortic stenosis, hypovolemia, peripheral vasodilation, and decreased venous return. Pulmonary embolism and metabolic abnormalities are rarer causes of noncardiogenic syncope.

Coma

Coma is a state of unresponsiveness from which the patient cannot be aroused. It arises from dysfunction of both cerebral hemispheres or of the brainstem reticular activating system. It can develop with mass lesions, metabolic encephalopathy, hypothermia, or seizures.

SIGNS & SYMPTOMS

The patient does not respond to verbal command or mechanical stimulation, although localizing movements or flexor or extensor posturing in response to pain may be present.

NEUROLOGY

DIAGNOSIS

Coma of acute onset is typical of a subarachnoid hemorrhage or a brainstem stroke. A progression to coma over minutes or hours occurs with intracerebral hemorrhage. Onset over days to a week suggests chronic subdural hematoma, tumor, or abscess. A coma that develops without focal signs of lateralization and that follows symptoms of delirium often is due to metabolic causes.

Pupil size can suggest the presence and location of an intracerebral mass. Pupils are slightly smaller than their normal 3- to 4-mm diameter during early transtentorial herniation with thalamic involvement. Dilated pupils (5 to 7 mm) nonreactive to light suggest damage at or below the midbrain. Pinpoint pupils of 1-mm diameter suggest a pontine lesion, opioid overdose, or some other exogenous toxin. In metabolic coma, the pupillary reflex remains intact, even when extraocular movements are impaired.

Motor response to pain also indicates the level of brain dysfunction. Localizing responses to pain occur in superficial coma. The decorticate response, with flexion at the elbow and leg extension, suggests a thalamic lesion of compression. The decerebrate response, characterized by elbow and leg extension, suggests a midbrain lesion (Figure 13-6). No response to pain occurs in patients with pontine or medullary compromise.

TREATMENT

Emergency management of the comatose patient involves the *ABCs,* with maintenance of *a*irway patency, *b*reathing, and *c*irculation. Blood must be analyzed for infection and metabolic abnormalities. Glucose, thiamine, and naloxone may be administered intravenously to treat several possible causes of coma. Anticonvulsants are given if seizures are present. The underlying cause of the coma should be rapidly identified and treated.

NEUROLOGY

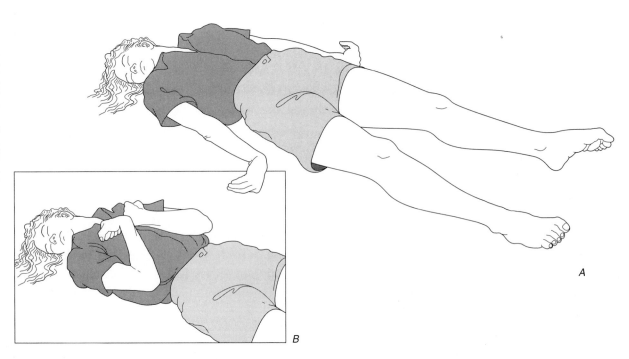

Fig. 13-6. A: Decerebrate posture. **B:** Decorticate posture. (Reprinted with permission from Caroline N: *Emergency Care in the Streets,* 5th ed. Boston, Little Brown, 1995, p 338.)

Vision Loss

Blindness

Visual acuity of 20/200 or worse with the best possible correction (e.g., glasses) is the legal definition of blindness. In the United States, prophylaxis of newborns with erythromycin to prevent chlamydia and gonococcal infection has effectively eliminated a major cause of blindness. Another preventable form of unilateral blindness, amblyopia (misalignment of the eyes), can often be corrected early in life with glasses or surgery. Finally, congenital cataracts, which are associated with a number of prenatal infections, such as rubella, may be prevented or treated early to maximize useful vision.

In adults, the major causes of blindness are glaucoma, cataracts, diabetic retinopathy, and macular degeneration. These disorders are discussed in more detail in the following sections.

Open-angle Glaucoma

Glaucoma refers to increased intraocular pressure, and open-angle glaucoma is the most prevalent form of the disease. It is characterized by a gradual, bilateral rise in intraocular pressure, leading to gradual loss of vision. The cause is unknown. Open-angle glaucoma is more common in elderly patients, diabetic patients, and African-Americans. It tends to be familial.

SIGNS & SYMPTOMS

Patients are asymptomatic initially, then experience gradual loss of peripheral vision, resulting in "tunnel vision." Eventually, central vision is lost as well. Patients may report "halos" around lights if the intraocular pressure is severely increased. On examination, cupping of the optic disk may be noted as an increase in the cup:disk ratio.

DIAGNOSIS

Tonometry (pressure testing), optic nerve visualization, and visual field testing confirm the diagnosis. One elevated pressure reading does not confirm or refute the presence of glaucoma because intraocular pressure varies throughout the day.

TREATMENT

Beta-adrenergic antagonists, such as timolol, and pilocarpine or other agents must be used daily. These medications decrease the production or facilitate the removal of aqueous humor, reducing the intraocular pressure. If medication is not effective, widening of the drainage canal by laser or surgical procedures may be necessary.

PREVENTION

All persons older than age 40 years should undergo tonometry and careful ophthalmoscopic evaluation every 3 to 5 years. Diabetics and individuals with a family history of glaucoma should begin testing at an earlier age.

Closed-angle Glaucoma

Closed-angle glaucoma is characterized by the rapid onset of increased intraocular pressure that is due to a blockage of the aqueous drainage of the eye. Approximately 1% of the population, predominantly Asians, elderly persons, and people with hyperopia (far-sightedness),

NEUROLOGY

have pre-existing narrowness of the anterior chamber angle; however, the majority of these individuals do not develop disease. Angle closure may occur with pupillary dilation (e.g., sitting in a darkened room or receiving a pharmacologic mydriatic during an eye examination).

Severe eye pain, blurred vision, and "halos" around lights are often accompanied by nausea and abdominal pain. The cause of the abdominal manifestations is unclear. On examination, patients have a red eye, a steamy-appearing cornea, and a dilated, nonreactive pupil. Increased pressure also causes the eye to feel "hard" on palpation.

Tonometry reveals a markedly increased intraocular pressure.

Administration of oral glycerin, mannitol, or acetazolamide will rapidly reduce intraocular pressure. Frequent administration of pilocarpine, which produces miosis, is also indicated. Permanent correction involves laser iridotomy or surgical iridectomy and is usually performed on the unaffected eye as well. Untreated acute-angle glaucoma usually results in permanent loss of vision within days.

Cataracts

Cataracts are a painless clouding of the lens. They are often bilateral. Cataracts may occur congenitally, after trauma, in systemic diseases, such as diabetes, with corticosteroid medications, or, most commonly, with increasing age. Cataract development is also associated with smoking.

Patients report painless and progressive blurring of vision, often over several months. Gray opacities of the lenses may be seen with ophthalmoscopic or slit-lamp examination. Red reflex may be absent.

The preceding signs and symptoms suggest the diagnosis.

Glasses may be helpful in early stages, but lens extraction and replacement surgery provide definitive treatment and are performed routinely.

Eye Infection

Conjunctivitis

Acute inflammation of the conjunctiva (the mucosal surface of the eye and eyelid) is typically caused by viruses, bacteria, or allergens. Adenoviruses are the most common cause, followed by staphylococci, streptococci, and *Haemophilus* species. *Neisseria gonorrhoeae* and

Chlamydia trachomatis may be involved in more severe infections. Conjunctivitis is highly transmissible and can develop after contact with infected hands, towels, and handkerchiefs.

Copious discharge in a red eye, accompanied by mild discomfort with little or no visual blurring, is the common presentation. On examination, the conjunctiva appears inflamed and injected. Bacterial conjunctivitis is accompanied by purulent discharge. Viral and chlamydial conjunctivitis may be associated with a tender preauricular lymph node and a follicular pattern of conjunctivitis. Allergic conjunctivitis is often itchy.

Gram's stain and culture of the discharge may provide the diagnosis of bacterial conjunctivitis. Most cases are diagnosed by the history and examination findings.

The majority of cases are self-limiting, but topical sulfonamide may speed recovery of bacterial conjunctivitis. Conjunctivitis caused by allergy may be treated with antihistamine or steroid solutions. The patient should wash his or her hands frequently to prevent the spread of infection.

Uveitis

Uveitis is characterized by inflammation of the uveal tract (iris, ciliary body, and choroid layer). Multiple diseases are associated with uveitis, including HLA-B27 collagen vascular diseases (e.g., Reiter's syndrome and ankylosing spondylitis), infections (e.g., herpes simplex virus, varicella zoster, and syphilis), GI diseases (e.g., Crohn's disease and ulcerative colitis), and diseases of unknown etiology (e.g., sarcoidosis).

Unilateral pain, redness, and photophobia are seen in cases of anterior uveitis (iridocyclitis). Subtle changes in vision, such as haziness or floating spots, are characteristic of posterior uveitis. Long-standing anterior uveitis can cause closed-angle glaucoma.

Slit-lamp examination in anterior uveitis shows cells and flare within the aqueous humor and cells with keratin precipitates on the corneal endothelium. In posterior uveitis, cells are visible within the vitreous, and retinal and choroid lesions may be evident. A "salt and pepper" fundus is characteristic of syphilis.

Topical corticosteroids and pupil dilation are useful in anterior uveitis. Systemic corticosteroids are useful in posterior uveitis. Patients should also be evaluated for signs of related systemic diseases such as ankylosing spondylitis and syphilis. Infections should be treated.

Retinal Disorders

Senile Macular Degeneration

Senile macular degeneration is the primary cause of vision loss in the elderly. It is caused by atrophic or exudative degeneration of the retina, resulting in retinal scarring and fibrosis and possible retinal pigment epithelium (RPE) detachment or serous retinal detachment. It is usually bilateral and may be hereditary.

Patients typically experience a gradual loss of visual acuity, especially of central vision, although acute changes occur with detachment and hemorrhage. Funduscopic examination shows hemorrhagic or pigmented areas in the macula (a normally yellow area of the retina near the optic disk) and may show retinal or RPE detachment. Yellow deposits in the macula signify drusen.

Fluorescein angiography may demonstrate the presence of neovascular membranes, the result of neovascularization between the RPE and Bruch's membrane, which cause permanent loss of vision.

Laser photocoagulation may arrest further loss of vision.

Central Retinal Artery Occlusion

Occlusion of the central retinal artery presents as the sudden, painless loss of sight in one eye. Common causes include thromboembolic disease and temporal arteritis. Examination may show a pale fundus with a "cherry-red spot" fovea (the central area of the macula and the sight of clearest vision) and the "boxcar" appearance of blood in the veins. Emergency referral to an ophthalmologist is essential. Treatment includes oxygen, ocular massage, acetazolamide, and fluid removal from the eye. Thrombolysis is sometimes used to treat embolic occlusion. High-dose corticosteroids are used to treat temporal arteritis.

Central Retinal Vein Occlusion

Occlusion of the central retinal vein typically occurs in elderly patients with atherosclerosis, but it is also associated with diabetes, glaucoma, hypertension, and hypercoagulable states. Unilateral painless impairment of sight tends to progress gradually. Examination shows swelling of the optic disk, cotton-wool spots, retinal hemorrhages, and tortuous, dilated veins. There is no widely accepted treatment; however, emergent ophthalmologic evaluation is important to distinguish this from any treatable causes of vision loss.

Diabetic Retinopathy

The development of diabetic retinopathy is related to the duration of diabetes. It is found in 20% of patients with type 2 diabetes at diagnosis and is seen frequently in type 1 diabetic patients. Damage to the retinal vasculature, including microaneurysms, ischemic changes, and neovascularization with abnormal vessels, is primarily responsible for the resulting vision loss.

SIGNS & SYMPTOMS

Vision is normal until later stages, when patients report decreased visual acuity. Other frequent symptoms include black spots, "cobwebs," and flashing lights. Ophthalmoscopic examination in nonproliferative retinopathy reveals microaneurysms, blot hemorrhages, infarcts, hard exudates, and macular edema. These changes occur early and do not tend to compromise vision until macular edema develops. In proliferative retinopathy, new tortuous vessels grow on the retina (neovascularization). These vessels are fragile and prone to hemorrhage. Fibrosis during healing can incite retinal detachment.

DIAGNOSIS

The preceding physical examination findings in a diabetic patient suggest the diagnosis.

TREATMENT

Laser photocoagulation or vitrectomy may decrease or eliminate neovascularization and hemorrhage.

PREVENTION

Good control of glucose levels reduces the risk of developing diabetic retinopathy but cannot reverse pre-existing damage. Diabetic patients should receive annual ophthalmologic examinations to monitor and treat asymptomatic development of retinal changes.

Retinal Detachment

The retina may separate from the pigment layer of the epithelium spontaneously or after acute trauma. Risk factors include myopia and cataract extraction. The accompanying unilateral, painless loss of vision is generally described as a "curtain" coming down over the eye. Funduscopic examination reveals a gray retina hanging within the vitreous humor. Because the area of retinal detachment increases quickly over time, treatment should be instituted quickly. Treatment options include laser photocoagulation, cryotherapy, and other techniques to close the retinal tears and reattach the retina.

Common Signs of Eye Disorders

Diplopia

Also known as "double vision," diplopia can occur in a number of contexts. Misalignment, cranial nerve dysfunction, and vascular disturbances may all be involved. Trauma resulting in damage to the muscles or orbit may also cause diplopia. Monocular diplopia (double vision when one eye is covered) is usually caused by lens abnormalities.

NEUROLOGY

Papilledema

Bilateral swelling of the optic disks because of increased intracranial pressure is termed papilledema. Patients are often asymptomatic but may report mild changes in vision, such as enlargement of the blind spot. Common causes include cerebral trauma or hemorrhage, meningitis, severe hypertension, and tumors.

Optic Atrophy

Degeneration of the optic nerve is often due to inflammation. The optic disk may be whitish or gray and often has indistinct edges. Loss of vision is generally proportional to the amount of degeneration. The presence of optic atrophy requires further investigation into its origin. In some cases (e.g., tumor removal), sight can be completely restored.

Audiovestibular Disorders

Hearing Loss

Hearing loss is divided into two major categories: **conductive hearing loss,** which is caused by damage to the middle or external ear canal; and **sensorineural hearing loss,** which results from damage to the inner ear or auditory nerve. Chronic ear infections and trauma are common causes of conductive hearing loss. Causes of sensorineural hearing loss include hair cell damage from noise, ototoxicity, and aging, as well as acoustic neuromas, stroke, and multiple sclerosis.

Two commonly used tests of hearing are Rinne's test and Weber's test. With Rinne's test, a vibrating tuning fork is held against the mastoid process and then in the air adjacent to the pinna to compare bone conduction and air conduction. Normally, the position in front of the pinna is perceived as louder; if not, the patient may have a conductive hearing loss. In Weber's test, the tuning fork is held against the midline of the forehead. A patient with unilateral conductive hearing loss hears the sound more loudly in the affected ear, whereas a patient with unilateral sensorineural hearing loss hears the sound more loudly in the unaffected ear. An audiometer can provide more specific information about the extent of hearing loss.

Presbycusis is the normal loss of hearing that occurs with aging. It is sensorineural in origin, resulting from stiffening and deterioration of the hair cells and basilar membrane. It initially affects high-frequency sounds, and it may be related to noise exposure. Men are more frequently affected than women. Amplification with a hearing aid and lip reading may be helpful.

Otitis Externa

Also known as "swimmer's ear," otitis externa is an infection most frequently caused by gram-negative rods such as *E. coli, Pseudomonas,* and *Proteus,* although *Staphylococcus aureus* may cause localized inflammation (a "furuncle"). Predisposing factors include frequent cotton swab use and recent water exposure.

Patients typically report itching, pain, and discharge from the affected ear. More severe cases result in hearing loss that is due to swelling of the ear canal. On examination, the external auditory canal appears red and swollen, and purulent discharge may be present. The patient characteristically reports tenderness on manipulation of the pinna.

The preceding symptoms and physical findings suggest the diagnosis.

After removal of superficial debris, topical antibiotics and corticosteroids are useful. If the infection is persistent, oral antibiotics that cover *Pseudomonas* are indicated, particularly in diabetics and immune-compromised patients, who are at risk for osteomyelitis of the skull base, termed malignant otitis externa.

Vertigo

Vertigo is an inappropriate sensation of rotational movement that is often associated with disturbances in balance and gait. Nystagmus is present during episodes of vertigo. Vertigo occurs in the context of a number of disorders, including Ménière's disease, but it may also be associated with inner ear disorders, such as benign positional vertigo, viral infections (labyrinthitis), and lesions of the eighth nerve and brainstem, such as multiple sclerosis and stroke. Neurologic examination of the cranial nerves and cerebellum is indicated. Meclizine is used for symptomatic treatment. Ménière's disease is described below. Benign positional vertigo is usually sudden in onset and can be provoked with head movement. It is currently believed that a loose otolith in a semicircular canal is responsible. Physical maneuvers designed to free the otolith from the canal appear to be effective. Labyrinthitis presents shortly after an upper respiratory infection (URI) with sudden onset and continuous vertigo and often is accompanied by hearing loss and tinnitus. It typically lasts up to a week and then gradually improves over weeks. Multiple sclerosis and stroke are described previously in this chapter.

Tinnitus

Tinnitus refers to the perception of noise without the presence of an exogenous source of the sound. The most commonly perceived sound is that of ringing, but buzzing, whistling, and roaring noises are also common. Brief episodes of tinnitus may be normal; more prolonged episodes may be associated with a multitude of disorders, including Ménière's disease, ear infection, ototoxic drug use, aspirin overdose, and excessive noise exposure. Pulsatile tinnitus, while quite rare, may indicate a vascular abnormality, such as an arteriovenous malformation, and requires careful workup. Treatment is directed at the underlying cause, and nortriptyline may be helpful in some cases.

Ménière's Disease

Ménière's disease, also known as endolymphatic hydrops, is a disorder characterized by severe, episodic vertigo, progressive sensorineural hearing loss, tinnitus, and a sensation of fullness in the ears. It is thought to be related to distention of the endolymphatic sac in the inner ear. It typically occurs in middle age.

Sudden attacks of vertigo, which may last up to 24 hours, are accompanied by nausea and vomiting, sensorineural hearing loss, tinnitus, and a sense of ear fullness. Over several years, significant hearing loss occurs. Tinnitus may be constant and often worsens during a vertiginous attack.

The preceding symptoms suggest the diagnosis.

Symptomatic relief of the vertigo is achieved through anticholinergics and antihistamines. Diazepam may also be effective. Diuretics and salt restriction are used to decrease endolymphatic fluid volume. Surgical intervention may be helpful if medical treatment is not sufficient.

Acoustic Neuroma

Also known as *vestibular schwannoma,* acoustic neuromas are benign tumors of the Schwann cells of the eighth cranial nerve that grow in the cerebellopontine angle and may expand and compress the eighth nerve, the cerebellum, and the brainstem.

Unilateral hearing loss, sustained mild dizziness, and tinnitus are common symptoms. On examination, the hearing loss appears sensorineural in origin. Unilateral facial palsy, decreased hemiface sensation, and ataxia may be present in more advanced cases.

Audiography demonstrates sensorineural hearing loss. MRI identifies the tumor and assesses its impingement on normal brain tissue.

Surgical excision.

Toxic Ear Damage

Toxic ear damage may occur as a result of intense noise or ototoxic drugs. Drugs most commonly associated with ear damage include aminoglycosides (e.g., gentamicin), furosemide, salicylates, quinine, and cisplatin. Prevention measures include ear protectors (for excessive noise) and avoidance of ototoxic drugs, especially in pregnancy or in patients with pre-existing hearing loss.

NEUROLOGY

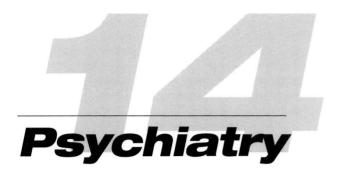

Psychiatry

Principles of Diagnosis

Psychiatric and medical disorders are classified on a multiaxis scheme.

Axis I   Clinical psychiatric disorders
Axis II   Personality disorders and development disorders
Axis III   Medical conditions
Axis IV   Psychosocial stress (6-point scale)
Axis V   Global assessment of functioning (90-point scale)

Diagnosis of psychiatric disorders (axis I and II) is based on specific sets of criteria, published in the *Diagnostic and Statistical Manual of Mental Disorders,* 4th edition (*DSM-IV*). Axis III is for the patient's medical conditions, whether they contribute to, result from, or are unrelated to the psychiatric disorder. Axis IV assesses stressors that significantly affect the current psychiatric disorder, and axis V is used to describe how well the patient has functioned in society during the past year, excluding the current exacerbation.

Emergency and Acute Care

Suicidal Ideation

Approximately 30,000 suicides occur every year in the United States. For every "successful" suicide, there are approximately ten attempted suicides. Risk factors for "successful" suicide include:

1. Age older than 45 years
2. Alcoholism
3. Rage and violent behavior
4. Prior suicide attempts
5. Male gender
6. Experiencing a recent loss or separation
7. Depression
8. Unemployment or retirement
9. Being single, widowed, or divorced

Patients who have a realistic suicide plan are at greater risk. Behaviors such as making a will or giving away personal property should be taken seriously. Hospitalization may not be required in patients who agree or "contract" to call in for help if their suicidal ideation worsens. In this case, someone must be available to the patient at all times. Involuntary hospitalization is clearly permitted for patients who may pose a danger to themselves. Alcohol addiction should be addressed. Medications, therapy, and electroconvulsive therapy should then be initiated as needed.

PSYCHIATRY

Homicidal Ideation

The possibility of causing danger to others is another clear indication for involuntary hospitalization. The patient may be restrained or sedated if necessary. Treatment directed at any underlying disorder should be initiated.

Neuroleptic Malignant Syndrome

Neuroleptic malignant syndrome is a serious complication of antipsychotic medications. It occurs within 1 to 3 days of starting medication and may last up to 2 weeks. Men have this reaction more frequently than women, and the mortality rate is as high as 25%. The pathology is not understood.

Extremely high fever and muscular rigidity develop, in addition to agitation, tachycardia, elevated blood pressure, tremor, incontinence, and an altered level of consciousness that may progress to coma.

Creatine phosphokinase and myoglobin are elevated because of muscle damage. This may lead to renal failure.

The presentation in the context of a new antipsychotic medication is usually sufficient for diagnosis.

Treatment involves immediately stopping the antipsychotic agent, cooling the patient, and maintaining acceptable vital signs and urine output. Dantrolene is a skeletal muscle relaxant that can relieve muscle rigidity and improve the prognosis.

Mood Disorders

Major Depressive Disorder

Depression is a very common condition. Women have a lifetime prevalence of as much as 25%, whereas men have a prevalence of approximately 10%. Mean age at onset is in the 40s. Patients have a high death rate, and many commit suicide. Risk of depression is not associated with socioeconomic status, education level, or ethnicity. There is a familial tendency toward major depressive disorder, as well as increased rates of alcohol dependence and attention-deficit hyperactivity disorder (ADHD) among first-degree relatives.

Major depressive disorder can be diagnosed in patients who have had at least one **major depressive episode** (described in box) without a history of manic episodes. Approximately one-half of patients have subsequent episodes later in life. When disease is recurrent, remissions may last for years but intervals tend to become shorter later in life.

A combination of psychotherapy and pharmacotherapy is most effective. Several effective antidepressant medications are available, but all of them take several weeks to take effect.

- **Tricyclic antidepressants** (TCAs) may induce a manic episode in susceptible individuals. Side effects include sedation and anticholinergic effects (e.g., dry mouth, constipation, blurred vision, urinary retention). Overdose causes cardiac arrhythmias, which may be fatal.
- **Selective serotonin reuptake inhibitors** (SSRIs), such as fluoxetine (Prozac), sertraline (Zoloft), and paroxetine (Paxil), are widely prescribed. Side effects include GI symptoms, headaches, and impotence. Overdose is not lethal.
- **Atypical antidepressants,** such as bupropion and venlafaxine, have few anticholinergic side effects and overdose is not lethal.
- **Monoamine oxidase inhibitors** (MAOIs) are particularly useful for patients with atypical depression. Foods containing tyramine (e.g., red wine, cheese) must be avoided, as they can precipitate a hypertensive crisis. Because of these food restrictions and the availability of SSRIs, MAOIs are now much less commonly used. Hypertensive crises may be treated with alpha-adrenergic antagonists, such as phentolamine and chlorpromazine.

Electroconvulsive therapy is used for refractory or very severe disease, or in patients who cannot tolerate medications. Electroconvulsive therapy is very effective when used properly and has few side effects except for short-term memory disturbance.

Major Depressive Episode

A major depressive episode is defined as a period of more than 2 weeks of either excessive sadness or anhedonia (inability to experience pleasure). Vegetative symptoms (change in appetite, weight, sleep, and psychomotor activity), low energy level, indecisiveness or lack of concentration, a sense of guilt or worthlessness, and suicidal ideation may also be present. Insomnia is much more typical than hypersomnia. Significant distress or impaired functioning must also result from the mood disturbance for the definition to apply. If untreated, a major depressive episode often lasts more than 6 months, but even these individuals may recover completely.

Dysthymic Disorder

Dysthymic disorder is characterized by a persistent feeling of depression that does not meet the criteria for major depressive disorder but lasts more than 2 years. Each year, approximately 10% of patients with dysthymic disorder develop major depressive disorder. Many patients also have evidence of personality disorders. Men and women are equally likely to have dysthymic disorder.

PSYCHIATRY

In addition to depressed mood, patients experience changes in appetite and sleep, decreased energy, inability to concentrate, hopeless feelings, and low self-esteem. Vegetative symptoms are less common than in major depressive disorder.

The patient must have a depressed mood on more days than not for 2 years and at least two of the associated symptoms.

Combination psychotherapy and cognitive therapy. Medications may be used for persistent symptoms.

Seasonal Affective Disorder

Actually a subtype of major depressive disorder, seasonal affective disorder involves depressive episodes that occur in winter, with improvement in spring and summer. Abnormal melatonin secretion may be responsible. Phototherapy and sleep deprivation therapy are useful in treatment.

Manic Episode

For at least 1 week, an individual experiences an abnormally euphoric, expansive, or irritable mood. At least three associated features must be present and may include grandiosity, decreased need for sleep, increased pressure or volume of speech, flight of ideas, increased distractibility, psychomotor agitation, increased goal-directed activity, and an increase in pleasurable activities that could have a high cost (e.g., extravagant shopping). Grandiose delusions and psychotic features may occur. Social, academic, or occupational functioning is impaired, and hospitalization is often necessary. If criteria of a major depressive episode are also present, the term **"mixed episode"** is used.

Bipolar Disorder

Bipolar disorder is a recurrent disease that involves features of both mania and depression. Each patient has an individual pattern of cycling. The natural history of the disease is typically approximately four episodes in a 10-year period, although a minority of patients are "rapid cyclers" with more than four episodes a year. Frequency increases as patients age. Most patients function normally between episodes, although approximately 25% continue to have deficits. Men and women have equal rates of bipolar disorder. Onset typically occurs in a person's 30s. Episodes may develop in women during their postpartum period. In patients older than 40 years, organic etiologies must be ruled out.

The patient must have a history of both mania (a manic, hypomanic, or mixed episode) and a major depressive episode for this diagnosis to apply (see boxes for specific symptoms).

Psychotherapy and cognitive therapy in combination with pharmacotherapy are often effective. Lithium may cause GI distress, weight gain, fatigue, and tremor. Toxicity causes vomiting, diarrhea, ataxia, and confusion, progressing to seizures and coma. The anticonvulsants carbamazepine and valproic acid are also effective in treating bipolar disorder. Some patients require antipsychotics.

Mood Disorder Due to Medical Conditions and Medications

A mood disorder can be caused by a medical disease. The mood change may be physiologic and not simply a result of the stress of having a serious medical condition. Common etiologies include neurologic conditions (e.g., multiple sclerosis, stroke), endocrine disorders (Cushing's disease), cancer, and autoimmune disease (e.g., rheumatoid arthritis). Medications used to treat nonpsychiatric disorders can also cause mood disorders that begin within 1 month of the initiation of the medication. Common culprits include β-blockers, steroids, oral contraceptives, and barbiturates. Alcohol may also cause depression.

Anxiety Disorders

Panic Attacks

A panic attack is defined as a period of extreme fear or anxiety, often with an overwhelming feeling of impending danger and an intense desire to escape. Associated symptoms include palpitations, sweating, trembling, shortness of breath, a sense of choking, chest discomfort, nausea, dizziness, derealization or depersonalization, fear of losing control, fear of dying, paresthesias, and chills or hot flushes. "Uncued" attacks occur without warning, whereas "cued" attacks occur in predictable situations.

Panic Disorder

In panic disorder, patients experience recurrent, uncued panic attacks and constantly worry about having another attack. The course of panic disorder varies greatly. It is generally chronic but episodic. Patients may have attacks regularly or in sporadic bursts with long asymptomatic periods. Panic disorder generally begins in late adolescence or early adulthood.

During an attack (see box on panic attacks), the patient may have elevated heart rate and blood pressure. Patients also may have generalized anxiety, worry, or low self-esteem. Major depressive disorder occurs in more than 50% of patients.

The patient has recurrent attacks and anxiety about having another attack. The diagnosis of panic disorder is classified as either with or without **agoraphobia,** which is an extreme fear and avoidance of any situation in which escape or help may not be immediately available.

SSRIs are most likely to be effective. Short courses of benzodiazepines, particularly alprazolam (Xanax), may also be useful. Cognitive and behavior therapy may help as well.

Specific Phobia

Previously called *simple phobia,* specific phobia is the fear of a particular object or situation. This may involve fear of being injured, of losing control, or of fainting. Most phobias have a childhood onset, and traumatic events or panic attacks may predispose the patient to developing a phobia. Women are diagnosed with this disorder more frequently than men.

The object or situation in question immediately provokes a panic attack or manifestation of excessive anxiety. The level of severity is related to the proximity of the object and to the patient's capacity to escape. Instead of panic attacks, some patients have vasovagal responses, particularly with phobias to blood, needles, or injury. Patients make efforts to avoid the phobic object, which can cause significant impairment in social or occupational functioning. Adult patients generally have some insight into the unwarranted nature of their fears.

Behavior therapy.

Social Phobia

Excessive fear of social or performance settings is accompanied by extreme anxiety when the patient is exposed to these situations. **Generalized social phobia** involves fear in most social interactions, and patients often have very severe impairments in their daily lives. Social phobia usually begins in the midteens, sometimes after an embarrassing incident. It lasts throughout the patient's life, with exacerbations during times of stress.

The response may be severe anxiety or a panic attack. Patients avoid the phobic situations and dread being embarrassed. Patients often have low self-esteem and may be underachievers. Anxiety may be evident with even minimal contact, and other anxiety or mood disorders are often present. Adults have insight that their fear is unwarranted, but children usually do not.

Behavioral therapy. MAOIs and antidepressants may also be useful. Beta-blockers can be used for stage fright, to block tachycardia and perspiration.

Acute Stress Disorder

During a traumatic event, the patient experiences a sense of detachment or numbed emotion, a lack of awareness, depersonalization, or dissociative amnesia. Dissociative symptoms follow the trauma, with numbed emotions, guilt, or an inability to experience pleasure. As in post-traumatic stress disorder (PTSD, see following section), the patient later relives the event and tries to avoid related stimuli. On physical examination, injury resulting from the recent trauma may be evident. Symptoms must last at least 2 days and less than 4 weeks, after which the diagnosis of PTSD applies. Supportive therapy may be helpful.

Post-traumatic Stress Disorder

The typical symptoms of PTSD develop after experiencing or witnessing a traumatic event. The syndrome generally develops within 3 months of the event. Half of patients recover completely within 3 more months, whereas others have symptoms for more than a year. PTSD may coexist with other anxiety disorders or with depression. Social supports and personal history can affect the development of PTSD, although it can occur in patients without any apparent predisposition.

SIGNS & SYMPTOMS

Dreams, memories, and flashbacks of the trauma are prominent. The resulting psychological distress is severe. Patients try to avoid settings that trigger memories, but may, at the same time, be amnestic of the trauma. They typically feel detached, unemotional, and unable to experience pleasure. Survivor guilt, self-destructive behavior, somatization, and social withdrawal are common. Anxiety and hypervigilance are often seen, and increased autonomic arousal (rapid heart rate and increased sweating) may be noted on examination.

DIAGNOSIS

For diagnosis to apply, a patient must have experienced a traumatic event and have felt intense fear, helplessness, or horror. Hypervigilance, mentally reliving the event, and avoiding associated stimuli occur for at least 1 month for diagnosis of acute PTSD and for more than 3 months for diagnosis of chronic PTSD.

TREATMENT

TCAs, MAOIs, and SSRIs may all be useful. Psychotherapy is also effective.

Generalized Anxiety Disorder

In generalized anxiety disorder, patients experience persistent anxiety and apprehension. Anxiety may concern normal daily events, and the worry is excessive relative to likely possible outcomes. Many patients are nervous or overly worried before the development of this disorder. Patients present in childhood, adolescence, or early adulthood, and symptoms continue throughout their lives. Generalized anxiety disorder is somewhat more prevalent in women than in men.

PSYCHIATRY

In addition to anxiety, the patient may experience restlessness, lack of concentration, easy fatigability, difficulty sleeping, irritability, and muscle tension or other musculoskeletal problems. Some somatic symptoms or stress-related conditions may be present.

Anxiety and worry persist at least 6 months with at least three of the preceding symptoms.

Psychotherapy and anxiolytics (benzodiazepines and buspirone) may be helpful. SSRIs are also used.

Obsessive-Compulsive Disorder

An **obsession** is a recurrent thought, feeling, idea, or image that is unpleasant and intrusive but cannot be controlled by the patient. Common obsessions concern contamination, order, frightening images or doubts, or disturbing sexual images. Patients try to suppress or counteract their obsessions. A **compulsion** is a repeated mental or motor behavior performed to lessen anxiety, usually following an obsessive thought. These acts are either excessive or clearly unable to accomplish the desired goal. Common compulsions are repetitive checking, washing, counting, and stereotyped ordering (e.g., alphabetizing soup cans).

The severe, recurrent obsessions or compulsions that characterize obsessive-compulsive disorder cause the patient significant distress and may require excessive time to complete. Obsessive-compulsive disorder begins in young adulthood. Men and women have equal rates of this diagnosis. Most patients have exacerbations at stressful times. There is a high rate of concordance with Tourette's syndrome and other tic disorders (see Chapter 8).

Patients may avoid settings that evoke obsessions or compulsions. Sleep disturbances, alcohol use, and feelings of guilt are common. Skin problems from cleaning compulsions may be found on physical examination.

Obsessions and compulsions must require excessive time or cause severe distress. Adult patients must have some degree of insight, realizing that the behaviors are unusual.

Clomipramine (a TCA), SSRIs, and behavioral therapy are often effective. Most patients improve, although one-third later develop major depression.

PSYCHIATRY

Anxiety Due to Medical Conditions and Medications

Anxiety and panic attacks can be caused by underlying medical disorders. Thyroid disorders, hypoglycemia, pheochromocytoma, chronic obstructive pulmonary disease (COPD), cardiac arrhythmias, and congestive heart failure (CHF) may all bring about symptoms of anxiety or panic. The diagnosis is supported by an appropriate temporal relation between the medical condition and the anxiety disorder.

Sympathomimetic substances such as amphetamine, cocaine, and caffeine may also cause symptoms of anxiety.

Schizophrenia and Other Psychotic Disorders

Schizophrenia

Schizophrenia is a devastating psychotic disorder with a poor prognosis. Onset is from the late teens to the early 30s, and it has a chronic course. The actual cause is unknown, although dopaminergic hyperactivity has been implicated. A genetic predisposition seems to exist as well, and first-degree relatives of schizophrenic patients have 10 times the rate of disease as the general population. Schizophrenia affects all socioeconomic and ethnic groups. The disproportionate number of poor and homeless people with schizophrenia is probably due to "downward drift," as these patients function poorly in society. Schizophrenic patients have an overall high mortality rate, and 50% attempt suicide.

Prognosis is best with a late, sudden onset in a patient with good premorbid functioning, especially when an obvious event precipitates the onset of symptoms. Patients with a family history of mood disorders and those who have primarily affective or **positive symptoms** (see Signs & Symptoms) tend to do better. Married patients with good support systems also have a better prognosis. History of perinatal trauma, family history of schizophrenia, personal history of aggressive behavior, presence of **negative symptoms,** and neurologic signs and symptoms are considered poor prognostic features.

SIGNS & SYMPTOMS

Onset may be abrupt, but most patients have a prodrome of increasingly bizarre behavior. Two categories of symptoms are present: **positive symptoms** (delusions, hallucinations, disorganized thoughts, and disorganized behavior) and **negative symptoms** (poverty of speech or thought content, flat affect, apathy, anhedonia, inattentiveness). The typical course involves psychotic episodes with periods of remission; however, the patient's baseline functioning deteriorates over time.

DIAGNOSIS

Symptoms must be present for at least 6 months.

TREATMENT

Antipsychotics (also called neuroleptics or major tranquilizers) are used, including dopamine-receptor antagonists (such as chlorpromazine, haloperidol) and serotonin-dopamine antagonists (such as clozapine, risperidone, olanzapine, and quetiapine). All medications require a trial period of at least 4 to 6 weeks.

PSYCHIATRY

Hospitalization may be needed to stabilize severe disease or for patient safety. Psychosocial therapy should be integrated into a comprehensive treatment plan.

Side effects of dopamine-receptor antagonists are numerous, including orthostatic hypotension, peripheral anticholinergic effects (dry mouth, blurry vision, constipation, urinary retention, mydriasis), and increased prolactin secretion (causing breast enlargement, galactorrhea, and impotence in men and amenorrhea and anorgasmia in women). Parkinsonian symptoms (cogwheel rigidity, pill-rolling tremor, and shuffling gait) may begin in 3 months, and **tardive dyskinesia** (often irreversible stereotypic movements, such as chewing) may develop after at least 6 months of use. Clozapine is usually used as a second-line treatment because of its side effects (seizures and agranulocytosis). Nonclozapine serotonin-dopamine antagonists have fewer side effects and are becoming the first-line treatment.

Schizophreniform Disorder

In schizophreniform disorder, the symptoms of schizophrenia have lasted more than 1 month but less than 6 months. If the patient has active symptoms for less than 6 months, schizophreniform disorder is applied as a provisional diagnosis because the criteria for schizophrenia may be met in the future. Antipsychotic medications or electroconvulsive therapy are used, and hospitalization may be needed for effective monitoring and treatment.

Schizoaffective Disorder

When the patient has a mood disorder and separate psychotic symptoms, the term schizoaffective disorder applies. The patient must experience delusions or hallucinations for at least 2 weeks without concurrent mood symptoms to establish the presence of separate psychotic features. Mania or depression may be present, and antimanic or antidepressant medications are the first line of treatment. Antipsychotics are used only when needed for acute management. Hospitalization and psychosocial approaches are appropriate as well.

Delusional Disorder

Delusional disorder involves the presence of one or more nonbizarre delusions in a patient without markedly impaired functioning. Nonbizarre delusions have a shred of plausibility, whereas bizarre delusions are outside accepted cultural possibilities.

SIGNS & SYMPTOMS

The delusion may be grandiose, jealous, erotomanic (when the patient believes that a certain individual, who may be entirely unconnected with the patient, is in love with him or her), or persecutory. Ideas of reference, in which random events are interpreted as having personal significance, are common. Auditory or visual hallucinations are not common. Tactile or olfactory hallucinations, on the other hand, may be prominent and may be related to the delusion. Otherwise, psychosocial functioning and behavior are not severely impaired.

DIAGNOSIS

Symptoms last at least 1 month. If delusions are bizarre, the diagnosis of schizophrenia or schizophreniform disorder applies.

Antipsychotic medications with hospitalization and psychotherapy. Half of patients recover completely.

Brief Psychotic Disorder

Formerly called *brief reactive psychosis,* patients with brief psychotic disorder have an abrupt onset of psychotic features, followed by complete recovery. Severe stress may trigger the disorder.

Symptoms of delusions, hallucination, and disorganized speech or behavior are present. Functional impairment may be extreme.

Symptoms are present for more than 1 day and less than 1 month. Diagnosis is specified as "with marked stressor," "without marked stressor," or "with postpartum onset."

Hospitalization, low-dose antipsychotics, and psychotherapy.

Shared Psychotic Disorder (Folie á Deux)

Shared psychotic disorder occurs when a patient becomes involved in the delusions of a psychotic person. The inducer, or primary case, is typically the dominant person in a close relationship. The inducer often has schizophrenia, and the delusions may be bizarre. If the relationship between the two is interrupted, the patient's delusional belief will diminish. Significant support is needed for this separation. Antipsychotics may be used, and family therapy is critical.

Psychotic Disorder Due to a General Medical Condition

In this disorder, prominent delusions or hallucinations are directly caused by another medical disorder. Common conditions include neurologic diseases (neoplasms, epilepsy, cerebrovascular disease, and dementias), endocrine or metabolic diseases, electrolyte imbalance, and renal disease. This diagnosis is supported by an appropriate temporal relation between the medical condition and the psychotic disorder, or by atypical features such as olfactory hallucinations.

PSYCHIATRY

Personality Disorders

When an individual's character traits deviate significantly from cultural norms, a diagnosis of personality disorder may apply. A personality disorder is pervasive and constant, causing serious distress or impaired functioning. The maladaptive patterns begin in adolescence or early adulthood. Some personality disorders lessen with time, whereas others continue throughout the patient's life. Personality disorders are Axis II diagnoses that fall into three clusters, discussed in the following sections.

Cluster A Personality Disorders

Patients with a cluster A personality disorder are eccentric or somewhat bizarre.

Paranoid personality disorder. Patients have a pervasive pattern of interpreting actions and events as malevolent or demeaning. They are suspicious of the motives of others, fear exploitation or deceit, and scrutinize peers closely. Other traits include reluctance to share personal information, frequent misinterpretation of benign comments, unwillingness to forgive others, frequent angry reactions, and pathologic jealousy. Alcohol and substance use are common, brief psychotic episodes are not unusual, and patients often develop major depressive disorder, agoraphobia, and obsessive-compulsive disorder.

Schizoid personality disorder. These patients are unable to form close relationships with others and have very restricted emotions. Patients do not attempt to achieve intimacy, prefer to be alone, have no close friends, show little interest in sexual activity, and do not enjoy most activities. Approval or disapproval from others is unimportant. Major depressive disorder may develop, and schizoid personality disorder may precede the development of delusional disorder or schizophrenia.

Schizotypal personality disorder. In addition to difficulty maintaining close relationships, patients have odd or distorted behavior, cognition, or perception. Suspiciousness and ideas of reference are common, as are interests in superstitions or the paranormal. Eccentric speech, inappropriate affect and behavior, lack of close relationships, and social anxiety are other features of this disorder. Increased psychotic features may result in the diagnosis of a psychotic disorder.

Cluster B Personality Disorders

Cluster B personality disorders involve dramatic or overemotional personality traits.

Antisocial personality disorder. Previously termed *psychopaths* or *sociopaths,* individuals with this disorder show disregard for social norms and the interests of others. They break laws, act aggressively or deceitfully, and lack remorse for their actions. Other diagnostic features include failure to plan, reckless patterns of behavior, and lack of responsibility. Conduct disorder may be present before age 18 years. Several disorders, such as anxiety, depression, substance use, and somatization disorder, are associated. The majority of these patients are men.

Borderline personality disorder. Patients experience unstable relationships, self-esteem, and emotions. They desperately fear being abandoned. Impulsivity, suicidal thoughts and actions, mood lability, uncontrolled anger, and feelings of boredom or emptiness are common features. Transient paranoid or dissociative symptoms may occur. Associated diagnoses include mood disorders, substance use, bulimia, PTSD, and ADHD. Approximately 75% of patients are women.

Histrionic personality disorder. Labile emotions and attention-seeking patterns of behavior characterize this disorder. Patients want to be the center of attention and often use seductive behaviors or physical appearance to achieve this goal. Shallow or labile emotions, dramatic speech and behavior, easily influenced opinions, and inappropriately perceived intimacy are common. Major depressive disorder, somatization, and conversion disorder may occur.

Narcissistic personality disorder. These self-centered patients have grandiose self-images, frequent fantasies of love and success, and a sense of entitlement. They expect admiration from others because they believe themselves to be superior. They lack empathy and may exploit, snub, or envy others. The majority of patients are men. Anorexia, substance use, and mood disorders may occur.

Cluster C Personality Disorders

Anxiety and fear characterize cluster C personality disorders.

Avoidant personality disorder. Patients avoid social situations for fear of rejection, and they make friends only when they are certain of being accepted. Fears of embarrassment lead to a reluctance to be open or to try new activities, a pattern of misinterpreting comments as critical, and the development of low self-esteem and feelings of inadequacy. Mood and anxiety disorders are common.

Dependent personality disorder. These needy patients require support and advice for everyday decisions and allow others to be responsible for their life choices. Conflict or disagreement is very difficult, as is personal motivation or initiative. Patients feel unable to care for themselves, so they fear being alone and seek out close relationships. Patients constantly try to have others nurture them. Mood and anxiety disorders are common. Men and women have equal rates of this diagnosis.

Obsessive-compulsive personality disorder. These perfectionistic and controlling patients may be overly conscientious to the point of missing deadlines. Their extreme devotion to work is accompanied by extreme preoccupation with petty details and rules and an inability to delegate tasks to others. Patients are inflexible and stubborn, miserly, and are often unable to discard old, unwanted objects. These patients do not typically meet criteria for obsessive-compulsive disorder. Mood and anxiety disorders are common. Men have this diagnosis more frequently than women.

Substance-related Disorders

Definitions

Intoxication. Reversible symptoms result from the use of a psychoactive substance because of its direct physiological effects on the CNS. Initial episodes of substance use and intoxication usually start in the teenage years and may develop into problems of abuse and dependence.

Abuse. Substance use continues, despite negative consequences that may include physical danger or harm, recurrent academic or occupational problems, legal problems, and impaired functioning in home or social environments.

Dependence. Dependence on a substance may be physical or psychological. In physical dependence, the patient uses the substance to avoid symptoms of withdrawal. Inhaled and injected agents, other rapidly acting agents, and substances with a short duration of action are more likely to cause physical dependence. In psychological dependence, patients experience a strong "craving" for the substance. Compulsive use is often present, including use of the substance in greater amounts than intended and excessive time spent in the acquisition or use of the substance. Other aspects of compulsive use include reduction in other activities in favor of substance use and continued use of the substance even when psychological or physical problems develop.

Withdrawal. Decreasing or stopping the prolonged use of a substance causes symptoms of withdrawal specific to that substance (see following sections). These may include behavioral, physiological, and cognitive changes that can cause severe distress.

Alcohol

Although the majority of Americans have used alcohol at some time in their lives, and many have experienced negative consequences, most do not go on to develop alcohol abuse or dependence. Those who do develop alcohol dependence often abuse other substances as well, and some have concurrent mood or anxiety disorders or schizophrenia. Alcohol-abusing and -dependent patients have increased rates of accidents, suicide, and criminal acts. A genetic predisposition is evident, with three to four times the prevalence in first-degree relatives of patients with alcohol dependence.

Alcohol intoxication involves slurred speech, decreased coordination, unsteadiness, nystagmus, and attention or memory deficits, and it may progress to stupor and coma. Many Asians do not have the enzyme aldehyde dehydrogenase and cannot metabolize alcohol properly. After intake, they experience flushing and palpitations.

Alcohol withdrawal begins approximately 12 hours after last intake in dependent individuals. Withdrawal involves increased autonomic activity (rapid pulse, diaphoresis), nausea and vomiting, hand tremor, difficulty sleeping, psychomotor agitation, anxiety, and even seizures. Transient hallucinations or illusions are common. **Delirium tremens** consists of grand mal seizures, delirium, and extreme autonomic activity. It can be life-threatening but occurs in a small minority of patients. Symptoms of withdrawal peak within 2 days and improve by 5 days, but some residual effects can last up to 6 months.

Alcohol intake eases symptoms of withdrawal but clearly does not address issues of abuse and dependence. Benzodiazepines, supportive measures, supplemental nutrition, and, occasionally, anticonvulsants are used in the management of withdrawal. Rehabilitation should address problems with alcohol use and any concurrent medical or psychological conditions.

Caffeine

Excessive caffeine use causes insomnia, restlessness, flushing, diuresis, twitches, nervousness, rambling thoughts and speech, tachycardia, and psychomotor agitation. Symptoms last 6 to 16 hours. Withdrawal can cause headaches, lethargy, and irritability.

Cannabis

Marijuana and hashish from cannabis leaves cause effects that are due to tetrahydrocannabinol (THC). Synthetic THC is used medically to relieve nausea from chemotherapy, anorexia from AIDS, and increased intraocular pressure from glaucoma. Intoxication causes feelings of elation, increased appetite, conjunctival injection, dry mouth, and tachycardia. Cannabis use and dependence, but not withdrawal, may develop.

Nicotine

All forms of tobacco use can contribute to dependence and withdrawal. Nicotine causes increased catecholamine release and is a CNS stimulant. The incidence of smoking is declining, with rates between 20% to 30% in the general population, although it is much higher among psychiatric patients.

Symptoms of withdrawal include depression, insomnia, irritability, anxiety, bradycardia, increased appetite, and difficulty with concentration.

Options for cessation include support groups, hypnosis, aversive therapy, nicotine gum, nicotine patches, and medications (bupropion, clonidine, or doxepin). Less than 25% of smokers are able to quit on their first attempt. Desire for a cigarette may last more than 6 months after quitting.

Cocaine

Cocaine can be snorted, smoked, or injected. Crack cocaine is a smoked form of cocaine that has extremely rapid onset. Because cocaine use evokes strong feelings of euphoria, dependence can develop quickly. A short half-life requires frequent dosing, and a great deal of money may be spent in a short period, leading to theft, prostitution, and drug dealing.

Intoxication produces euphoria, hyperactivity, anxiety, grandiosity, and impaired judgment. Tachycardia, pupillary dilation, nausea and vomiting, psychomotor agitation, and chest pain or cardiac arrhythmias are possible physical manifestations. Withdrawal symptoms include dysphoric mood, fatigue, unpleasant dreams, insomnia or hypersomnia, and psychomotor retardation.

Hospitalization is often necessary to remove the patient from the drug source. Psychological intervention and medical treatment with bromocriptine and desipramine may be useful.

Amphetamine

Amphetamine and amphetamine-related compounds are generally purchased illegally but may be prescribed for obesity, ADHD, and narcolepsy.

Intoxication causes hyperactivity and a sense of physical or mental strength. Physical manifestations include rapid heart rate, dilated pupils, high blood pressure, nausea and vomiting, and sweating or chills. With increased use, paranoia or psychosis may develop. Withdrawal occurs several hours to a few days after last use. Patients develop depression, hypersomnia, and increased appetite.

Supportive treatment and antipsychotics may be used to manage withdrawal.

Lysergic Acid Diethylamide

Lysergic acid diethylamide (LSD) is one of many available hallucinogens. There is no syndrome of physical dependence or withdrawal, but psychological dependence occurs.

The patient feels a sense of heightened awareness and may experience hallucinations and feelings of depersonalization. A "bad trip" results in feelings of paranoia, depression, or psychosis. Physical symptoms (which can help distinguish between substance-induced and organic psychosis) include tachycardia, pupillary dilation, sweating, and tremors.

Protect the patient from injury until the drug is metabolized. Antipsychotics are occasionally necessary.

Phencyclidine

Phencyclidine (PCP, angel dust) is a synthetic drug that can be ingested, inhaled, or injected. The drug's half-life is long (20 hours). True physical dependence is rare.

The patient feels euphoric and may have the sensation of floating or depersonalization. Users typically have a distorted body image, may exhibit unusual strength, and often become combative or violent. Nystagmus, hyperthermia, hyperreflexia, and hypertension are common physical signs.

TREATMENT

Hospitalization, ideally in a dim, quiet environment, may be necessary to protect the patient and others. Restraints should be avoided, as they may lead to rhabdomyolysis. Benzodiazepines and antipsychotics may be helpful.

Opioid

The term *opioid* includes morphine, heroin, codeine, hydromorphone, methadone, and other synthetic opiates. Opioid use is associated with drug-related crimes, antisocial personality disorder, and PTSD. Intravenous heroin users are at risk for HIV, hepatitis B, and hepatitis C.

SIGNS & SYMPTOMS

In addition to euphoria, intoxicated patients have slurred speech, pupillary constriction, deficits in attention and memory, and stupor or coma. Withdrawal causes dysphoria, tearing, runny nose, muscle aches, nausea and vomiting, pupillary dilation, diarrhea, yawning, insomnia, and fever.

TREATMENT

Methadone is an oral synthetic opioid used to stabilize dependent patients. It is then tapered down and withdrawn. Clonidine can be used for symptomatic relief. Opioid antagonists, such as naloxone, are used to treat overdose. Therapeutic communities are the best option for rehabilitation, although dropout and relapse rates are high.

Sleep Disorders

Stages of Sleep

Sleep can be categorized into rapid eye movement (REM) sleep and four stages of non-REM sleep. Relaxed wakefulness, with alpha waves on the EEG, precedes stage 1, or light sleep. Half of human sleeping time is spent in stage 2 sleep, in which K complexes and sleep spindles appear on the EEG. Together, stages 3 and 4 comprise slow-wave sleep, with an increasing appearance of delta waves as the patient falls into deeper sleep. Children have more slow-wave sleep than do adults. Dreams occur during REM sleep, which accounts for approximately one-fourth of sleep time. During REM sleep, brain and physiologic activity are similar to activity during wakefulness, but muscle activity is inhibited. These stages cycle in 90-minute intervals throughout the night, with more REM sleep and less slow-wave sleep occurring as the night progresses.

Insomnia

Insomnia may manifest as difficulty getting to sleep or staying asleep. Negative conditioning may occur, in that patients are so accustomed to having difficulties falling asleep that they expect and reinforce these problems. Mood and anxiety disorders are commonly associated. Sleep studies often show increased stage 1 sleep and insufficient slow-wave sleep.

PSYCHIATRY

Sleep usually becomes lighter and more easily disturbed with aging, so elderly patients are prone to insomnia. Insomnia usually begins suddenly during a time of stress, but it may persist after the stressful episode ends. Untreated, the disorder typically worsens for a few months, then stabilizes, sometimes persisting for years.

Insomnia is best treated by improving "sleep hygiene," which involves avoiding any substances with CNS effects (e.g., caffeine, alcohol, tobacco), maintaining regular sleeping and waking times, avoiding daytime napping, and developing strategies for relaxation. If unsuccessful, short courses of benzodiazepines, chloral hydrate, or antihistamines may be useful; however, sedatives put elderly patients at risk for falls, and antihistamines may cause urinary retention, acute confusion, or cognitive slowing.

Sleep Apnea Syndrome

Sleep apnea syndrome is characterized by periodic cessations of breathing (apnea) during sleep, which result in reduced oxygenation of the blood and arousal from sleep. **Obstructive sleep apnea** (OSA), caused by upper airway obstruction, is most often seen in obese, middle-aged men and in young children with tonsillar enlargement.

Patients present with excessive daytime somnolence that is due to frequent arousals and disrupted sleep patterns during the night. Morning headache, memory problems, and sexual dysfunction are also common symptoms. In OSA, bed partners often report loud, crescendo snoring. Alcohol may worsen symptoms.

Apneic episodes and subsequent arousals are documented during sleep studies, and time spent in slow-wave and REM sleep is diminished. Apneic episodes cause hypoxia.

Continuous positive airway pressure to relieve airway obstruction is administered using a nasal mask and a machine that can be used at home. Weight loss is helpful. Nasal or palatal surgery to widen the airway may be necessary.

Narcolepsy

Narcolepsy is a disorder of REM sleep. Clinical onset is typically during adolescence.

Sudden bouts of daytime sleep and cataplexy (loss of muscle strength and tone triggered by emotional reactions) are typical symptoms. Attacks last 10 minutes to 1 hour and may occur several times a day. Intense dreams and temporary paralysis may occur during transitions between wakefulness and sleep.

Sleep studies show that REM sleep is present at sleep onset, rather than 90 minutes after sleep onset, as is the case in normal sleep patterns.

Scheduled naps may improve symptoms dramatically. Medical treatment involves amphetamines.

Circadian Rhythm Sleep Disorder

Circadian rhythm sleep disorder occurs when the patient's internal clock does not match that of occupational or societal requirements. Patients may be sleepy during the day and wakeful at night. Jet lag and shift work may be contributory. (This disorder is an occupational hazard of medical internship.)

Parasomnias

Parasomnias generally occur in children and involve unusual phenomena during sleep. Treatment is rarely required and these disorders tend to resolve, but diazepam can lessen symptoms somewhat.

- In **nightmare disorder,** patients have terrifying dreams that awaken them to an alert state. The dreams usually occur during REM sleep in the second half of the night. Onset is between 3 and 6 years old.
- **Sleep terror disorder** involves sudden, frightened awakenings from slow-wave sleep. This usually occurs early in the night and is accompanied by a scream or cry. Up to 10 minutes of panicked behavior and difficulty waking follow. Children with this disorder do not have an increased incidence of other mental disorders, but adults may have an associated anxiety or personality disorder. Symptoms typically begin in 4- to 12-year-old children and remit during adolescence.
- **Sleepwalking disorder** may include a variety of complex behaviors and occurs during slow-wave sleep. The individual is unresponsive, unable to be awakened, and later, cannot recall the event. Sleepwalking in children usually begins around 4 years of age, peaks at age 12 years, and resolves by age 15 years. In children, sleepwalking is not associated with other disorders, but adults may have mood, anxiety, and personality disorders.

Somatoform and Factitious Disorders

Somatization Disorder

The multiple, recurring physical problems experienced in somatization disorder cannot be explained by the presence of a general medical condition but are not produced intentionally. Symptoms usually involve clinically significant pain with serious impairment. Frequent medical visits, diagnostic procedures, and unnecessary surgeries may result. Female patients are much more prone to this disorder.

PSYCHIATRY

In addition to pain, patients may have nausea, bloating, diarrhea, vomiting, and vague neurologic symptoms. Women often have menstrual irregularities, and men may report sexual dysfunction.

Significant somatic symptoms begin before age 30 years and last several years. For the diagnosis to apply, the patient must have experienced two gastrointestinal symptoms, one sexual symptom, one pseudoneurologic symptom, and four different sites of pain during the course of the illness. Laboratory tests do not support the physical symptoms.

Psychotherapy. Frequent, scheduled visits with a single primary care provider may keep the syndrome under control.

Conversion Disorder

In conversion disorder, patients develop deficits in sensation or voluntary movement without evidence for an underlying organic etiology. "Conversion" historically reflects the redirection of an unconscious psychological conflict into physical symptoms, and the symptoms reported may reflect local or cultural ideas of expressions of distress. Symptoms are exacerbated by stress, implicating psychological factors, but they are not intentional or factitious.

Physical symptoms affecting voluntary motor or sensory function seem to suggest a neurologic disorder. Common motor problems include paralysis, aphonia (loss of voice), and swallowing difficulties. Sensory symptoms may involve blindness, deafness, or decreased skin sensation. Pseudoseizures may occur. Symptoms may be inconsistent, physiologically implausible, and not supported by physical examination or laboratory findings.

Motor or sensory deficits cause significant impairment in functioning, without a medical explanation. This diagnosis should be considered tentative early on, because medical diagnoses may become clear years later.

Psychotherapy and reassurance. Symptoms usually resolve within a month.

Hypochondriasis

Patients with hypochondriasis misinterpret minor physical symptoms and develop excessive fears about having serious disease. They often have a history of childhood illness or serious disease in close family members. Women and men have equal rates of this disorder, usually with onset in middle age. The course is typically chronic except in children, who often recover completely.

Symptoms are multiple and typically involve GI or cardiac function. Physical examination and laboratory evaluation do not show signs of a serious medical disorder, but the patient's concern is not eased. Symptoms continue to cause significant stress or impaired functioning on an episodic basis for months or years.

For diagnosis, the preceding constellation of symptoms must persist for at least 6 months.

Regularly scheduled visits to the doctor may reassure the patient. Patients are typically unwilling to undergo psychotherapy but group therapy may be useful.

Factitious Disorder

Patients with factitious disorder, also known as **Münchhausen syndrome,** intentionally produce physical or psychiatric symptoms. Unlike **malingering,** in which feigning illness allows realization of an external goal (e.g., monetary gain), factitious disorder is a means for the patient to assume a "sick role." This disorder is more common in men than in women.

Feigned or exaggerated symptoms may be complicated by self-inflicted injury. Abuse of prescription medications, particularly analgesics and sedatives, is common.

No effective treatment is known. Try to avoid unnecessary diagnostic procedures.

Sexual and Gender Identity Disorders

Sexual Dysfunctions

The spectrum of sexual dysfunction includes loss of sexual desire, sexual aversion, failure of genital response (erection in men and vaginal lubrication in women), orgasmic dysfunction, premature ejaculation, vaginismus (spasm of the perivaginal muscles), and dyspareunia (pain with sex). Any symptoms may be generalized or situational, total or partial, and lifelong or acquired.

Diagnosis requires that the patient is unable to participate in sexual relations as she or he wishes and that the dysfunction has been present for at least 6 months. A physical cause for the dysfunction should be investigated before the symptoms are attributed to psychological causes.

PSYCHIATRY

After addressing any medical issues, couples therapy, hypnotherapy, and behavioral therapy may be useful. Antianxiety agents may help, and testosterone is occasionally used to increase libido.

Paraphilias

Patients with paraphilias experience recurrent sexual fantasies or arousal that involve either inanimate objects, children, unconsenting adults, or physical and psychological pain. These occur primarily in men and begin before age 18 years. Severity peaks at approximately 20 years of age and then declines somewhat. Patients often have several paraphilias.

Symptoms depend on the type of paraphilia:

- **Pedophilia,** the most common paraphilia, involves sexual acts with a young child by a patient at least 5 years older.
- Patients with **exhibitionism** expose their genitals to strangers and may masturbate while exposed.
- **Fetishism** involves arousal from the use of inanimate objects, such as women's clothing.
- Patients with **frotteurism** are aroused by sexually touching an unconsenting adult.
- Sexual **masochism** is characterized by arousal from acts of humiliation or physical aggression against oneself.
- Sexual **sadism** involves arousal by humiliating or being physically aggressive toward others.
- **Transvestic fetishism** involves arousal from cross-dressing.
- Patients with **voyeurism** are aroused by "peeping" at unknowing victims who are undressing or are involved in sexual activity.

Psychotherapy and behavioral therapy. Antiandrogens seem to be helpful with some hypersexual paraphilias.

Gender Identity Disorders

Discomfort about one's gender and a persistent desire to be the other gender are characteristic of gender identity disorder.

Boys often dress in women's clothing and are involved in traditionally female pastimes. Girls show an aversion to traditionally feminine things, may urinate standing up, and plan to grow a penis or develop into a man. Peer conflicts are common. As adults, these patients may be heterosexual or homosexual and may attempt to live as a member of the other sex.

A strong identity with the other sex causes distress or impaired functioning. The diagnosis of gender identity disorder may be made in children or in adults.

Play therapy is used in children, but parental counseling may be more beneficial. Psychotherapy and surgical sex change are used as treatment for adults.

Other Psychiatric Disorders

Bereavement Versus Major Depression

Bereavement is the period of grief that follows the death of a loved one. Normal symptoms include sadness, difficulty concentrating, preoccupation with thoughts of the loved one, poor appetite, and insomnia. It is not uncommon to dream about the deceased or even to hear the person's voice or sense his/her presence. In normal bereavement, however, the survivor realizes that these impressions are not real. The onset of bereavement may be delayed by several months, particularly if the death was unexpected, and normal bereavement may last a year or more.

Many symptoms of bereavement are also symptoms of depression, but generally a major depressive episode (see box earlier in this chapter) is not diagnosed until at least 2 months after the acute loss. Signs of depression above and beyond bereavement may include intense guilt, preoccupation with death, feelings of worthlessness, hallucinations, psychomotor retardation, and inability to function normally in society. The depressed mood is relatively constant, whereas normal grief comes in waves.

Adjustment Disorder

Within 3 months of a psychological stressor, a patient develops emotional or behavioral changes that are far in excess of what would be expected but do not include delusions or hallucinations. The symptoms resolve within 6 months, unless the stressor continues. Acute and chronic adjustment disorders are more prevalent in poor urban communities, where violence and poverty are constant stressors. This diagnosis does not apply to normal bereavement.

Dissociative Disorder

Dissociative disorders are characterized by a sudden disruption in the normal integration of cognitive functions, including identity, state of consciousness, memory, and perception. These disorders are generally but not always transient and reversible. Dissociation, repression, and denial are the major defense mechanisms used. There are four major dissociative disorders.

- **Dissociative amnesia,** the most common, involves partial or complete amnesia about a stressful or traumatic event. This diagnosis does not apply to symptoms caused by drug use or head trauma. Spontaneous recovery is usually abrupt and complete. Barbiturates may precipitate the recovery of memory.

PSYCHIATRY

- **Dissociative fugue** involves amnesia about the past in a patient who has unexpectedly traveled away from home. Heavy use of alcohol, mood disorders, and personality disorders may be predisposing factors. Episodes may last months, with spontaneous but not always complete recovery.
- **Depersonalization disorder** involves constant or recurrent feelings of ego-dystonic detachment from the patient's internal identity. A perception of being estranged and mechanical is accompanied by insight and intact reality testing. This diagnosis can only be made in the presence of severe distress or impaired functioning. Stress and physical or mental illness may precede or exacerbate this disorder.
- **Dissociative identity disorder,** previously called *multiple personality disorder,* occurs when patients have at least two distinct personalities. The personalities alternate control of the body, and deficits in memory result. Abuse in childhood, usually sexual, precipitates the development of this chronic disorder. Hypnosis or an amobarbital interview may elicit hidden personalities. Hypnotherapy and psychotherapy are used for treatment.

Delirium

Delirium may be an organic mental syndrome, a manifestation of medical illness, or a result of substance intoxication. It reflects widespread brain dysfunction that is most often reversible.

Decreased attention, disorganized thinking, and some change in level of consciousness, orientation, memory, or perception are present.

The preceding symptoms develop over hours to days and fluctuate. An underlying cause should be established; if one cannot be found, the diagnosis is an organic mental syndrome.

Identify and treat the underlying cause.

Dementia

In dementia, chronic progressive cognitive and intellectual deficits cause severely impaired functioning without any change in consciousness. Two major causes of dementia are Alzheimer's disease (see Chapter 13) and multi-infarct dementia. Alzheimer's develops gradually over time, while multi-infarct dementia progresses in a step-wise fashion.

Impaired memory, cognition, and judgment are present, in addition to some deficits in language, motor skills, or sensory function. Personality changes may occur.

PSYCHIATRY

The preceding symptoms develop over weeks to months. An underlying disorder should be sought, including potentially reversible causes of dementia, such as vitamin B12 deficiency, thyroid disease, and normal pressure hydrocephalus.

Symptomatic and psychosocial support are helpful. Treatment should be directed to the underlying disorders. In some cases, early diagnosis may guide risk-factor reduction and limit progression of disease.

PSYCHIATRY

15

Injury and Poisoning

Accidental Injury

Death from accidental injury accounts for a significant proportion of the mortality in younger age groups. After approximately age 45 years, chronic diseases, such as cancer and cardiovascular disorders, become more important causes of mortality (Table 15-1).

By far the largest cause of accidental death is motor vehicle accidents, which account for almost half of all childhood injuries. However, the incidence of childhood automobile deaths is declining because of regulations requiring car seat and seat belt use. Motor vehicle accidents often involve alcohol and are particularly common in adolescents. Suicide and homicide are also seen primarily in teens, whereas falls, drownings, and fires are more common in younger age groups. Alcohol and cigarettes are frequently associated with residential fires.

Drowning

Approximately 4500 people drown each year in the United States. The distribution of drowning deaths is bimodal, with the first group consisting of children younger than age 5 years and the second group consisting of male teenagers. Teenage drowning victims are most often boys. The accident usually occurs in a large body of water, such as a lake or river, and alcohol is frequently involved.

Infants younger than age 2 years are at risk for drowning in bathtubs and buckets, and children between ages 2 and 5 years are at greatest risk of drowning in swimming pools. Often, the child may have escaped supervision for only a few minutes. Mandatory pool fencing is being considered in some states, as this measure reduces the drowning rate by more than 80%.

Once submersion occurs, there are two mechanisms by which hypoxemia results. Flooding of the alveoli with fluid may impair gas exchange. Also, hyperventilation and a "panic" response may lead to laryngospasm and glottic closure. Noncardiogenic pulmonary edema results from direct pulmonary injury as well as cerebral hypoxia. The hypoxemia and decreased perfusion result in metabolic acidosis.

Treatment of drowning victims involves the establishment of a patent airway and assisting ventilation. Removal of water through postural drainage or the Heimlich maneuver has not been proven to improve oxygenation. Possible hypothermia should also be addressed; all near-drowning victims should be warmed to 86–90°F before cardiopulmonary resuscitation (CPR) attempts are made.

Once patients are transported to medical facilities, supplemental oxygen should be provided and a nasogastric tube should be placed to prevent further aspiration. Fluid resuscitation may be necessary if the patient is in noncardiogenic pulmonary edema. Chest radiographs may appear normal or may show pulmonary edema and do not necessarily correlate with the patient's oxygenation status. Antibiotics and steroids have not been shown to alter the clinical course and should not be given routinely.

Aspiration

Most cases of foreign body aspiration occur in children ages 6 months to 3 years. Common high-risk objects include small toys, hard candy, peanuts, and pieces of hot dogs.

INJURY

Table 15-1. Leading causes of death by age group

Age	Causes of death
Birth to 1 year	Congenital anomalies
	Low birth-weight/preterm birth
	Sudden infant death syndrome
	Maternal causes
	Respiratory distress syndrome
1 to 4 years	Accidents
	Congenital anomalies
	Homicide
	Neoplasms
	Heart diseases
5 to 14 years	Accidents
	Neoplasms/cancer
	Homicide
	Congenital anomalies
	Heart diseases
15 to 24 years	Accidents
	Homicide
	Suicide
	Cancer
	Heart diseases
25 to 44 years	Accidents
	Cancer
	Heart diseases
	Suicide
	HIV infection
45 to 64 years	Cancer
	Heart diseases
	Accidents
	Cerebrovascular disease
	Diabetes
	Chronic obstructive pulmonary disease
	End-stage liver disease
65 years and older	Heart diseases
	Cancer
	Cerebrovascular disease
	Chronic obstructive pulmonary disease
	Pneumonia
	Diabetes mellitus
	Accidents
	Kidney disease
	Alzheimer's disease

INJURY

The common triad of symptoms is choking, coughing, and wheezing.

DIAGNOSIS

Diagnosis may be difficult, because parents may not notice that aspiration has occurred. Plain chest x-ray may suggest the site of the foreign body. Because of the position of the bronchi, most aspirated objects fall into the right middle lobe.

TREATMENT

Diagnosis and removal may require bronchoscopy. Sequelae of foreign-body aspiration include atelectasis, lung abscess formation, and pneumonia.

PREVENTION

Parents should be counseled on the risks of giving small objects to children in this age group.

Bites and Stings

In the United States, the most common poisonous **snake bites** come from pit vipers, such as rattlesnakes, water moccasins, and copperheads. Without treatment, swelling, pain, coagulopathy, and respiratory distress ensue, and death usually occurs within 6 to 8 hours. First aid includes splinting of the affected area and transporting the patient to a medical facility. Tourniquets, ice packs, and incision and suction by mouth are not recommended. Once hospitalized, specific antivenin is administered.

The most clinically important spider bites are from black widow spiders and brown recluse spiders. **Black widow bites** cause vomiting, abdominal pain, and shock. These symptoms may mimic an acute abdomen, but they are generally not lethal. Calcium gluconate and methocarbamol are effective therapies, but local bite treatment is not useful. **Brown recluse spider bites** are slightly more dangerous. The bite develops into a black scab that is associated with rash, fever, vomiting, and jaundice. Fatal disseminated intravascular coagulation can occur. Treatment includes dexamethasone, dapsone, colchicine, and total excision of the lesion.

Most **insect stings** result from bees, wasps, and ants. The resulting local pain, redness, and swelling are best treated with removal of insect tissue (the "stinger") and cool compresses. Rapid onset of urticaria, respiratory distress, and hypotension indicates the development of anaphylaxis, an allergic reaction in a sensitized individual. Immediate treatment for anaphylaxis consists of intubation and epinephrine injection, which may be followed by administration of bronchodilators and IV fluids. Patients who are known to be allergic to stinging insects should carry anti-anaphylaxis kits.

Dog and cat bites are quite common, especially in young children. Wound care includes high-volume, high-pressure saline irrigation, wound debridement, and tetanus prophylaxis. Rabies prophylaxis may also be necessary if the animal has not been vaccinated. Likely organisms from dog and cat bites include *Pasteurella multocida,* staphylococci, streptococci, and anaerobes. Antibiotic treatment is indicated if there are signs of infection, but prophylaxis is not recommended.

Rabies

Rabies is an acute viral disease that is transmitted by a bite from an infected animal. Rabid dogs provide the greatest risk to humans worldwide, but wild animals are the primary source of infections in the United States. The rabies virus travels from the site of inoculation through peripheral nerves to the spinal cord and brain. It proliferates in the brain and then spreads by efferent nerves to the salivary glands.

The incubation period after being bitten ranges from 30 to 50 days. Patients experience malaise, fever, and restlessness initially, and symptoms rapidly progress to extreme excitement and painful laryngeal and pharyngeal spasms. Death is from asphyxia, exhaustion, or paralysis and usually occurs within 2 weeks of initial symptoms.

Any animal that bites a human should be isolated. If the animal appears normal after 10 days of observation, it was probably not infectious at the time of the bite. If it becomes rabid, its brain must be analyzed for the virus, and the patient must begin prophylactic therapy. Viral testing of patients once symptoms begin confirms the diagnosis.

Thorough cleaning of the wound reduces the likelihood of contracting rabies. In patients bitten by a rabid animal or by a high-risk animal not available for observation, prophylaxis involves passive immunization with rabies immunoglobulin and active immunization with vaccine. Aggressive symptomatic treatment of patients who develop rabies may help; without treatment, mortality is 100%.

Thermal Burns

Burn injuries are generally classified by their extent and depth. The extent of the burn describes the amount of body surface area affected. In adults, the **"rule of nines"** divides the body surface into areas consisting of approximately 9% of the total area. In children, the surface of one side of the child's hand can be used to approximate 1% of body surface area. The "rule of nines" is shown in Figure 15-1.

The depth of the burn is classified by degree. **First-degree burns** affect only the epidermis. They are red or gray and do not blister (due to lack of dermal injury). **Second-degree burns** appear hyperemic and generally blister because of partial-thickness injury to the dermis. **Third-degree burns** involve full-thickness injury to the dermis. They may appear leathery or pearly. These burns are numb to the touch because of destruction of nerve endings in the dermis.

Initial treatment of the patient includes airway management, cooling, and IV fluid resuscitation for burns of more than 25% of body surface area. The Parkland formula suggests giving lactated Ringer's solution at a rate of 3 to 4 mL per kg of body weight for each 1% of body surface burned. This volume should be administered over the first 24 hours, with half of the solution given in the first 8 hours. Complications of burns include paralytic ileus, which requires placement of a nasogastric tube to prevent aspiration, and stress gastritis, which requires treatment with IV H_2 receptor antagonists.

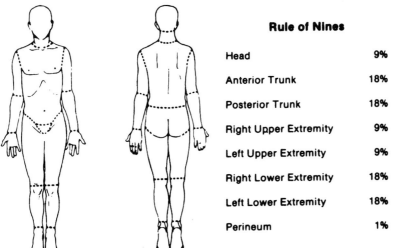

Rule of Nines

Head	9%
Anterior Trunk	18%
Posterior Trunk	18%
Right Upper Extremity	9%
Left Upper Extremity	9%
Right Lower Extremity	18%
Left Lower Extremity	18%
Perineum	1%

Fig. 15-1. Rule of nines. (Reprinted with permission from Rippe J, Irwin R, Fink M, Cerra F: *Intensive Care Medicine,* 3rd ed. Boston, Little, Brown, 1996.)

Infections are a common and extremely serious complication of burn injuries. Burn patients are particularly at risk for infection with *Pseudomonas aeruginosa* and may develop sepsis. Systemic antibiotics are generally not effective in full-thickness burns because of lack of vascularity, so topical antibiotics, particularly silver sulfadiazine, are used. All patients should receive tetanus immunoglobulin and tetanus toxoid if they have not received a tetanus booster within 5 years. Large burn wounds require analgesia and debridement, as well as evaluation for possible skin grafting.

Burns are an important cause of injury and death in children, most commonly as a result of scalding injuries. Parents can adjust water heater thermostats to below 54°C to minimize this risk. Cigarette use causes a large number of building fires. Smoke detectors and fire alarms should be installed and maintained in all buildings.

Electrical Injuries

The passage of high-voltage electricity through body tissue results in thermal injury. These injuries are sometimes known as "fourth-degree" burns to denote damage to the muscle and bone, often despite relatively normal skin appearance. Patients typically have a charred area of skin where the current entered the body and an "exit wound" that resembles the explosive exit wound from a projectile injury.

Several organ systems are affected after an electrical injury. Ventricular fibrillation can occur with exposure to even small amounts of electrical current, and respiratory failure can result due to thoracic wall and diaphragmatic tetany. Other sites of damage include neurologic damage resulting in seizures as well as corneal burns resulting in cataract formation. Renal failure due to rhabdomyolysis and local areas of hemorrhage and compartment syndrome may also be seen.

CPR is key in the initial treatment of these patients. IV fluid administration is also necessary to prevent shock and maintain urine output in the face of myoglobinemia. Surgical evaluation should be performed, as small areas of superficial burns may conceal larger areas of necrosis that require debridement.

INJURY

Prevention measures include installing grounding structures and disconnecting circuit breakers whenever work is done on electrical appliances. Injuries in children can be prevented by unplugging appliances not in use and installing safety guards in electrical outlets.

Chemical Burns

Chemical burns are common in both household and industrial settings and can be caused by a variety of chemicals, including lyes (drain cleaners, paint removers), cleansers (disinfectants, toilet bowl cleaners), and pesticides. The face, eyes, and extremities are most commonly affected.

Initial treatment involves stopping any ongoing burning by removing soaked garments and diluting or neutralizing the remaining chemical. Irrigation with water or saline is appropriate, although certain chemicals, such as carbolic acid or sodium metal salts, may be activated and cause further damage.

After irrigation and debridement, patients may require fluid resuscitation similar to that required in thermal burns. Treatment with analgesics, antihistamines, and antibiotics may also be indicated.

Lye ingestion (swallowing drain cleaner) is a common cause of poisoning because most drain cleaners are odorless and tasteless. Lye ingestion causes liquefaction necrosis, which primarily affects the esophagus and can result in ulceration and perforation. Insertion of a nasogastric tube for dilution is controversial, as it may result in perforation. Endoscopy is necessary as soon as the patient is stable since the extent of oropharyngeal damage is not indicative of esophageal injury. Areas of severe necrosis may require surgery. The most common delayed complication is stricture formation, which can result weeks or years after the ingestion. Esophageal cancer is 1000 times higher in these patients than in the general population.

Shock

Shock can be caused by several different mechanisms, each with its own presentation (Table 15-2). Diagnosis depends on the clinical scenario and careful physical examination. The basic treatment of shock is the ABCs:

- **Airway:** Ensure that the patient has a patent airway, and intubate if necessary.
- **Breathing:** Use bag or ventilator.
- **Circulation:** Ensure adequate circulation.

Treatment depends on the type of shock.

Poisoning

Childhood Poisoning

Unintentional poisoning occurs most often in children younger than age 6 years who ingest common household products, such as analgesics and cosmetics. Iron poisoning from

INJURY

Table 15-2. Characteristics of different types of shock

	Hypovolemic	Septic	Cardiogenic	Neurogenic
Etiologies	Hemorrhage	Infection	Arrhythmias	Spinal cord injury
	Burns	Gangrene	Myocardial infarction	Drug overdose
	Diarrhea	Necrosis	Congestive heart failure	
	Vomiting		Cardiovascular obstruction	
			Cardiovascular compression	
Skin	Pale	Pale/pink*	Pale	Pink
Neck veins	Flat	Flat	Distended	Flat
Pulse	High	High	High	Normal/low
Vascular resistance	High	High/low*	High	Low
Treatment	Rehydration		Medications	
	Transfusions	Fluid	Pacemaker	Fluid
	Medications	Antibiotics		Medications
		Medications		

*Septic shock varies depending on whether it is low-output (late) or high-output (early) septic shock.

vitamin overdose is a particular hazard because many parents are under the mistaken impression that vitamins are harmless and therefore do not seek timely medical attention. Prevention measures include childproof cupboard latches and childproof medication bottles.

Emergency treatment is essential and depends on the poison ingested. Parents with small children should always have syrup of ipecac and activated charcoal readily available for use. These remedies should not be administered if the patient is unconscious or if the poison is corrosive. Ipecac induces vomiting, whereas activated charcoal helps to adsorb many poisons. Gastric lavage or dialysis may be necessary.

Organophosphate and Carbamate Poisoning

Organophosphates and carbamates are found in insecticides and inhibit cholinesterase molecules in both the central and peripheral nervous systems, resulting in paralysis. Absorption occurs through the skin and mucous membranes. The symptoms that result can be recalled by the mnemonic SLUDGE (*s*alivation, *l*acrimation, *u*rination, *d*iarrhea, *g*astrointestinal cramping, and *e*mesis). Severe exposure can result in confusion, seizures, and coma. Diagnosis is made clinically and by history, as labs that assess cholinesterase activity cannot be done on a timely basis. Treatment involves maintaining an airway, decontamination, and administration of atropine or pralidoxime.

Methemoglobinemia

Methemoglobinemia usually occurs as an adverse reaction to the administration of certain medications, typically topical anesthetics (benzocaine) and sulfonamides. Because methemoglobin is incapable of binding with oxygen, patients become hypoxic and may appear cyanotic. Administration of oxygen will not reverse the patient's cyanosis and venous blood will appear chocolate brown. Treatment is with administration of methylene blue, which reduces the methemoglobin.

Carbon Monoxide Poisoning

Carbon monoxide poisoning occurs through exposure to combusted materials and typically results from improperly vented heating systems as well as exposure to engine exhaust and methylene chloride-containing paint thinners. Carbon monoxide binds to hemoglobin, blocking oxygen binding and resulting in hypoxia. Symptoms begin with headache and dizziness and can progress to seizures, hypotension, and coma. Pulse oximetry and arterial blood gas measurements are not useful, and diagnosis must be made by measuring blood carboxyhemoglobin levels. Treatment is with 100% oxygen.

Common Poisons and Antidotes

Table 15-3 contains several common chemicals that can result in overdose or poisoning, as well as the symptoms of toxicity and the antidotes (if available).

Table 15-3. Common poisons and antidotes

Chemical	Symptoms of toxicity	Antidote/treatment
Acetaminophen	Nausea, anorexia, liver failure	N-acetylcysteine
Benzodiazepines	Slurred speech, drowsiness, respiratory depression	Flumazenil
Beta-blockers	Hypotension, bradycardia, AV block, pulmonary edema, hypoglycemia	Glucagon, atropine, temporary pacemaker
Cyanide	Headache, nausea and vomiting, confusion	Nitrite or hydroxycobalamin
Digoxin or foxglove plants	Anorexia, nausea and vomiting, visual disturbances, arrhythmias	Digoxin-specific antibodies
Ethylene glycol (antifreeze)	Ataxia, hallucinations, seizures, tachycardia	Ethanol
Heparin	Bleeding	Protamine sulfate
Isopropyl alcohol	CNS depression, coma	Supportive care
Methanol	Visual disturbances, headache, dizziness, seizures	Ethanol
Salicylates	Nausea and vomiting, tinnitus, hyperventilation, anion gap metabolic acidosis	GI decontamination, charcoal, correct metabolic abnormalities, hemodialysis
Strychnine	Convulsions	Supportive care
Tricyclic antidepressants	Anticholinergic effects (dry mouth, urinary retention, tachycardia, agitation), cardiac toxicity with QRS widening	Sodium bicarbonate
Warfarin	Bleeding	Vitamin K, fresh frozen plasma

INJURY

Mechanisms of Injury

Motor Vehicle Accidents

During a motor vehicle collision, three types of impacts occur. First, the vehicle is brought to a stop. Next, the occupants, previously traveling at vehicular speed, collide with part of the stopped vehicle. Finally, the organs within the occupants' bodies collide with the body's frame (Figure 15-2). Injuries in head-on collisions are listed in Table 15-4. Rear-end collisions typically cause whiplash injuries to the neck. Lateral collisions frequently cause multiple fractures and cervical-spine injuries.

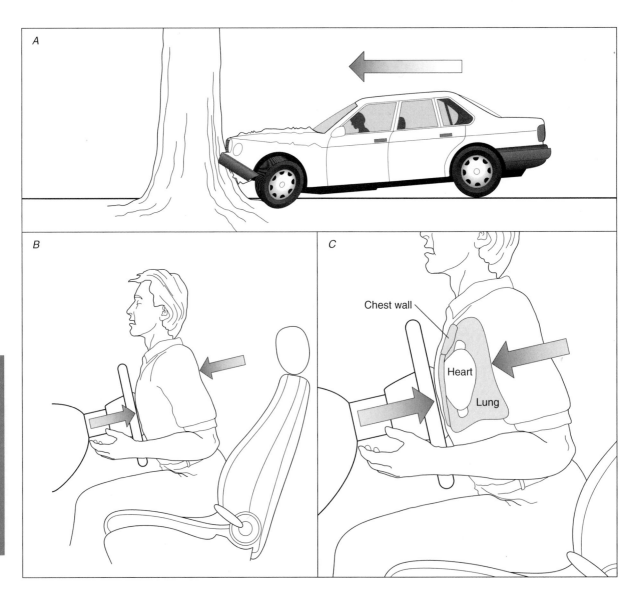

Fig. 15-2. Collisions injury pattern. **A:** The automobile collides with the tree. **B:** The occupant collides with structures inside the automobile. **C:** The organs of the body collide with body walls. (Reprinted with permission from Caroline N: *Emergency Care in the Streets,* 5th ed. Boston, Little, Brown, 1995, p 290.)

Table 15-4. Injuries in head-on collisions

Steering wheel injuries	Dashboard injuries	Windshield injuries*
Mouth/chin lacerations	Knee injury	Scalp/facial lacerations
C-spine injuries	Hip dislocation	C-spine injuries
Tracheal rupture	Femur fracture	Brain injury
Cardiac trauma		
Pneumothorax/hemothorax		
Aortic shearing		
Abdominal trauma		

*If windshield injury occurs, the patient is assumed to have a cervical spine (C-spine) injury until proven otherwise.

Pedestrian Injuries

In most pedestrian-versus-car accidents, the person is struck by the car's bumper. Injuries are caused by a threefold impact pattern. First, the bumper hits the pedestrian's leg. Next, the chest hits the front grill. Finally, the head hits the ground (Figure 15-3). In adults, this series of impacts causes leg fractures and head injury. In children, abdominal and thoracic injury accompanies head injury.

Fall Injuries

Fall injuries depend on the height of the fall, the landing surface, and the position of the body on impact. Children tend to fall head first because of their higher center of gravity. They tend to sustain head injuries as well as wrist and upper extremity fractures as they attempt to break their fall. Adults sustain heel fractures, vertebral compression fractures, and femoral and pelvic fractures, as well as pulmonary contusions and spleen and liver rupture.

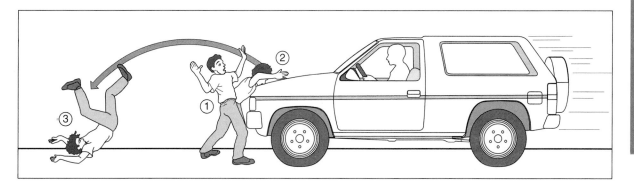

Fig. 15-3. Pedestrian injury pattern. First the leg is struck by the car bumper (*1*); next the chest is struck by the grill (*2*); finally, the head hits the ground (*3*). (Reprinted with permission from Caroline N: *Emergency Care in the Streets,* 5th ed. Boston, Little, Brown, 1995, p 293.)

Gunshot Wounds

Bullet wounds produce damage by crushing the tissue in the bullet's path. Travel through the tissue results in the formation of a cylindrical "permanent cavity" of the same diameter as the bullet. Bullets may tumble or oscillate, resulting in a larger permanent cavity. The size of entrance and exit wounds depends on the type of bullet used, but the exit wound is generally the larger one. Bits of hair and skin may accompany the bullet on its path, resulting in contamination of the wound.

Stab and Puncture Wounds

Stab and puncture wounds may not cause significant external injury, but internal injuries may be severe. If the knife or object remains in the wound, do not remove it, as this may cause hemorrhage and further damage. Instead, attempt to stabilize the item until it can be surgically removed. If careful inspection reveals a superficial wound that will not require deep surgical repair, it may be treated as a simple laceration. This generally requires local anesthetic, debridement, and suturing. Avoid vasoconstricting anesthetics, such as those containing epinephrine or cocaine, on the digits, nose, ear, and penis.

Injuries by Anatomic Site

Traumatic Injury to the Head

Head injury is the leading cause of death in males younger than 35 years old. Brain tissue may be damaged at the point of impact (**coup**) or opposite the point of impact (**contrecoup**). Skull penetration and fractures can lead to tissue damage and to hematoma formation. The presence of a skull fracture should be assumed until ruled out in any patient who sustained significant head trauma. Clinical signs of skull fracture include **Battle's sign** (discoloration over the mastoid bone), blood drainage from the ears, bruising of the orbit, cranial nerve palsies, and CSF leakage from the ears and nose. Skull fractures may require surgical treatment.

Intracranial injury is a blanket term covering subdural and epidural hematomas, cerebral contusion, and cerebral laceration.

Acute Subdural Hematoma

Acute subdural hematoma occurs from rapid bleeding between the dural and arachnoid layers of the meninges, usually as a result of tearing of the bridging veins. It is a common cause of death in patients with head injury.

SIGNS & SYMPTOMS

Symptoms progress more slowly with this venous bleed than with arterial hemorrhage. Spastic hemiplegia with increased deep tendon reflexes may be present. Signs of transtentorial herniation may develop, including deepening coma with decorticate and then decerebrate posturing and midposition or dilated fixed pupils.

INJURY

CT or MRI is diagnostic. Lumbar puncture is contraindicated because the procedure may precipitate brainstem herniation.

Surgical drainage of the hematoma.

Chronic Subdural Hematoma

Chronic subdural hematoma is the delayed or slowed formation of a subdural clot. This condition is particularly common in the elderly and in alcoholics. Symptoms may develop weeks after a head injury, with a progressive, daily headache, fluctuating consciousness, and mild hemiparesis. CT or MRI reveals the lesion. Treatment is with surgical drainage, and prognosis is good.

Epidural Hematoma

Epidural hematomas, bleeding between the dura and the skull, are not as common as sub-dural hematomas. Epidural hematomas typically arise from injury to arteries, most commonly the middle meningeal artery. Because it is an arterial bleed, an epidural hematoma can cause rapid brain compression with permanent neurologic sequelae or death.

Patients typically experience a brief lucid interval after a severe head injury, followed by progressive headache, decreasing level of consciousness, motor deficits, and pupillary abnormalities. Temporal fracture lines may be noted on examination.

CT or MRI is diagnostic and may reveal a coexisting skull fracture.

The extradural clot must be quickly removed. In the absence of imaging devices, burr holes through the cranium provide both diagnosis and treatment.

Concussion

Concussion refers to injury to the brain that is due to blunt trauma without evidence of significant lesions or sequelae.

INJURY

Transient loss of consciousness typically lasts seconds to minutes. Although unconscious, the patient has intact brainstem function without signs of hemiplegia or decerebrate reflexes. Afterward, the patient may experience a post-traumatic confusional syndrome, with transient retrograde and anterograde amnesia, and longer-lasting headache, vertigo, and mild cognitive dysfunction.

Clinical presentation.

Careful observation for development of more severe signs is all that is necessary.

Cerebral Contusion and Laceration

Cerebral contusions and lacerations are often associated with skull damage and depressed fragments of bone. They may result in brain edema and transtentorial herniation, leading to coma, decorticate or decerebrate posturing, and death. Signs of brainstem injury suggest a poor prognosis. The clinical presentation usually suggests the diagnosis, which is confirmed by CT or MRI scan. Depressed skull fractures should be repaired, and supportive care is critical.

Facial Trauma

Facial trauma may lead to nasal and maxillary injuries. The most common facial fracture is a broken nose. Symptoms include tenderness, swelling, bleeding, and crepitus (a crackling sensation). Treatment requires pressure and cold packs to reduce bleeding and swelling. Reduction may be necessary.

Blunt eye trauma may cause periorbital ecchymosis ("black eye"), hemorrhage into the anterior chamber of the eye (hyphema), and edema. Fracture of the orbital bone is called a *blowout fracture*. Severe injury should be seen by a specialist, and daily ophthalmologic examinations should be performed until the symptoms resolve. Aspirin or other anticoagulants are contraindicated.

After blunt ear trauma, an auricular hematoma ("cauliflower ear") may develop. It requires prompt drainage to prevent dissolution of the cartilage.

Injuries to the Neck and Back

The most common cause of paraplegia and quadriplegia is spinal cord injury from vertebral fractures, often after motor vehicle or diving accidents. Emergency treatment includes immobilization and ensuring an airway. Cervical-spine protectors should be kept in place until cross-table neck x-rays show that no injury has occurred. Compression fractures of the vertebral bodies are also frequently seen in elderly men and women as a result of osteoporosis and degenerative joint disease.

Injuries to the Chest

Injuries to the thorax can result in hemothorax, pneumothorax, and aortic rupture, all of which may be rapidly fatal. Cardiac tamponade is another commonly seen injury, discussed in Chapter 2. Blunt trauma to the heart may also result in myocardial injury. Injuries below the level of the nipples are considered abdominal injuries because of the presence of the liver and the spleen directly under the diaphragm.

Cardiac Trauma

Traumatic injury to the heart occurs frequently in motor vehicle accidents. Cardiac tamponade and myocardial contusion can result.

Depending on the nature of the injury, the patient may be asymptomatic or may show symptoms of tamponade or myocardial contusion. Symptoms of contusion are similar to those of infarction.

The mechanism of injury is consistent with cardiac trauma.

The first priority is to stabilize the patient. Surgical decompression may be necessary.

Traumatic Injury to the Lung

Injury to the chest can result in numerous pulmonary complications, including hemothorax, pneumothorax, and flail chest. **Open pneumothorax** from penetrating chest injury occurs when air is sucked into the pleural space, forcing the lung to collapse. **Tension pneumothorax** can occur from blunt trauma. Tissue damage of the lung itself allows air to enter the pleural space and not escape. **Flail chest** describes the unstable condition that occurs after several ribs and the sternum are fractured.

Reduced breath sounds and hyperresonance to percussion are noted. In open pneumothorax, air being sucked into the lung through the chest may be heard. In flail chest, the portion of the rib cage that has broken moves paradoxically in comparison to the rest of the chest during breathing.

History of trauma combined with evidence of the preceding. Chest x-ray will show a mediastinal shift away from the affected side in tension pneumothorax.

INJURY

Chest tube or valve placement may allow equalization of pressures and expansion of the lung in pneumothorax.

Injuries to the Abdomen

Blunt abdominal trauma, typically a result of motor vehicle accidents, usually causes damage to the solid organs (liver, spleen, pancreas, and kidneys) and can cause massive internal bleeding. Penetrating abdominal injuries usually result in perforation of the intestines because they occupy the largest volume in the abdomen.

Physical examination findings depend on the type and degree of injury. Large intestinal perforation will cause peritonitis and may lead to septic shock, but smaller perforations may not initially cause peritoneal irritation. A developing fever and elevated WBC count are important clues. Massive hemorrhage will cause hypotension or shock, but small, retroperitoneal bleeds may be initially contained and stable. Hematuria is evidence of damage to the kidneys or urinary tract.

In any situation for which the diagnosis is not immediately apparent, serial abdominal examinations are critical. Peritoneal lavage, in which a catheter is placed into the peritoneal cavity so fluid can be instilled and removed for analysis, is a standard test to identify peritoneal bleeding and organ rupture. It can be performed on a patient who is not stable enough for CT. CT is better able to detect retroperitoneal injuries but often misses small perforations.

Patients with peritonitis or hypovolemia despite fluid resuscitation should undergo an exploratory laparotomy. Generally, all abdominal stab wounds should also be surgically explored to rule out intestinal perforation because a delay in diagnosis can lead to severe sepsis. Blunt trauma victims without abnormalities on CT or peritoneal lavage may be observed for signs of decompensation.

Sprains

Sprains refer to injuries of the ligaments or other soft tissues surrounding a joint. Severe sprains may involve the complete separation of a ligament from the bone, resulting in joint instability. The most commonly affected joints are the ankle and the knee. Symptoms can range from slight loss of function to severe swelling and pain.

Treatment guidelines for the first 24 to 48 hours are remembered with the mnemonic *RICE:*

- *R*est: Immobilize the joint for 24 to 48 hours. Use crutches if necessary.
- *I*ce: Apply cold packs immediately to reduce pain and swelling.
- *C*ompression: Wrap with an elastic bandage to immobilize and compress the joint.
- *E*levation: Keep the afflicted limb above the level of the heart whenever possible to help reduce swelling.

In addition, NSAIDs may be helpful for their analgesic and anti-inflammatory properties. After 2 to 3 days, the patient may begin bearing weight on the joint as tolerated.

Fractures

Types of Fractures

Open (compound) fracture: A fracture with an associated open skin wound.

Closed (simple) fracture: A fracture with no associated skin wound.

Greenstick fracture: A fracture through only one side of the cortex that generally occurs in children.

Spiral fracture: A fracture involving a twisting breakage of the bone.

Comminuted fracture: A fracture with multiple bone fragments.

The most common wrist fracture is a Colles fracture in which the distal radius is broken and displaced posteriorly. It typically results from an attempt to "break" a fall using an outstretched hand. This fracture is seen commonly in postmenopausal women.

Elbow fractures generally occur in children younger than age 10 years after a fall on an outstretched hand with the elbow in extension. They can result in compression of the radial and median nerves or the brachial artery. Improper care can lead to the development of **Volkmann ischemic contracture,** in which the fingers are permanently contracted.

Patients with **tibial fractures** are at risk for developing **compartment syndrome,** in which bleeding into the tight muscle compartments causes compression of the blood supply, leading to muscle ischemia. The "six Ps" of compartment syndrome are **pain, pallor, pulselessness, poikilothermia** (cool temperature), **paresthesias,** and **paresis** (weakness) or paralysis. Surgical opening of the compartment is necessary to prevent permanent muscle and nerve damage.

Simple **rib fractures** are the most common thoracic injury and are typically caused by direct blows to the chest. The fifth through ninth ribs are most often injured because the lower "floating" ribs are more flexible and resilient to trauma. Patients typically experience localized pain that worsens on deep breathing. A pneumothorax may be present. Splinting the fracture may help control pain.

Pelvic fractures occur primarily as a result of motor vehicle accidents. Bleeding is a common cause of death in these patients, as more than 30% of a patient's blood volume can be lost to the pelvic cavity. ABCs (airway, breathing, and circulation) should be established, and these patients should be managed as shock victims. Pelvic x-rays should be obtained in all cases of major trauma.

Hip fractures are a major cause of disability and death in the elderly. Osteoporosis weakens bones, which can then be broken in a minor fall. More than 200,000 hip fractures occur in the United States annually, and 10% to 20% lead to death. Many of the survivors require long-term care. Avascular necrosis of the femoral head may occur if displacement of the femoral head compromises blood flow. Treatment usually includes surgery within hours of the injury. A prosthetic hip may be implanted to increase stability. Prevention includes safety measures to prevent falls, such as handrails in the tub and nonslip bath mats, as well as estrogen replacement therapy and calcium supplementation to prevent bone loss in women.

INJURY

General Guidelines for the Treatment of Limb Fractures

- Splint fracture and elevate above the heart, if possible.
- Apply ice to reduce swelling.
- Perform a neurologic examination and check that both sensory and motor pathways are intact.
- Check that pulses are present with no compromise of vascular supply.
- Administer anesthesia and reduce fracture if necessary.
- Immobilize with a cast or splint.

Dislocation

Dislocation refers to the disruption of joint placement, sometimes associated with tearing of the ligaments. Shoulders, elbows, fingers, hips, knees, and ankles are the most common sites of dislocation injury. They are often treated by manipulation and traction but may require surgery.

Hip dislocation commonly occurs as a result of motor vehicle accidents. If the knee hits the dashboard at high speed, posterior displacement of the femoral head from the acetabulum may result. This may damage the blood supply, causing avascular necrosis of the femoral head. Additionally, compression of the sciatic nerve may occur, leading to an abnormal gait and footdrop.

Sternoclavicular dislocation (posterior dislocation of the clavicle at the sternum) may be seen after strong pressure to the chest. It is a typical football injury. Symptoms include a sensation of choking and a sensory deficit in the upper extremity. Complications include damage to the mediastinal structures, including the trachea and the esophagus.

Intentional Injury

Child Abuse

More than 2.4 million reported incidents of child abuse occur annually. Child abuse may include physical and emotional abuse, sexual abuse, or neglect. Physicians must report suspected abuse and may be held legally liable if they do not. Confidentiality of the physician's identity is maintained. The increase of mandatory reporting laws has made clinicians more aware of the signs of child abuse, although many cases are still missed.

The clinician should look for a history of multiple injuries, regardless of how "nice" the family may appear. Children should be interviewed alone, if possible. Also, evaluate whether the extent of trauma matches the injury history. Common child abuse injuries include burns, fractures, abdominal trauma, and head trauma.

On examination, the distribution of an injury often suggests whether it was intentional or not. For example, splash marks tend to accompany accidental scald burns, whereas clearly demarcated lines without splash marks indicate intentional injury. A small circular area that is spared also suggests intentional injury, if the abuser used that area to hold and "dunk" the child. Injuries to a child's front are generally accidental, whereas trauma to the back may be intentional. Signs of neglect include dehydration, poor weight gain, hypervigilance, and depression.

Clinicians should document all lesions, and any remarks by the child or parent that suggest abuse must be recorded verbatim. Photographs and x-rays are allowed in most states without parental permission if abuse is suspected. Reporting to the department of social services should be done as soon as possible by phone, and a written report should be sent within 48 hours. If in doubt, it is always better to report suspected cases of abuse.

Sexual Abuse

Sexual abuse is any nonconsensual sexual activity and includes exposure, genital manipulation, oral sex, and intercourse. Physical contact is not required. A child cannot give informed consent and may not even understand that what is occurring is considered abusive.

Dysfunctional behavior in children, such as clinging, unusual fears about other people, and recurrent nightmares, may reflect abuse. Chronically abused children often display poor self-esteem and depression.

In a clinical setting, questions should focus on living and caretaking arrangements and on possible touching or hurting of any body part. Proceed from head to toe; do not focus solely on the genital area. The physical examination should occur with another health care worker in the room, and the child should be reassured that he or she has not done anything wrong. A supine, frog-legged position is best for the genital examination, and any bruises, swelling, or lacerations should be noted. An enlarged horizontal diameter of the hymen may indicate that penetration has occurred, although a normal examination does not exclude abuse. The anal area, scrotal area, and penis must be examined. Gonorrhea and chlamydia cultures should be taken, and any unusual discharge must be investigated. Throat cultures should also be performed in cases of suspected oral sex. As with other forms of child abuse, all observations should be recorded clearly and reported to the department of social services as soon as possible.

Spouse Abuse

Spouse abuse is the deliberate physical, sexual, or emotional assault by one romantic partner on another. Most commonly, men abuse their female partners; however, women may be batterers, and spousal abuse may occur in homosexual relationships as well. Other problems associated with spousal abuse include child abuse and alcoholism. As many as 10% of battered women attempt suicide.

Battering is the most common cause of injury for which women seek medical attention. Clinicians should be aware that patterns of repeated emergency room or clinic visits may be a sign of domestic violence. As with child abuse, the history may not match the severity of injury. In addition to symptoms related to their injuries, victims of battering may manifest symptoms of depression, post-traumatic stress disorder, or pelvic disorders.

If spousal abuse is suspected, the patient should be interviewed alone and asked direct questions in a supportive manner. Plans for intervention are made according to the patient's wishes and may include safety plans, hot lines, shelters, or family therapy. The patient may choose not to take action. If so, clinicians should continue to provide support and information about possible alternatives.

INJURY

Elder Abuse

Elder abuse is broadly defined as physical or emotional abuse and neglect of persons aged 65 years or older, typically occurring in a domestic setting. A caretaker or family member is often the perpetrator, and patients are reluctant to report abuse for fear of losing their only support. As the American population ages, elder abuse is becoming an increasingly common problem.

Clinicians should be aware of unusual or frequent bruises, welts, and fractures. Evidence of poor nutrition, dehydration, social isolation, and depression should also arouse suspicion. Currently, all 50 states have mandatory reporting laws. Protective services may evaluate the patient's competence and make recommendations for alternate guardianship.

Rape

Rape is forced sexual assault. In the United States, roughly 1 in 10 women will be raped in her lifetime. Current estimates indicate that only 20% of rapes are reported to the authorities, and many rapes are perpetrated by an acquaintance or family friend.

Patients need emotional support as well as clinical attention. They should be treated respectfully and nonjudgmentally. History-taking should include details of the assault as well as activities such as bathing that may have been performed afterwards. Physical examination must document traumatic injuries anywhere on the body, including external and internal genital, anal, and oral areas. A Pap test may show sperm, and vaginal fluid should be collected by cotton swab and placed on slides and in glass tubes. Wood lamp examination of the patient's body is useful because seminal fluid will fluoresce. The pubic area should be combed, and material collected should be saved as possible evidence. Fingernail scrapings and pubic hair samples may also be useful. Any sites penetrated should be checked for sexually transmitted diseases, including gonorrhea, chlamydia, and *Trichomonas*. VDRL tests should be performed on blood to check for syphilis. Follow-up examinations should include HIV and pregnancy testing. Prophylactic protocols include penicillin, tetracycline, and tetanus immunization.

It is important to ensure that the patient has social support systems and follow-up examinations, both for physical as well as psychological evaluation.

INJURY

16

Research, Adult Care, and Ethics

Statistics

Measures of Central Tendency

The **mean** (or average) is calculated by adding all observations and dividing by the number of observations.

Example: Data set {1, 1, 1, 2, 3, 5, 8}

$$\text{Mean} = \frac{(1 + 1 + 1 + 2 + 3 + 5 + 8)}{7} = \frac{21}{7} = 3$$

The **median** is the "middle" observation, obtained by ordering all data and finding the center value. (With an even number of observations, the middle two values are averaged to obtain the median value.) The median is not affected by extreme values, as is the mean.

Example: Data set {1, 1, 1, 2, 3, 5, 8}

Median = center-most value = 2

The **mode** refers to the most frequent observation. Some data sets may have more than one mode (bimodal) or may have no mode (i.e., all observations are different).

Example: Data set {1, 1, 1, 2, 3, 5, 8}

The mode = most common value = 1

Measures of Variability

Measures of variability describe the spread of data from the center values. The common measures are range, variance, and standard deviation.

The **range** is simply the difference between the maximum and the minimum values.

Data set: {1, 3, 5, 5, 6}

Range = maximum value − minimum value = 6 − 1 = 5

The **variance** (known as s^2) is obtained by adding the squares of each point's deviation from the mean, and dividing by sample size minus one.

Data set: {1, 3, 5, 5, 6}

$$\text{Variance} = \frac{(1-4)^2 + (3-4)^2 + (5-4)^2 + (5-4)^2 + (6-4)^2}{(5-1)} = \frac{16}{4} = 4$$

The **standard deviation** is the square root of the variance. The units of standard deviation are the same as the original units of measurement.

Data set: {1, 3, 5, 5, 6}

PUBLIC HEALTH

Standard deviation $= \sqrt{4} = 2$

Gaussian (bell-shaped) distributions have a mean = median = mode. Approximately 68% of the population falls within one standard deviation of the mean, 95% of the population falls within two standard deviations, and 99% of the population falls within 2.5 standard deviations (Figure 16-1).

Probability and Distribution

Probability distributions allow evaluation of the likelihood of a particular event by its location on a graph. Many biological variables (e.g., albumin level, height) follow bell-shaped or "normal" distributions. If the tail of the curve is on the right side (toward higher $\times$ values), the curve is said to be **skewed right,** whereas a curve with a tail to the left is **skewed left** (Figures 16-2 through 16-4). The further a patient's data point is from the peak of the graph, the less likely it is to be a normal variant.

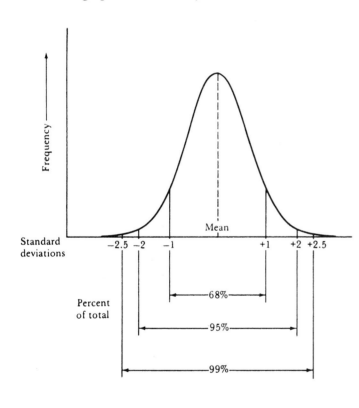

Fig. 16-1. Percentage of measurements within various standard deviations of the mean. (Reprinted with permission from Hennekens C, Buring J: *Epidemiology in Medicine.* Boston, Little, Brown, 1987, p 238.)

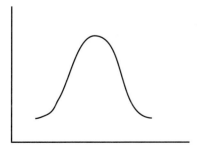

Fig. 16-2. Normal distribution.

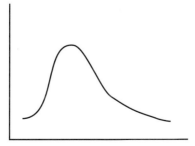

Fig. 16-3. Distribution with right skew.

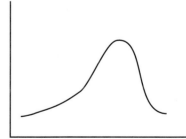

Fig. 16-4. Distribution with left skew.

PUBLIC HEALTH

Incidence and Prevalence

$$\text{Incidence} = \frac{\text{Number of \textbf{newly} reported cases of a disease}}{\text{Total population}}$$

$$\text{Prevalence} = \frac{\text{Number of \textbf{existing} cases of a disease at a given time}}{\text{Total population}}$$

Prevalence depends on the incidence and the natural history of the disease. If patients survive a long time after diagnosis, prevalence will be higher than incidence.

Disease Frequency

$$\text{Disease frequency} = \frac{\text{Number of people with disease}}{\text{Population at risk}}$$

Remember to think about which individuals are at risk. For example, pregnancy (which is not technically a disease) only affects reproductive-aged women, so this is the population that must be used in the denominator.

Case Fatality Rate

$$\text{Case fatality rate} = \frac{\text{People who die from the disease in a given period}}{\text{Number of people with disease}}$$

This is sometimes mistakenly used as a measure of risk. The case fatality rate will tell you only what percentage of people who have the disease die, not the risk of disease faced by the general population.

Relative Risk

Relative risk (RR) is the risk of developing a particular disease for people with a known exposure compared with the risk of developing the same disease without the exposure. An RR greater than one implies a positive association between the exposure and the disease, whereas an RR less than one implies a negative association. An RR of one shows no association between the exposure and the disease, with an equal risk of the disease in both populations (Table 16-1).

RR can be calculated only from **cohort** studies.

$$\text{RR} = \frac{a/(a+b)}{c/(c+d)} = \frac{\text{Disease in exposed population}}{\text{Disease in unexposed population}}$$

Odds Ratio

Odds ratio (OR) is the odds of exposure among cases compared with the odds of exposure among controls. It is also used to measure the strength of association between a particular exposure and disease. This is an *estimate* of RR that can be calculated from **case-control** trials.

PUBLIC HEALTH

Table 16-1. Calculating relative risk and odds ratio

		Disease			
		Present	Absent		
Exposure	Present	a	b	a + b	$RR = \dfrac{a/(a + b)}{c/(c + d)}$
	Absent	c	d	c + d	$OR = \dfrac{a/c}{b/d}$
		a + c	b + d	a + b + c + d = N	

OR, odds ratio; RR, relative risk.

$$OR = \frac{a/c}{b/d} = \frac{ad}{bc}$$

Standardized Mortality Rate

Mortality rates are the number of people dying per year within a certain population. Mortality rates are often used to assess differing risks for populations living in different areas. If, however, the age distributions of the two populations are different, then the mortality rate may be expected to be different. Adjusting the mortality rate according to the age distribution results in standardized mortality rates, which can then be compared with assessed risk.

Attributable Risk

Attributable risk, or risk difference, is the difference in rates of disease between exposed and unexposed populations. It is an estimate of the percentage of disease attributable to a certain risk factor. For example, if nonsmokers have a lung cancer rate of 5 per 100,000 and smokers have a lung cancer rate of 180 per 100,000, the attributable risk is $180 - 5 = 175$ per 100,000. Thus, for a population of 100,000, 175 out of 180 lung cancer deaths would be "attributable" to smoking.

Sensitivity

The sensitivity of a test is the probability that results will be positive in patients who actually have the disease (mnemonic: **positive in disease, or PID**). It reflects the test's ability to diagnose accurately all cases of the disease. If a person is disease-free but has a positive test result, the result is termed false-positive (Table 16-2).

$$\text{Sensitivity} = \frac{a}{a + c}$$

Typical sensitivity rates for medical tests used to diagnose disease are around 80%–90%.

PUBLIC HEALTH

Table 16-2. Calculating sensitivity and specificity

		Disease			
		Present	Absent		
Test results	Positive	a	b	a + b	$\text{Sensitivity} = \dfrac{a}{a + c}$
	Negative	c	d	c + d	$\text{Specificity} = \dfrac{d}{b + d}$
		a + c	b + d	a + b + c + d = N	

Specificity

The specificity of a test is the probability that the test results will be negative in those without the disease (mnemonic: **negative in health, or NIH**). If a person has the disease but has a negative test result, the result is termed **false-negative.**

$$\text{Specificity} = \frac{d}{b + d}$$

Typical specificity rates for medical tests used to diagnose disease are around 85%–95%.

Positive Predictive Value

The positive predictive value (PPV) of a test is the probability that an individual who has a positive test result actually has the disease.

$$\text{PPV} = \frac{a}{a + b}$$

Negative Predictive Value

The negative predictive value (NPV) of a test is the probability that an individual who has a negative test result does not have the disease.

$$\text{NPV} = \frac{d}{c + d}$$

Decision Analysis

Decision analysis is a process in which quantitative methods are applied to a medical problem in an attempt to determine the best course of action. This technique involves the use of decision trees and estimation of probabilities for each possible outcome.

PUBLIC HEALTH

Accurate Versus Precise Measurements

An **accurate** measurement provides true information that matches a particular standard. For example, if a patient weighs 140 pounds, and a scale provides the same information, the measurement is accurate. A **precise** measurement refers to the size of units used for measurement. For example, a scale may provide the information that a patient weighs 145.75 pounds, which is a precise measurement. However, if the patient in reality weighs 140 pounds, this precise measurement is also inaccurate.

Valid Versus Reliable Measurements

A **valid** measurement is one that provides true and genuine information about the subject being measured. For example, blood pressure is a valid measure of risk of hypertension. A **reliable** measurement is reproducible, so it will result in similar results if repeated. Blood pressure measurements may not be reliable from one measure to the next, depending on changes in the patient's position or stress level.

Hypothesis Generation and Test Statistics

Hypotheses are generated from clinical observation and descriptive epidemiology (case reports, case series, and cross-sectional surveys). They are tested by conducting analytic studies (case-control, cohort, and intervention studies) and assessing the statistical significance of the results by using test statistics (chi-squared tests, z-tests, and t-tests). In general, the null hypothesis (H_0) states that there is no association between the exposure and the disease, whereas the alternative hypothesis (H_1) states that an association is present.

The *P* value is the probability of obtaining the results of a study by chance alone, assuming the null hypothesis is true. By convention, the null hypothesis is rejected when the likelihood of a particular result occurring by chance alone is less than 5% ($P < .05$). Thus, a *P* value less than .05 supports a true difference between the two groups being studied. A **type I error** occurs when the null hypothesis is rejected even though it is true (Table 16-3). A **type II error** occurs when the null hypothesis is not rejected even though it is false. **Statistical power** is defined as the probability of being able to reject the null hypothesis when it is false. A larger sample size has more statistical power and will reduce the likelihood of type I and type II errors.

Confidence Intervals

A confidence interval provides the range of values that is statistically consistent with a particular study's data. If the 95% confidence interval for an OR or RR estimate spans 1.0, then the data do not support the hypothesis that the factor in question is associated with an increased risk of disease. This is the same as having a $P > .05$, and the null hypothesis is not rejected.

PUBLIC HEALTH

Table 16-3. Possible errors in hypothesis testing

		Truth	
		H_0 is true	H_0 is false (H_1 is true)
Decision based on study	Accept H_0	Correct decision	Type II error False-negative
	Reject H_0 (assume H_1 is true)	Type I error False-positive	Correct decision

H_0, null hypothesis; H_1, alternative hypothesis.

Research Issues

Case Series

A case series is a report of the characteristics of a group of individuals with a particular disease. A case series may raise hypotheses about risk factors for a disease but cannot be used to test these hypotheses. A well-known case series reporting an unusual occurrence of *Pneumocystis carinii* pneumonia among gay men in Los Angeles was the first published report about the AIDS epidemic.

Cross-sectional Studies

Cross-sectional studies assess risk factors and disease status in a group of people at one point in time. They are useful for correlating disease prevalence with exposure prevalence, but no conclusive statement can be made about whether a risk factor precedes the onset of a disease. As a case series, the purpose of a cross-sectional study is to raise hypotheses.

Case-Control Studies

Case-control studies compare a group of individuals who have a particular disease (cases) with a group of individuals without the disease (controls). The frequency of various exposures is assessed in the two groups. From this information, the **odds ratio** (see section on odds ratio) can be calculated, which is an approximation of the **relative risk.** Case-control studies are relatively quick and inexpensive to conduct and may not require many subjects. Case-control studies are ideal for studying diseases that are rare or have long latent periods. Disadvantages include the need to rely on a subject's memory to assess exposure (recall bias) and the inability to calculate rates of disease incidence.

PUBLIC HEALTH

Cohort Studies

Cohort studies begin by classifying a group of individuals by exposure status. Studies that follow a group over time to identify those who develop disease are **prospective cohort studies.** In **retrospective cohort studies,** exposure and disease have both already occurred. For example, work records from shipyards in World War II describe exposure to asbestos. Death records of men who worked in the shipyards can be used to assess the number of cancer deaths, and data from this study can be used to calculate the increased health risk associated with exposure to asbestos.

The advantages of cohort studies include the ability to calculate the **relative risk** (see section on relative risk) and the ability to study more than one effect of an exposure. Recall bias is minimized in prospective studies because exposure status is established before the disease develops. Disadvantages include the need to study large numbers of people to ensure an adequate number of subjects with a disease. It is virtually impossible to use a cohort to study a rare disease because any given population will have very few cases, making calculations unreliable. Other disadvantages include time (it may take years to get enough data to analyze) and expense.

Clinical Trials

A **double-blind, placebo-controlled clinical trial** is the gold standard for testing the effectiveness of a new drug or treatment for a particular condition. Subjects are randomly divided into a treatment group (which receives the intervention) and a control group (which does not receive the intervention). If an effective treatment is already available, the new treatment may be compared with the current standard of care; otherwise, the control group should receive a placebo. After a period, the treatment outcomes of the two groups are compared. To decrease the bias, it is important to carry out these trials in a blinded fashion, so that neither the patients nor the clinicians know which patients are receiving treatment.

Community Intervention Trials

Community intervention trials are experiments in which a community is the unit of intervention. For example, fluoridated water may be supplied to one community, and the average number of dental caries per child in that community is compared with a community that does not receive fluoridated water. In structuring these interventions, it is important to ensure that the members of the community will not be exposed to any significant risk of illness. Animal testing may be required before testing in humans.

Quality of Research Data

Guidelines for screening and treatment are formulated after the data for or against a particular recommendation are assessed and balanced. The quality of the data is typically ranked along the following continuum:

PUBLIC HEALTH

I: Evidence obtained from at least one properly randomized controlled trial.

II-1: Evidence obtained from well-designed controlled trials without randomization.

II-2: Evidence obtained from well-designed cohort or case-control analytic studies, preferably from more than one center or research group.

II-3: Evidence obtained from multiple time series with or without the intervention. Dramatic results in uncontrolled experiments (such as the results of the introduction of penicillin treatment in the 1940s) could also be regarded as this type of evidence.

III: Opinions of respected authorities, based on clinical experience; descriptive studies and case reports; or reports of expert committees.

Well-designed and well-conducted **meta-analyses** (statistical analyses in which the data from several different studies are pooled) are also considered and graded according to the quality of the studies on which the analyses were based (e.g., grade I if the meta-analysis pooled properly randomized controlled trials).

For example, practice guidelines based on type I and II data are considered more **evidence-based** than recommendations based on type III data.

Bias

Investigator Bias

Investigator bias is the bias that results when the measurement of outcome depends upon subjective interpretation by the person performing the study. This does not necessarily imply fraud, but results from the natural tendency that people will interpret data to see what they expect or would like to see. Due to the widespread presence of this type of bias, most studies are **blinded**—that is, the people collecting the data are kept unaware of whether the subjects that they are interviewing are in the intervention group or the control group.

Lead-Time Bias

Lead-time bias results when a comparison is made from the time of diagnosis to an outcome (such as death) in a group that is studied and compared with a group that is not studied. The classic example of lead-time bias is the fact that asymptomatic smokers who undergo screening chest x-rays appear to have longer survival after a diagnosis of lung cancer when compared with smokers diagnosed during routine medical care. Although it may appear that the screened group has an improved prognosis, this may simply be an artifact of earlier detection without any actual prolongation of life.

Length Bias

Length bias occurs when a disease has both a slowly progressive and a rapidly progressive form (as is seen in many types of cancer). When a comparison is made between screened and nonscreened groups in these types of diseases, it may appear that persons who were screened and diagnosed earlier have a longer survival than those who present with symptoms. In actuality, it may be that the cases detected by the screening are more likely to be slowly progressive to begin with, and thus the survival advantage is conferred by the type of disease detected by the screening, not the screening itself.

PUBLIC HEALTH

Publication Bias

Publication bias results because there is a greater tendency to publish studies that show a difference between two groups than studies that show no difference between the groups. Also, the ability of a study to detect a difference between two groups depends upon the power of the study, and the power of a study depends upon the number of subjects enrolled in the study. Thus, smaller studies are less likely to show a difference between two groups than larger studies and are therefore less likely to be published. This type of bias is of greatest concern in a **meta-analysis,** in which the data of several studies are pooled together. The data available for meta-analyses may be biased because unpublished data that showed no effect may not be available for inclusion in the analysis.

Recall Bias

Recall bias describes the fact that people with more dramatic outcomes may be more inclined to recall (or think they recall) adverse events preceding the outcome. For example, women who have children with birth defects may be more likely to recall minor illnesses or conditions they experienced during pregnancy than women who bear children without birth defects.

Reporting Bias

Reporting bias describes the tendency of people to report their history differently, depending upon the perceived importance or sensitivity of the issue. For example, people who are diagnosed with sexually transmitted diseases (STDs), which may result in serious outcomes (such as HIV), are more likely to report the names of all sexual partners than people diagnosed with less serious STDs (such as trichomonas).

Investigator, recall, and reporting bias are all forms of assessment bias.

Selection Bias

Selection bias occurs whenever there is a difference between the subjects of the intervention and the control group that is likely to affect the results. For example, teenage girls using oral contraceptives may be more likely to contract STDs than girls not using oral contraceptives. However, if the teenage girls using oral contraceptives are more likely to be sexually active than the control group, then the differences in the rates of STDs may have to do with differences in the behaviors of the two groups and may not be associated with the use of oral contraceptives at all. To avoid this type of bias, the subjects are usually randomly selected (or **randomized**) to participate in either the intervention or the control group.

Self-selection bias refers to the fact that people who seek out clinical studies, screening tests, or participation in research may also have certain characteristics that can affect the outcome. For example, subjects who volunteer for studies may be more compliant with medications or dietary regimens than the average patient, and therefore the outcome may be different when the results are generalized to the population at large.

Research Design

Subject Selection

If a study's results are to be generalizable to the population of interest, the subjects in the study must be representative of that population. Any systematic variation from the population (e.g., being more or less ill, more willing to volunteer, of a different SES) may introduce bias that will reduce the validity of the study. A randomly selected population is usually ideal.

Sample Size

If the sample size of a study is too small, an observed difference between the exposed and unexposed may not be statistically significant. Standard formulas for sample size determination allow for choice of a proper sample.

Consent

In a research context, a subject must be clearly informed about the interventions and possible consequences, and the subject must give definite agreement and permission.

Placebos

Placebos are substances that have no known pharmacologic activity. However, many patients experience improvement of symptoms after receiving placebo medications because of psychological interactions in the perceptions of symptoms and pain. Whenever the efficacy of a medication is tested, results should be compared with a control group receiving placebos, unless the current existence of a helpful treatment makes the use of placebos unethical.

Conflict of Interest

Conflicts of interest occur when what is best for the patient is not best for the experiment. For example, an investigator may have to choose between keeping a subject in the experiment or treating his or her newly diagnosed diabetes. The patient's best interests are always considered most important.

Vulnerable Populations

Research protocols using populations that are unable to give informed consent (e.g., children or the mentally ill) or that may be subject to coercion (e.g., prison inmates) should be carefully monitored.

Normal Adulthood and Aging

Prevention

Preventive measures can be directed against a health problem at several different points in its development.

- **Primary prevention** refers to actions that decrease the incidence of a health problem before it develops (e.g., immunization).
- **Secondary prevention** involves intervention at an early stage of a health problem to limit further development (e.g., diabetes screening and Pap tests).
- **Tertiary prevention** refers to intervention to treat the health problem itself and to prevent further morbidity or mortality (e.g., coronary artery bypass graft).

PUBLIC HEALTH

Well-Adult Care

Table 16-4 provides a brief summary of recommended adult screening and preventive care requirements. These guidelines apply only to adults with no history of related diseases and no family history for these diseases; patients at higher risk may require more frequent screening.

Stress Management

Stress has been implicated in the development of many medical conditions, including hypertension and heart disease. Both positive and negative events can cause stress. The ten most stressful life events are:

Table 16-4. Adult preventive health measures

		Preventive measure	*Frequency*	*Age (yrs)*
Immunizations		Tetanus booster	Every 10 yrs	18+
		Influenza vaccine	Every yr	65+
		Pneumococcal vaccine	Once	65+
Cardiovascular		Blood pressure	Every 2 yrs	21+
		Cholesterol	Every 5 yrs*	35–65 (men)
				45–65 (women)
GI		Obesity (weight and height for BMI <27)	1–3 yrs	
		Stool for occult blood OR	Every yr	50+
		Sigmoidoscopy OR	Every 5 yrs	50+
		Colonoscopy OR	Every 10 yrs	50+
		Barium enema	Every 5–10 yrs	50+
Men				
	Prostate	Digital rectal examination	Every yr*	50+
		PSA	Every yr*	50+
	Testicles	Testicular examination	Every 3 yrs*	20–40
Women				
	Breast	Breast self-examination	Monthly**	20+
		Provider breast examination	Every 3 yrs*	20–50
			Every yr	50+
		Mammography	Every 1–2 yrs*	40–50
			Every 1–2 yrs	50–69
	Pelvic	Pelvic examination	Every 1–3 yrs	18–40
			Every yr	40+
		Pap test	Every year	18+ or earlier if sexually active
			Every 3 yrs	After two normal tests

*Controversial. **No data to support this recommendation.

BMI, body mass index (weight in kg over height squared in meters); PSA, prostate-specific antigen.

Adapted from U.S. Preventive Services Task Force Guidelines and American Cancer Society Guidelines.

- Death of a spouse or child
- Divorce
- Marital separation
- Institutional detention (e.g., jail)
- Death of close family member
- Major personal injury or illness
- Marriage
- Loss of job
- Marital reconciliation
- Retirement
- Taking the Step 2 exam

Stress management techniques include:

- Counseling
- Social support
- Biofeedback
- Hypnosis
- Relaxation techniques
- Antianxiety medications
- Health-promoting strategies, including a healthy diet, exercise, and recreational activities

Normal Aging

Some slowing in physical and mental ability is a natural part of aging; however, clinicians should rule out treatable illnesses before accepting a decrease in function in an older patient. More than 80% of people older than age 65 years have one or more chronic illnesses, and the average number of prescription drugs taken ranges from three to five. In fact, drug interactions account for more than 10% of hospital admissions in this age group. Assessment of the capacity to perform activities of daily living (e.g., bathing, eating, dressing) may provide more specific information on functional status.

Some decrease in memory and intellectual capability is normal, but it is incorrect to assume that senility is a normal part of aging. Clinicians should investigate other causes, such as depression. Decreasing mental function because of "old age" should be a diagnosis of exclusion. Only 10% of patients older than age 65 years have significant dementia; this increases to approximately 40% in patients older than age 85 years. Comparatively, 15% to 25% have significant depression.

Psychosocial Adaptations of Aging

Most older persons attempt to maintain their previous level of social activity, but isolation, loss of family and friends, health problems, and changes in living situation can all lead to depression. Depression in the elderly is associated with insomnia and loss of appetite, as well as memory impairment. The elderly also have a high incidence of suicide. Unmarried, widowed, and divorced patients are at greater risk of developing depression than married patients. In a clinical setting, physicians should assess the full range of issues in the elderly, including physical, psychological, and social functioning. Possible approaches to increas-

PUBLIC HEALTH

ing socialization and combating depression include therapy, senior day care centers, volunteering, and support groups.

Nutrition with Aging

Aging is associated with a lower caloric requirement that is due to decreased muscle mass, although this may depend on the patient's activity level. Some elderly persons may be malnourished because of difficulties in obtaining and preparing food, cost, difficulty with teeth or dentures, or depression. Reductions in fluid intake may make elderly patients prone to dehydration. Dehydration is one of the most common causes of acute confusional states in the elderly.

Epidemiology of Neoplastic Disease

Although cardiovascular disease is the primary cause of death in the United States, accounting for 36% of deaths each year, cancer is the second leading cause of death, responsible for 22% of deaths each year. Age is the most important predictor of cancer incidence, with the incidence of cancer generally rising with increasing age. Overall, the mean age of diagnosis is 65 years.

Certain cancers are more prevalent in some racial groups than in others. For example, the rate of prostate cancer is much higher in African-American men than among any other group. Lifestyle and habits are well-known factors contributing to the development of neoplastic disease. For example, 90% of lung cancers are attributed to tobacco use. Men are more likely to develop lung cancer than women because of the higher rates of smoking among men. Gender and socioeconomic status (SES) may be independent risk factors for disease. In addition, lower SES may be associated with poor access to medical care, delayed diagnosis, and therefore poorer prognosis. Some cancers and their associated risk factors are listed in Table 16-5.

Death and Dying

The emotional states that people experience when informed of a terminal illness have been described in detail by Elizabeth Kübler-Ross. A brief overview of the five stages are as follows:

- **Denial** is the phase in which the patient may be in a state of shock and reject the diagnosis or the presence of physical impairment.
- The next stage is **anger.** The patient may be upset and frustrated and ask, "Why me?"
- The patient may **bargain,** making promises of good behavior and charity to family, physician, or God in exchange for a cure.
- Patients often experience some amount of **depression;** however, serious depression should not be accepted as a normal response and should receive appropriate psychiatric treatment. Mild depression, which may include insomnia and a sense of hopelessness, is a normal part of accepting death.
- Ultimately, patients should reach the stage of **acceptance,** realizing that death is inevitable and coming to terms with their prognosis.

Table 16-5. Risk factors for cancer

Risk factor	Associated cancer
Tobacco	Lung
	Head and neck
	GI
	Kidney and bladder
	Pancreas
	Cervix
Alcohol	Liver
	GI
	Head and neck
Ionizing radiation	Leukemia
	Lymphoma
	Thyroid
	GI
	Bladder
Sun exposure	Basal and squamous cell skin cancers
	Malignant melanoma
DES exposure	Cervix
	Vagina
Infectious agents	
Epstein-Barr virus	Burkitt's lymphoma
Hepatitis B and C viruses	Liver
Human papillomavirus	Cervix
Schistosomiasis	Bladder
Nutritional factors	
High fat and low fiber	Colon
Aflatoxins (from fungi)	Liver

DES, diethylstilbestrol.

Chronic Care

Pain management is a critical issue in the chronic care of a dying patient. Addiction is not a concern for terminally ill patients, so narcotics should not be withheld if needed for pain control. Regular dosing schedules, rather than "as needed" administration, are used to maintain an adequate level of analgesia and to avoid episodes of breakthrough pain.

Infections occur frequently in patients with cancer as a result of immunosuppressive therapies, the effects of chronic disease, and chemotherapy-induced bone marrow suppression. The decision to give antibiotics should be based on the potential to improve both quantity and quality of life. Hospitalization with isolation may be necessary if patients become neutropenic.

Although nutrition is often a concern in the terminally ill patient, enteral or "forced" feedings are generally not recommended. The decreased food intake may be a necessary result of progressing illness, and excess food may cause discomfort and reduce the quality of life.

PUBLIC HEALTH

Hospice Care

Hospice care can be given to patients with terminal illnesses, usually during their last 6 months of life. It is provided in many settings, including private homes, hospitals, nursing homes, and specially designed hospice facilities. Hospice care focuses less on invasive medical treatments for prolonging life and more on physical and emotional comfort. It does not encourage euthanasia or assisted suicide but attempts to provide the support that a patient needs to die comfortably and with dignity.

Medical Ethics

Competency and Decision-making Capacity

A competent patient is capable of making his or her own decisions about care. Competent patients may refuse medical interventions at any time, not solely in the case of terminal illness. The basis of competency is the idea of **patient autonomy**—that the patient's self-determination and individual right to make decisions about his or her care are respected. Exceptions may be made in some cases of communicable disease, when patients must be treated or quarantined. Issues regarding pregnant women, whose decisions may threaten the life of the fetus, are currently under debate, and legal precedents in these cases have been contradictory.

How is a person's "decision-making capacity" assessed? Consider the following:

- The mental status examination is used to ensure that decisions are not a product of delusional beliefs or hallucinations.
- The patient must understand the situation enough to give informed consent (see section below).
- The patient's decision should be relatively stable over time and consistent with the patient's values and goals.

In general, decisions concerning children should be made with the child's best interests in mind and with the child's preferences taken into consideration. Parents are presumed to be the appropriate decision makers for their children, except in emergencies (when physicians may provide care without explicit parental instruction) or when parents themselves lack decision-making capacity. The courts may overrule the parents' decision if it is not thought to be in the best interest of the child, but most physicians prefer not to resort to this option unless it is absolutely necessary.

Full Disclosure and Medical Errors

In general, the physician has the responsibility to inform the patient about his or her condition in a manner that the patient can understand. When family members ask that a patient not be told about a diagnosis or test results, the physician should ask about their specific fears and concerns. Ascertain if it is the family's wish or the patient's wish, and focus on how to tell the patient in an appropriate way, not whether to tell the patient. One ap-

PUBLIC HEALTH

proach is to discuss the issue with the patient early in the diagnostic workup. ("Some patients want to know everything about their medical condition, whereas others do not. What are your feelings about this?") Also, try to be aware of cultural issues regarding the disclosure of diagnoses.

Medical errors occur and are sometimes unavoidable. Physicians generally have ethical and moral obligations to disclose these errors to the patient. However, physicians are not obligated to inform patients of errors performed by others.

Informed Consent

Informed consent is a process through which decision-making power is shared between doctor and patient. The required components are as follows:

- The pertinent information is discussed with the patient, including the nature of the proposed interventions, the risks, the benefits, any available alternative treatments, and the expected consequences of receiving no medical treatment. All the patient's questions are answered.
- The patient decides whether to proceed with the treatment plan.
- There is no coercion from any party.

Informed consent is not required when the patient lacks decision-making capacity. In this case, an appropriate surrogate must make decisions. In an emergency, there is a **doctrine of implied consent,** and the physician is permitted to intervene in a manner presumed to be in the best interests of the patient.

Involuntary Confinement

Involuntary confinement involves hospitalization or detainment of a patient against the patient's wishes. It may be invoked when the patient is thought to pose an immediate danger to himself or herself or to others. Confinement may also be enforced if the patient is unable to care for himself or herself (e.g., by providing food, clothing, and shelter).

Confidentiality

Confidentiality, the idea that all communication between a patient and physician is private, is integral to the patient-doctor relationship. The rules of confidentiality do not apply if the following occurs:

- The patient waives confidentiality and allows the doctor to discuss the condition with the family, partner, or other persons.
- There is serious potential harm to the patient or a third party (such as suicidal or homicidal plans).
- The patient is a teenager with a condition that may result in serious adverse health consequences. In these cases, the physician may breach confidentiality and involve the parents.

PUBLIC HEALTH

Public Reporting

The Centers For Disease Control and Prevention require the reporting of several infectious diseases (Table 16-6).

Reporting of a medical impairment to public officials may also be required for the following conditions, but this varies from state to state:

- Impaired drivers (e.g., those prone to loss of consciousness)
- Elder and child abuse

If possible, discuss the fact that you will be breaching confidentiality with the patient before you report the illness.

Abortion

In the United States, approximately one induced abortion occurs for every five live births. The U.S. Supreme Court has upheld that abortion cannot be denied to women in the first

Table 16-6. The 52 Notifiable Infectious Diseases in the United States

Acquired immunodeficiency syndrome (AIDS)	Anthrax
Botulism	Brucellosis
Chancroid	*Chlamydia trachomatis,* genital infection
Cholera	Coccidioidomycosis
Congenital rubella syndrome	Cryptosporidiosis
Diphtheria	Encephalitis, California serogroup viral
Encephalitis, eastern equine	Encephalitis, St. Louis
Encephalitis, western equine	*Escherichia coli* 0157:H7
Gonorrhea	*Haemophilus influenzae,* invasive disease
Hansen disease (leprosy)	Hantavirus pulmonary syndrome
Hemolytic uremic syndrome, postdiarrheal	Hepatitis A
Hepatitis B	Hepatitis C; non-A, non-B
HIV infection, pediatric	Legionellosis
Lyme disease	Malaria
Measles (rubeola)	Meningococcal disease
Mumps	Pertussis (whopping cough)
Plague	Poliomyelitis, paralytic
Psittacosis	Rabies, animal
Rabies, human	Rocky Mountain spotted fever
Rubella (German measles)	Salmonellosis
Shigellosis	Streptococcal disease, invasive, group A
Streptococcus pneumoniae, drug-resistant	Streptococcal toxic-shock syndrome
Syphilis	Syphilis, congenital
Tetanus	Toxic-shock syndrome
Trichinosis	Tuberculosis
Typhoid fever	Yellow fever

3 months of pregnancy. However, poor women and women in isolated areas may not, in truth, have access to abortion. Methods of abortion induction include suction curettage, surgical curettage, and intra-amniotic instillation. In France, the abortion drug mifepristone (RU486), which acts as a progestin analogue, is commonly used; mifepristone is now legal in the United States but is only minimally used. Methotrexate and misoprostol have been used as abortifacients and may be used more frequently in the future. Dilation and evacuation and induction are techniques used in termination of second-trimester fetuses.

Disclosure of abortions to the biological father is controversial, and rules regarding this vary from state to state.

Maternal-Fetal Conflict

Maternal-fetal conflict arises during pregnancy when a treatment or request that benefits one party may be harmful to the other. Two common issues are surgical interventions and maternal behavior that may be toxic to the fetus.

Surgical intervention (e.g., cesarean section) against the mother's will is extremely controversial. Some courts have upheld that forcing a woman to undergo a cesarean section (and forcing a Jehovah's Witness to accept a blood transfusion during the procedure) is acceptable if the child's life would otherwise be lost. Other courts have disagreed, however, stating that it is a violation of patient autonomy. Judges generally rule in favor of the intervention (especially after it has already been performed).

Another area of controversy is the maternal use of known fetotoxic substances, such as drugs and alcohol. Most cases are tried under child abuse laws without success because most child abuse laws do not include "prenatal conduct or omissions." Some states are adopting more specific laws in the hope of prosecuting these cases successfully.

Euthanasia and Assisted Suicide

Euthanasia is the act of ending the life of a patient to avoid the prolongation of pain and suffering. Assisted suicide is the act of providing the means for a patient to commit suicide. **Assisted suicide** and euthanasia are currently illegal in the United States. Although a few states have successfully passed euthanasia and assisted-suicide initiatives, these laws are still being challenged in court.

What if a patient requests assisted suicide? Here are some recommendations:

- Do not impose your own values or become judgmental of the patient.
- Try to find out reasons for the request (e.g., inadequate pain control, fears, feelings of hopelessness).
- Try to relieve the patient's distress, if possible.
- Reaffirm the patient's control over medical decisions (e.g., no treatment will be forced on the patient).

Advance Directives

Advance directives allow patients to indicate their preferences for medical interventions and appoint a surrogate to act on their behalf should they lose their decision-making ca-

PUBLIC HEALTH

pacity. Directives can take the form of an oral or written statement. In **living wills** (not available in all states), the patient can ask that life-sustaining treatment be withheld in specified circumstances. Patients may also have a **durable power of attorney,** which appoints a particular person to act as a surrogate to make decisions if decision-making capacity is lost.

Advance directives can be limited in duration (e.g., 5 years) and to the situations in which they are enforceable (e.g., during an upcoming surgery).

Do-Not-Resuscitate Orders

Do-not-resuscitate (DNR) or "no code" orders are written to withhold cardiopulmonary resuscitation (CPR) if cardiac arrest occurs. (Even with CPR, more than 85% of patients requiring intervention do not survive.) The physician should discuss CPR preferences with patients and ensure that patients understand all options. Patients may choose to request limited DNR orders, which allow CPR for a specified period or allow only certain parts of the code. DNR orders are appropriate if

- The patient refuses CPR.
- The patient does not have decision-making capacity, and the surrogate refuses CPR on the patient's behalf.
- CPR would be futile. There is currently much debate on the exact definition of "futility," but the general meaning implies that the overall long-term status of the patient would not be improved with emergent resuscitation, as is often the case with end-stage terminal illness.

Life Support

Patients on life support may have left instructions regarding their desire for such medical care or may have previously appointed a surrogate to make these decisions. Without such instructions—although it is still legally challenged from state to state—physicians are generally allowed to discontinue a respirator. Discontinuation of nutrition and hydration, however, has been seen in many cases as "morally different" from the discontinuation of mechanical ventilation. Patients are able to refuse nutrition and hydration, but discontinuing this support in an unconscious patient generally depends on the patient's previously stated wishes or the decision of the surrogate. Some cases of prolongation of maternal life support in order to allow continued fetal development have also been documented.

Organ Donation

The **Uniform Anatomical Gift Act,** adopted in all 50 states, allows any competent adult to allow or forbid use of his or her organs through a written statement (usually a donor card). If no donor card has been provided, a surrogate may make the decision. If a donor card exists, however, physicians may procure organs over the objection of the family, although this is rarely done in practice for fear of lawsuits. In 1986, the U.S. government enacted a law requiring all hospitals that receive Medicare payments (essentially all of them) to perform a "required request" for organs, in which the family of a suitable deceased patient is asked to donate the patient's organs.

Diagnosing Death

Believe it or not, this is more confusing than you might think. Several different and competing definitions are used to diagnose death. "Heart death" is defined as the moment at which a spontaneous heartbeat cannot be restored. Usually, however, "brain death" is considered better grounds for a determination of death. Brain death is generally defined as an irreversible coma with no brainstem reflexes present (e.g., absent pupillary, corneal, vestibular, gag, and respiratory reflexes) for at least 6 hours. It may also involve the absence of EEG tracings for a specified amount of time, but this has been challenged by people who have recovered from drug overdoses who had previously shown flat EEGs. In any case, cessation of spontaneous respiration is not generally considered enough to diagnose death in a medical setting. Finally, a patient must be warmed to normal body temperature before death is definitively diagnosed, as some patients with hypothermia have "come alive" after warming.

Autopsy

Autopsy is the postmortem examination of a body, usually to determine the cause of death. Autopsies may be mandatory when intentional death is suspected, but if this is not the case, consent must be obtained from the patient's surrogate. Families may request autopsies, and some find that the objective information is helpful during the grieving process.

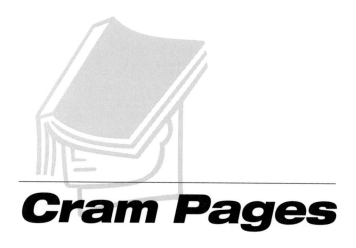

Cram Pages

This section contains charts of facts and word associations that often appear on the Step 2 exam. For some, the association may not be completely obvious; we suggest that you refer to earlier chapters or to more detailed medical texts if you are unfamiliar with the topic.

These pages are for you to tear out, write on, and personalize as much as you want, and we encourage you to add your own cram facts. After the exam, write to us (using the form in the back of the book) with your favorite cram facts, and we will try to include them in the next edition.

GASTROENTEROLOGY

Vitamins

Vitamin A	Night blindness
Vitamin D	Rickets
	Osteomalacia
Vitamin K	Clotting deficiency with long prothrombin time
Thiamine (B$_1$)	Beriberi
	Peripheral neuropathy
	Cardiomyopathy
	Wernicke-Korsakoff
	Confabulation
Niacin	Pellagra
	Diarrhea
	Dermatitis/stomatitis
	Dementia
Pyridoxine (B$_6$)	Neuropathy
	Deficiency associated with isoniazid
Cobalamin (B$_{12}$)	Macrocytosis
	Pernicious anemia
Folate	Macrocytosis
	Common in alcoholics
Vitamin C	Scurvy
	Bleeding gums

Esophagus and Stomach Disorders

Achalasia	Dysphagia for solids and liquids
	Absent peristalsis and tight lower esophageal sphincter
	Beak-like esophagus on x-ray
Esophageal cancer risk factors:	Smoking
	Alcohol use
	Gastroesophageal reflux
	Barrett's esophagus—adenocarcinoma
Gastritis: risk factors	Nonsteroidal anti-inflammatory drugs
	Alcohol use
	Helicobacter pylori
Peptic ulcer disease	*H. pylori* infection
Zollinger-Ellison syndrome	Gastrinoma
	Recurrent ulcers
Gastric cancer	Risk factor is *H. pylori* gastritis
	Virchow's (supraclavicular) node

Intestinal Disorders

Indirect inguinal hernias	Infants
	Persistent processus vaginalis
Direct inguinal hernias	Adults
	Weakness in Hesselbach's triangle
Crohn's disease	Can affect entire GI tract
	Terminal ileum most common
	Transmural
	Skip lesions
	"Cobblestoning"

Ulcerative colitis	Colon and rectum without skip lesions
	"Lead pipe" appearance on x-ray
Toxic megacolon	Children: Hirschsprung's disease
	Adults: inflammatory bowel disease
Ischemic colitis	Pain much greater than examination findings
Colon cancer	"Apple core" on x-ray
	Right-sided lesion: anemia
	Left-sided lesion: pencil stools

Gastroenteritis

Viral enteritis	Norwalk virus
	Rotavirus in young children
Staphylococcal enteritis	Onset in 3 to 6 hours
	"Church picnic" epidemic
Cholera	Fecal-oral transmission
	"Rice water" stools
Vibrio parahaemolyticus	Oysters
Shigella dysentery	Very small bacterial dose needed
	Blood and mucus in stools
Salmonella enteritis	Undercooked poultry
Hemorrhagic colitis	*Escherichia coli* H7:O157
Pseudomembranous colitis	*Clostridium difficile*
	Associated with antibiotics

Pancreatic Disorders

Acute pancreatitis	Pain radiates to back
	Gallstones, alcoholics
	Ranson's criteria
Chronic pancreatitis	Alcoholics
	Causes malabsorption and diabetes

Hepatobiliary Disorders

Cholelithiasis	"Female, fertile, forty, fat"
Cholangitis	Charcot's triad
	Biliary colic
	Jaundice
	Fever
Hepatitis A	Fecal-oral transmission
Hepatitis B	Blood-borne and sexually transmitted
	Hepatitis B surface antigen in early infection and carrier state
	Hepatitis B core immunoglobulin G present for life
Hepatitis C	Post-transfusion hepatitis, IV drug use
Hepatocellular carcinoma risk factors	Hepatitis B virus
	Hepatitis C virus
	Alcoholic cirrhosis
	Aflatoxins

CARDIOVASCULAR

Vascular Disorders

Secondary hypertension	Estrogen
	Renal or renovascular disease
	Hyperaldosteronism
	Pheochromocytoma
	Coarctation of the aorta
Aortic aneurysms	Abdominal
	Pulsatile mass on examination
	Atherosclerosis, smoking, hypertension
	Thoracic
	Marfan's, syphilis
Aortic dissection	Pain radiates to back
	Weak pulses
Peripheral vascular disease	Weak pulses
	Atrophic skin
	Little hair growth
	Nonhealing ulcers

Vasculitis/Inflammatory Disorders

Raynaud's phenomenon	Pallor, cyanosis, erythema of fingers
	Most cases idiopathic; others related to collagen vascular disease
Giant cell arteritis	Visual loss, high ESR
	Treat with steroids
Bacterial endocarditis	New heart murmurs
	Splinter hemorrhages under fingernails
	Osler's nodes (nodules on digits)
	Roth's spots (retinal hemorrhages)

Valvular Disorders

Mitral stenosis	Most caused by rheumatic fever
	Loud S_1 and opening snap after S_2
	Low-pitched diastolic rumble
Mitral regurgitation	Midsystolic click
	Harsh, blowing, holosystolic murmur
Aortic stenosis	Angina
	Syncope
	Left-sided heart failure
	Crescendo-decrescendo systolic murmur radiating to carotids
Aortic regurgitation	Decrescendo murmur
	Widened pulse pressure
	"Water hammer" pulse
	"Pistol shot" over femoral artery

Arrhythmias

Supraventricular tachycardia	Sudden attacks due to re-entrant rhythm
	P waves hidden in T waves on ECG
Atrial flutter	"Sawtooth" pattern on ECG
Atrial fibrillation	Absent P waves and irregular baseline on ECG
	Irregularly irregular pulse
Ventricular tachycardia	Three or more consecutive premature ventricular contractions
	Independent P waves on ECG
Ventricular fibrillation	No definable waves on ECG
	No pulse

CRAM PAGES

Lipid Metabolism

Familial hypercholesterolemia	Autosomal dominant
	Xanthomas and xanthelasmas
	Myocardial infarctions in 40s
Familial hypertriglyceridemia	Autosomal dominant
	Pancreatitis
	Milky serum
Familial combined hyperlipidemia	Autosomal dominant
	Increased cholesterol or triglycerides
	No xanthomas

Heart Disease

Myocardial infarction	ST elevation, T wave inversion on ECG
	Creatinine phosphokinase of myocardial origin peaks after 12 to 40 hours
	Serum LDH peaks after 3 to 6 days
Left-sided failure	Dyspnea on exertion
	Orthopnea
	Paroxysmal nocturnal dyspnea
Right-sided failure	Neck vein distention
	Liver enlargement
	Edema
Heart failure signs	S_3 due to rapid ventricular filling
	S_4 due to noncompliant ventricle
Congestive cardiomyopathy	Alcohol use

Pericardial Disease

Acute pericarditis	Pansystolic "friction rub"
Chronic pericarditis	Causes right-sided heart failure
	Kussmaul's sign present
Pericardial effusion	Friction rub
	Distant heart sounds
	"Water bottle" appearance on x-ray
Cardiac tamponade	Pulsus paradoxus
	Kussmaul's sign absent

RESPIRATORY DISORDERS

Upper Respiratory Infections

Streptococcal pharyngitis	High fever, red pharynx with exudate
	Associated with rheumatic fever and acute glomerulonephritis
Peritonsillar abscess	Displaced uvula
	Painful swallowing
	Trismus (cannot open mouth)
Influenza	Annual vaccine for at-risk people
Sinusitis	Yellow-green discharge
	Viral, *Streptococcus pneumoniae, Haemophilus influenzae*

Lower Respiratory Infections

Viral pneumonia	Flu-like prodrome
	Patchy infiltrates on x-ray
	Most common pneumonia in children

S. pneumoniae pneumonia	Red-brown "rusty" sputum Lobar pneumonia Gram-positive diplococci
H. influenzae pneumonia	Chronic obstructive pulmonary disease (COPD) patients Small gram-negative rods
Klebsiella pneumonia	Alcoholics, aspiration "Currant jelly" sputum Encapsulated gram-negative rods
Staphylococcal pneumonia	Pink "salmon-colored" sputum Often nosocomial Gram-positive cocci in clusters
Mycoplasma pneumonia	Young adults X-ray looks worse than patient does
Pseudomonas pneumonia	Cystic fibrosis and immunocompromised patients
Legionella pneumonia	CNS and GI symptoms
TB	Fever Night sweats Weight loss Bloody sputum

Chronic Obstructive Pulmonary Disease

Emphysema	Destruction of alveolar walls
	Risk factors
	    Smoking
	    Alpha$_1$-antitrypsin deficiency

Chronic bronchitis	Smoking, chronic asthma

CRAM PAGES

Neoplasms

Laryngeal cancer	Squamous cell
	Due to alcohol and smoking
	Vocal hoarseness
Lung cancer	Squamous cell (40% to 50%)
	Adenocarcinoma (35%)
	Small cell (25%)
	Associated with smoking, paraneoplastic syndrome, Horner's syndrome, superior vena cava syndrome

Interstitial Lung Disease

Sarcoidosis	Increased calcium
	"Ground glass" appearance on x-ray
Asbestosis	Increased risk of lung cancer and mesothelioma
	Construction or shipyard workers
Silicosis	Increased risk of TB
	Metal mining

Other Lung Disorders

Pulmonary embolism	Most arise from deep venous thrombosis in leg
	$\dot{V}/\dot{Q}$ scan and CT scan useful for diagnosis, angiography is gold standard
Pulmonary hypertension	Accentuated P_2 component of S_2
	Cyanosis and clubbing
Pleural effusion	Exudates
	>3 g/dL protein
	Pleural/serum protein >0.5
	Pleural/serum LDH >0.6
	Caused by neoplasms and infection

CRAM PAGES

Transudates

>   <3 g/dL protein

>   Pleural/serum protein <0.5

>   Pleural/serum LDH <0.6

>   Caused by congestive heart failure, cirrhosis, nephrotic syndrome

| **Pulmonary edema** | Pink, frothy sputum
"Kerley B" lines on x-ray |

ENDOCRINE DISORDERS

Thyroid

Hypothyroidism	Weight gain Lethargy Coarse hair and dry skin Irregular menses Cold intolerance Myxedema
Hyperthyroidism	Weight loss despite good appetite Nervousness Sweating Tachycardia Heat intolerance Arrhythmias
Thyroid nodule: cancer risk factors	Previous neck irradiation Hoarse voice "Cold" nodule on thyroid scan
Thyroid cancer	Papillary (most common, best prognosis) Follicular Medullary [calcitonin-producing cells, multiple endocrine neoplasia (MEN) type 2a and 2b] Anaplastic (worst prognosis)

CRAM PAGES

Diabetes

Diabetes symptoms   Polyuria

Polydipsia

Polyphagia

Diabetic complications
  Acute   Diabetic ketoacidosis

Hyperosmolar nonketotic coma

  Chronic   Retinopathy

Nephropathy

Neuropathy

Vascular disease

Parathyroid

Hypoparathyroidism   Tingling

Tetany

Chvostek's sign/Trousseau's sign

Hyperparathyroidism   "Bones, stones, abdominal groans, and psychic moans"

Pituitary/Hypothalamic Disorders

Diabetes insipidus   Lack of antidiuretic hormone (ADH)

Polyuria and polydipsia

Syndrome of inappropriate ADH secretion   Tumor, trauma, pulmonary disease, drugs

Hyponatremia

Concentrated urine

Treat by restricting water

Acromegaly	Bone and tissue enlargement
	Glucose intolerance
	Osteoarthritis

Adrenal

Addison's disease	Decreased cortisol
	Weight loss and fatigue
	Skin pigmentation
	Eosinophilia
Cushing's syndrome	Increased cortisol
	Buffalo hump, moon facies, central obesity
	Easy bruising and striae
	Osteoporosis
	Cushing's disease due to adrenocorticotropic hormone from pituitary adenoma
Pheochromocytoma	Headache, palpitations, anxiety, hypertension
	Diagnosis by urinary catecholamines

Other Endocrine Disorders

Hemochromatosis	Autosomal recessive
	Excessive iron accumulation
	Cirrhosis
	Diabetes
	Bronze skin
Wilson's disease	Autosomal recessive
	Excessive copper accumulation
	Ataxia and dementia
	Kayser-Fleischer rings on cornea

CRAM PAGES

MEN 1	Parathyroid tumors
	Pituitary tumors
	Pancreatic tumors
MEN 2a	Parathyroid tumors
	Thyroid tumors (medullary)
	Pheochromocytoma
MEN 2b	Neuromas
	Thyroid tumors (medullary)
	Pheochromocytoma
	Marfanoid habitus

GENITOURINARY DISORDERS

Urinary System

Cystitis	Usually *E. coli*
	Frequency, urgency, dysuria
Bladder carcinoma: risk factors	Smoking
	Schistosomiasis
	Aniline dyes
Renal artery stenosis	Cause of secondary hypertension
	Fibromuscular dysplasia (young women)
	Atherosclerosis (older patients)
Glomerulonephritis	Hematuria
	Proteinuria
	RBC casts
Nephrotic syndrome	Proteinuria
	Edema
	Hypoalbuminemia

CRAM PAGES

Acute tubular necrosis	Due to ischemia or toxins
	Resolves in several weeks
	May need dialysis
Uremic syndrome	CNS changes
	Asterixis
	Pericarditis
	Nausea and vomiting
	Yellow-brown skin
Polycystic kidney disease	Autosomal dominant
	Hematuria
	Hypertension
	Urinary tract infections (UTIs)
Alport's syndrome	X-linked
	Deafness and renal failure

Electrolyte Disorders

Hypernatremia	>155 mEq/L
	Often due to dehydration
	CNS depression
Hyponatremia	<135 mEq/L
	Central pontine myelinolysis if corrected too rapidly
Hyperkalemia	>5.5 mEq/L
	Muscular weakness
	Cardiac arrhythmias
Hypokalemia	<3.5 mEq/L
	Muscular weakness
	Cardiac arrhythmias
	Respiratory failure

CRAM PAGES

Male Reproductive System

Urethritis	Classified as "gonococcal" and "nongonococcal" (chlamydial)
	High rate of coinfection
Epididymitis	Induration and tenderness
	Support relieves pain
Torsion of the testes	Adolescent boys
	Swelling and tenderness
	Support does not relieve pain
	Emergent surgery required
Hydrocele	Painless lump
	Can be transilluminated
Varicocele	"Bag of worms"
	Associated with infertility
Seminoma	Painless lump
	Does not transilluminate
	Undescended testis at higher risk, even after surgical correction
Benign prostatic hypertrophy	Enlarged, rubbery prostate
	Urinary retention
Prostatic carcinoma	Firm, nodular, irregular prostate
	Bone metastases

GYNECOLOGY

Sexually Transmitted Diseases

Pelvic inflammatory disease (PID)	Cervical motion tenderness
	Purulent discharge
	Associated with ectopic pregnancy and infertility

Trichomonas vaginitis	Yellow-green, bubbly discharge
	"Strawberry patches" and petechiae
	Motile, flagellated organisms
	Metronidazole for patient and partner
Syphilis	Painless ulcer with rolled edges and punched-out base
	Penicillin
Venereal warts	Human papillomavirus (HPV) 6, 11
	Not associated with cervical cancer

Other Infections

Candida	"Cottage cheese" discharge and red vulva
	Pseudohyphae on slide
	Associated with diabetes and antibiotics
Bacterial vaginosis	Copious discharge with fishy odor
	"Clue cells" on microscopy
	Metronidazole for patient
UTI	Usually caused by *E. coli*
	Dysuria, frequency, urgency
	Trimethoprim-sulfamethoxazole
Toxic shock syndrome	*Staphylococcus aureus* exotoxin
	Rash
	High fever

Neoplasms

Vulvar cancer	Squamous cell
	Usually after menopause
	Pruritus
Cervical cancer	HPV 16, 18, 31
	Sexually transmitted
	Postcoital bleeding

CRAM PAGES

Uterine myoma (fibroid)	Heavy, prolonged menses
	Anemia
Endometrial cancer risk factors	Unopposed estrogen
	Obesity
	Nulliparity
	Early menarche
	Late menopause
Breast fibroadenoma	Common in young women
Breast cancer: risk factors	Family history
	Nulliparity
	Early menarche
Breast cancer	Painless lump
	Nipple retraction
	Most are in upper outer quadrant
	More than 90% are "invasive ductal" type

Other Gynecologic Conditions

Endometriosis	Ectopic endometrial tissue
	Dysmenorrhea
	Dyspareunia
	Infertility
Polycystic ovary syndrome	High luteinizing hormone (LH) and low or normal follicle-stimulating hormone (FSH)
	Hirsutism and obesity
	Menstrual irregularities
	Infertility
Menopause	High LH and FSH
	Hot flashes
	Atrophic vaginal epithelium

OBSTETRICS

Alpha-fetoprotein	Increased levels
	Neural tube defects
	Abdominal wall defects
	Multiple gestation
	Fetal demise
	Decreased levels
	Down syndrome
Amniocentesis	Performed at weeks 16 to 20
	Recommended in women older than 35 years
Gestational diabetes	Macrosomia
	Respiratory distress syndrome
	Congenital abnormalities
Preeclampsia	Hypertension
	Proteinuria
	Edema
Hydatidiform mole/ choriocarcinoma	Preeclampsia in first half of pregnancy
	Very high beta–human chorionic gonadotropin (β-hCG)
	"Snowstorm" appearance on ultrasound
Ectopic pregnancy	β-hCG rises slowly
	Amenorrhea, spotting, and pain
	Empty gestational sac on ultrasound
	Ampulla of fallopian tube is most common site
Polyhydramnios	Duodenal atresia
	Tracheoesophageal fistula
	Anencephaly
Oligohydramnios	Renal agenesis
	Pulmonary hypoplasia
Premature rupture of membranes	Pooling of fluid in vagina
	Positive Nitrazine test
	Positive ferning test
	Risk of endometritis

CRAM PAGES

Labor: first stage	From regular, painful contractions to complete cervical dilation
Labor: second stage	From cervical dilation to birth
Labor: third stage	From birth to delivery of placenta
Fetal cardiac monitoring: early decelerations	Normal Occur with contractions
Fetal cardiac monitoring: late decelerations	Begin after contraction begins Indicates fetal hypoxia Deliver as soon as possible
Fetal cardiac monitoring: variable decelerations	Variable onset Occur due to cord compression Change maternal position

PEDIATRICS

Congenital Infections

Congenital toxoplasmosis	IUGR Seizures Jaundice Retinitis
Congenital rubella	IUGR Cataracts Mental retardation and hearing loss Cardiac defects Purpura
Congenital cytomegalovirus (CMV)	IUGR Microcephaly "Blueberry corn muffin" appearance

CRAM PAGES

Congenital syphilis	Jaundice
	Hepatosplenomegaly
	Rash on palms and soles
	"Snuffles"
Congenital varicella	Limb hypoplasia and scars
	Retinitis
	Cortical atrophy

Substance-exposed Infants

Fetal alcohol syndrome	IUGR
	Microcephaly
	Short palpebral fissures
	Cardiac anomalies
Fetal narcotic exposure	Hypertonicity
	Sweating
	Stuffy nose
Fetal cocaine exposure	Limb reduction malformations
	Intestinal atresia
	Jitteriness and tremors
	Vomiting and diarrhea

Gastroenterology

Tracheoesophageal fistula	Congenital defect
	Coughing and cyanosis when feeding
Pyloric stenosis	Projectile vomiting in neonates
	"String sign" on x-ray
Meconium ileus	Associated with cystic fibrosis

Hirschsprung's disease   No autonomic nerves in colon

Obstipation

Megacolon

Cardiovascular

Atrial septal defect	Widely split and fixed S_2
Ventricular septal defect	Pansystolic murmur
Pulmonic stenosis	Early systolic click
	High-pitched systolic ejection murmur
	Soft or absent S_2
Patent ductus arteriosus	Continuous "machinery" murmur
Coarctation of the aorta	Hypertension in arms but not legs
	Murmur heard on back
Tetralogy of Fallot	Ventricular septal defect
	Right ventricular hypertrophy
	Pulmonic stenosis
	Overriding aorta

Respiratory Disorders

Respiratory distress syndrome	Usually <34 weeks gestation
	Test for lung maturity. Mature if:
	Lecithin/sphingomyelin ratio >2
	Positive phosphatidyl glycerol
	Corticosteroids hasten maturity
Neonatal pneumonia	Group B streptococcus
	E. coli
	Chlamydia

Epiglottitis	*H. influenzae* type b
	Inspiratory stridor
	Dysphagia with drooling
	Must intubate
Laryngotracheitis (croup)	Parainfluenza virus
	Barking cough
	Stridor
Bronchiolitis	Respiratory syncytial virus
Cystic fibrosis	Autosomal recessive
	COPD
	Pancreatic insufficiency
	High chloride in sweat

Genitourinary Disorders

Wilms' tumor	Children younger than 4 years of age
	Hematuria
	Abdominal mass

Neurology

Neonatal meningitis	Group B streptococcus
	E. coli
	Listeria

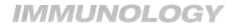

IMMUNOLOGY

Human Immunodeficiency Virus/Acquired Immunodeficiency Syndrome

Human immunodeficiency virus (HIV) infection	Flu-like illness Antibodies 1 to 6 months after infection
Acquired immunodeficiency syndrome (AIDS)-related infections: viruses	CMV Herpes simplex virus (HSV) Varicella-zoster virus (VZV) Epstein-Barr virus
AIDS-related infections: mycobacteria	*Mycobacterium tuberculosis* *M. avium*-complex
AIDS-related infections: fungi	*Candida* Coccidioides Histoplasma *Cryptococcus*
AIDS-related infections: protozoa	Pneumocystis carinii *Toxoplasma* *Cryptosporidium* *Giardia*

Congenital Immunodeficiency

DiGeorge's syndrome	Thymic aplasia Absent T cells "Poor George has no thymus"
Wiskott-Aldrich syndrome	X-linked No antibodies against encapsulated bacteria
Chronic granulomatous disease	Autosomal recessive Recurrent bacterial and fungal infections

CRAM PAGES

Chédiak-Higashi syndrome	Autosomal recessive
	Recurrent streptococcal and staphylococcal infections
Bruton's disease	X-linked
	No B cells or antibodies

HEMATOLOGY

Anemia

Microcytic anemia [mean corpuscular volume (MCV) <80]	Iron deficiency
	Chronic disease
	Lead poisoning
	Thalassemia
Normocytic anemia (MCV 80 to 100)	Hemolysis
	Chronic disease
	Bone marrow suppression (drugs, leukemia)
Macrocytic anemia (MCV >100)	Vitamin B_{12} or folate deficiency
	Liver disease
	Hypothyroidism

Genetic Disorders

α-Thalassemia	Acanthocytes
	Target cells
	Very low MCV but mild anemia
β-Thalassemia	Basophilic stippling
	Nucleated RBCs
	Very low MCV but mild anemia

CRAM PAGES

Sickle cell anemia	*Salmonella* osteomyelitis
	S. pneumoniae sepsis
	Penicillin prophylaxis
Hemophilia	X-linked factor VIII (A) or IX (B) deficiency
	Joint and soft-tissue bleeding
von Willebrand's disease	Autosomal-dominant deficiency of factor VIII and von Willebrand's factor
	Epistaxis
	Menorrhagia
	Bruising

Other Hematologic Disorders

Eosinophilia	NAACP
	Neoplasms
	Asthma/allergies
	Addison's disease
	Connective tissue disorders
	Parasites
Thrombotic thrombocytopenic purpura	Adults more than children
	Platelets consumed in clotting reactions
	Fluctuating neurologic deficits
Idiopathic thrombocytopenic purpura	Children more than adults
	Autoimmune destruction of platelets
	Purpura and petechiae
	Epistaxis and menorrhagia
Hemolytic-uremic syndrome	Usually caused by *E. coli* strain 0157:H7
	RBC fragments on smear

CRAM PAGES

Neoplasms

Acute lymphocytic leukemia	80% of childhood leukemias 80% is B cell Abundant blasts on smear
Acute myelocytic leukemia	More common in adults Auer rods (red intracellular inclusions) on smear May be stable for several years
Chronic myelocytic leukemia	Very high count (>150,000) Philadelphia chromosome May be stable for several years
Chronic lymphocytic leukemia	B cells Numerous, small, mature-appearing lymphocytes on smear No "blast crisis"
Hairy cell leukemia	B cells Pancytopenia on smear
Hodgkin's lymphoma	Macrophages Painless cervical lymphadenopathy Reed-Sternberg cells
Non-Hodgkin's lymphoma	Worse prognosis than Hodgkin's Smear normal with increased mature cells
Burkitt's lymphoma	B cell lymphoma Associated with Epstein-Barr virus
Multiple myeloma	Plasma cells Paraproteins seen on SPEP RBCs in Rouleau formation
Waldenström's macroglobulinemia	B cell Monoclonal IgM overproduction RBCs in Rouleau formation
Mycosis fungoides	CD4 T cells Skin lesions may look like eczema or dermatitis
Polycythemia vera	Overproduction of all three cell lines Treated with phlebotomy

DERMATOLOGY

Allergic contact dermatitis	Type IV hypersensitivity reaction Poison oak, poison ivy, nickel
Seborrheic dermatitis	Red skin with greasy scales on face
Psoriasis	Silvery-scaled plaques Pitted fingernails HLA-B27
Atopic dermatitis	Pruritic, dry lesions, asthma, allergic rhinitis
Acne vulgaris	Inflammation of hair follicles *Propionibacterium acnes*
Herpes simplex	Periodically activated from neurons of sensory ganglia
Chickenpox	Contagious 10 days after exposure Pneumonia in adults
Herpes zoster	VZV (chickenpox) reactivated One dermatome affected
Necrotizing fasciitis	Group A β-hemolytic streptococcus
Gas gangrene	Crepitus in subcutaneous tissues *Clostridium* species
Dermatophytoses	Scaly round lesions with raised borders
Pilonidal cyst	Hair-lined tract in sacral area
Actinic keratoses	Firm, yellow scale May lead to squamous cell cancer
Skin cancer	Basal cell more common than squamous cell Associated with sun exposure
Malignant melanoma	Change in size, shape, color of mole Itching and ulceration Common in multiple dysplastic nevi syndrome

MUSCULOSKELETAL AND CONNECTIVE TISSUE DISORDERS

Degenerative joint disease	Common in old age
	Distal interphalangeal (DIP) and proximal interphalangeal (PIP) joints
	Also affects hips, knees, spine
Osteoporosis: risk factors	Postmenopause
	Whites and Asians
	Smoking
	Alcohol
	Corticosteroids
Gout	Affects big toe, pinna of ear
	Negatively birefringent crystals
Lyme disease	*Borrelia burgdorferi*
	Ixodes tick
	Arthralgias
	Rash with central clearing
	CNS changes 1 month after exposure
Systemic lupus erythematosus (SLE)	Young African-American women
	Malar "butterfly" rash
	Arthralgias
	Antinuclear antibodies test is sensitive (most patients positive)
	Anti-dsDNA is specific (only positive in SLE)
Polymyositis and dermatomyositis	Violet discoloration of eyelids ("heliotrope" rash)
	Elevated muscle enzymes
Rheumatoid arthritis (RA)	Symmetric
	PIP and metacarpophalangeal (MCP) joints
	Subcutaneous nodules
	75% have positive rheumatoid factor
Ankylosing spondylitis	"Bamboo spine" on x-ray
	Associated with HLA-B27

CRAM PAGES

Bone metastases: **common primary sites**	Breast
	Lung
	Prostate
	Kidney
	Thyroid
Shoulder-hand syndrome	Pain and swelling in hand and stiffness in shoulder
	Occurs 1 month after myocardial infarction
Paget's disease	Frontal "bossing" and shortened spine
	Elevated alkaline phosphatase
	"Cotton-wool" appearance on skull x-ray

NEUROLOGY AND SPECIAL SENSES

Headache

Migraine	More women than men
	Family history
	Nausea and vomiting, photophobia
	Aura in classic migraine
Cluster headache	Same time each day
	Periorbital
	Unilateral Horner's or rhinorrhea and tearing
Tension headache	Constant, bilateral, viselike
Giant cell arteritis	Temporal artery tenderness may be present
	Jaw claudication, fever
	Elevated ESR
	Immediate steroids prevent blindness
Trigeminal neuralgia	Lightning-bolt pain in V1 and V2 distribution
Tumor-associated headache	Dull headache steadily increasing
	Worse in a.m. or with position changes

CRAM PAGES

Increased intracranial pressure	Usually due to resistance to venous or CSF outflow
	Rarely due to increased CSF production
	Papilledema, bradycardia, elevated systolic blood pressure

Epilepsy/Seizures

Partial seizures	Begin with localized symptoms
Simple partial	Consist of a focal symptom
	May be motor, sensory, or psychomotor
	Consciousness retained
Complex partial	Complex, stereotyped psychomotor symptoms
	Frontal or temporal epileptic focus
	Consciousness impaired
	Postictal state

Generalized seizures	
Absence seizures	Brief loss of consciousness without postictal state
Tonic-clonic seizures	Tonic contraction followed by clonic movements
	Postictal state
Status epilepticus	Multiple seizures without periods of regained consciousness

Cerebrovascular Disease

Transient ischemic attacks	Brief period of reduced blood flow to brain
	Focal neurologic symptoms lasting <24 hours
	Usually <1 hour

Ischemic Stroke	Infarction of brain tissue due to ischemia
Middle cerebral	Most common
	Contralateral weakness and sensory loss; arm worse than leg
	Contralateral homonymous hemianopsia
	Aphasia if dominant hemisphere affected
	Sensory neglect or apraxia if nondominant hemisphere affected

CRAM PAGES

Ophthalmic	Ipsilateral vision loss
Anterior cerebral	Contralateral leg weakness
	Behavioral changes
Posterior cerebral	Contralateral homonymous hemianopsia
Vertebrobasilar	Frequently fatal
	Cranial nerve abnormalities
	Ataxia
	Decreased consciousness
Congenital berry aneurysms	Associated with polycystic kidney disease and aortic coarctation
Intracerebral hemorrhage	Usually due to hypertension, stimulant abuse, or rupture of arteriovenous malformations
Subarachnoid hemorrhage	"The worst headache of my life!"
	Berry aneurysms, arteriovenous malformations, trauma
	CT, then lumbar puncture
Cavernous sinus thrombosis	Infection can result from bacterial sinusitis
	Papilledema, cranial nerve palsies, exophthalmos

Toxic Neurologic Disorders

Toxic vestibulopathies	Alcohol, aminoglycosides, salicylates
Toxic neuropathies	
Lead	Multiple motor mononeuropathy
	Acute encephalopathy in children
Organophosphates	Delayed motor neuropathies, cholinergic crisis
Alcohol	Bilateral distal sensorimotor neuropathy
	Wernicke's encephalopathy
	Korsakoff's syndrome
Isoniazid	Sensory polyneuropathy
	Prevented by pyridoxine (vitamin B_6) administration
Metabolic encephalopathy	Pupillary reflex intact despite coma

CRAM PAGES

Infections

Bacterial meningitis
  Infants younger   Group B streptococci
    than 1 month   *E. coli*
  Babies and children   *Neisseria meningitidis*
                      S. pneumoniae
  Adults   *S. pneumoniae*
  All ages   *N. meningitidis*
                      Associated with petechial rash
  Brudzinski's sign   Neck flexion while supine causes hip and knee flexion
  Kernig's sign   Knee extension with hip flexed is painful

Aseptic meningitis   Milder disease caused by viruses
                      High CSF lymphocyte count

Subacute meningitis   TB, *Cryptococcus,* CMV, sarcoidosis, syphilis, Lyme disease

Encephalitis
  Sporadic   VZV, HSV, mumps
  Epidemic   Coxsackie virus, polio, echovirus, arboviruses

Brain abscess   Streptococci, staphylococci, anaerobes

Neurosyphilis   Argyll-Robertson pupil
                      Tabes dorsalis

Polio   Affects motor neurons
                      Sensation not affected

Botulism   *Clostridium botulinum*
                      Cranial nerve palsies

Neoplasms

Adults   Meningioma (benign)
                      Glioblastoma multiforme (malignant)
                      Metastatic

CRAM PAGES

| **Children** | Cerebellar astrocytoma |
| | Medulloblastoma |

Degenerative Disorders

Alzheimer's disease	Slowly progressive dementia
	Elderly (older than 80 years)
	Trisomy 21
	Familial
Multi-infarct dementia	Pseudobulbar palsy common
	Stroke risk factors
	Multiple cortical and subcortical infarcts
Huntington's disease	Chorea and dementia
	Onset in middle age
	Autosomal dominant
Parkinsonism	Pill-rolling tremor, decreased movement, mask-like facies, cogwheel rigidity, postural instability
	Loss of dopaminergic cells in substantia nigra
Amyotrophic lateral sclerosis	Loss of upper and lower motor neurons
	Multiple, asymmetric, upper and mower motor neuron findings in extremities and face

Demyelinating Disorders

Multiple sclerosis	Progressive demyelination with exacerbations
	Optic neuritis
	Acute idiopathic polyneuropathy
Guillain-Barré syndrome	Progressive symmetric proximal leg weakness extending to arms and face
	Follows viral illnesses or vaccinations
	CSF shows protein

Miscellaneous Disorders

Myasthenia gravis	Easy muscle fatigability
	Autoimmune antibodies against acetylcholine receptor in neuromuscular junction
	Transient relief of symptoms with edrophonium
	Possible thymoma
Lambert-Eaton syndrome	Weakness that improves with sustained activity
	Autoimmune antibodies against voltage-gated calcium channels of the neuromuscular junction presynaptic terminal
	Often associated with malignancy
Peripheral neuropathy	
Mononeuropathy	Trauma, entrapment, compression
Multiple mono-neuropathy	Collagen vascular disorders (SLE, RA), vasculitis, diabetes, HIV
Polyneuropathy	Diabetes, nutritional deficiencies (B_1, B_{12}), Guillain-Barré syndrome, paraproteinemias, toxins, hereditary conditions
Gait abnormalities	
Cerebellar lesions	Broad-based, unsteady gait with poor turning
Corticospinal lesion	One leg circumducts
Extrapyramidal	Festinating gait
Motor system lesion	Footdrop, waddling, etc., depending on lesion
Sensory deficit	Steppage gait
Coma	
Decorticate	Arm flexion, leg extension
	Suggests thalamic lesion
Decerebrate	Arm and leg extension
	Suggests midbrain lesion

Vision Loss

Open-angle glaucoma

Gradual increase in intraocular pressure

Tunnel vision, halos, cupping of optic disk

Closed-angle glaucoma

Blockage of aqueous drainage causes rapid pressure increase

Occurs with pupillary dilation

Conjunctivitis

Adenovirus

Staphylococcus, Streptococcus, Haemophilus species

Gonorrhea, chlamydia

Uveitis

Inflammation of iris, ciliary body, choroid layer

Associated with

Collagen vascular diseases (RA, Reiter's syndrome)

Infections (TB, CMV, syphilis)

Inflammatory bowel diseases

Retinal Disorders

Senile macular degeneration

Loss of central vision because of atrophic or exudative retinal degeneration

Central retinal artery occlusion

Sudden, painless blindness in one eye

Cherry-red spot fovea, boxcar veins

Central retinal vein occlusion

Gradual, painless blindness in one eye

Tortuous, dilated veins

Diabetic retinopathy

Neovascularization, cotton-wool spots

Retinal detachment

Curtain coming down over one eye

Retinoblastoma

Child with abnormal white (not red) reflex

Disorders of the Ear

Otitis externa	*E. coli, Pseudomonas, Proteus, S. aureus*
Mastoiditis	Sequelae of untreated otitis media
Ménière's disease	Distention of endolymphatic sac Severe vertigo, hearing loss, tinnitus
Acoustic neuroma	Schwannoma of the eighth cranial nerve Sensorineural hearing loss, vertigo, tinnitus

PSYCHIATRY

Delirium	Decreased, fluctuating level of consciousness Often due to substance abuse or medical illness Reversible
Dementia	Chronic, progressive decrease in memory and cognition Often irreversible
Schizophrenia	Delusions, hallucinations, disorganized behavior over more than 6 months Genetic predisposition
Schizophreniform disorder	Symptoms of schizophrenia lasting <6 months
Schizoaffective disorder	Schizophrenia and a mood disorder
Schizoid personality	Unable to form close relationships Blunted or absent emotions
Neuroleptic malignant syndrome	Occurs days after starting neuroleptics Hypertension and muscle rigidity Fever

CRAM PAGES

Tardive dyskinesia	Stereotypical oral movements
	Associated with long-term neuroleptic use
	Irreversible
Somatization disorder	Multiple, vague, recurrent somatic problems
	May be related to personality disorder
Conversion disorder	Somatic expression of a specific psychological conflict
Factitious disorder	Feigned illness to assume sick role
Malingering	Feigned illness for external gain

INJURY AND POISONING

Burns: classification	First-degree: red-gray only
	Second-degree: red with blistering
	Third-degree: leathery, numb
Burns: management	Remember "Rule of 9s"
	Fluid replacement at 3–4 mL/kg for each percent burned
Skull fractures	Battle's sign (discoloration over mastoid)
Colles fracture	Distal radial fracture from falling on outstretched hand
Compartment syndrome	Associated with tibial fractures
	Pain
	Pallor
	Pulselessness
	Poikilothermia
	Paresthesias
	Paresis

RESEARCH, ADULT CARE, AND ETHICS

Relative risk	$\dfrac{a/(a + b)}{c/(c + d)}$
Odds ratio	$\dfrac{a/c}{b/d} = \dfrac{ad}{bc}$
Sensitivity	$\dfrac{a}{a + c}$
Specificity	$\dfrac{d}{b + d}$
Positive predictive value	$\dfrac{a}{a + b}$
Negative predictive value	$\dfrac{d}{c + d}$

Index

Note: Page numbers followed by *f* indicate figures; page numbers followed by *t* indicate tables.

Student Rating & "Cram Fact" Form

What were your overall impressions of *Prescription for the Boards: USMLE Step 2,* third edition? _____

_____

_____

_____

_____

_____

_____

Was there anything on the test that was not covered in the book? _____

_____

_____

_____

Was there anything in the book you could have done without? _____

_____

_____

_____

Comments: _____

_____

_____

_____

_____

Suggested additional topics or "cram facts": _____

_____

_____

_____

_____

THANKS! Your input is appreciated, and it is necessary to help keep the book fresh and appropriate for a new generation of students. Include your name, address, and phone number. If we use your comments in promotion materials, we'll send you a coupon for $10 toward any Lippincott Williams & Wilkins medical book!

Name: _____

School/Affiliation: _____

_____

Address: _____

City/State/Zip: _____

Phone: _____

Send to:

Prescription for the Boards: Step 2
c/o Lippincott Williams & Wilkins
Scott Lavine
351 West Camden Street
Baltimore, MD 21201

Return Address

_____

_____

_____

Postage required

Prescription for the Boards: Step 2
c/o Lippincott Williams & Wilkins
Scott Lavine
351 West Camden Street
Baltimore, MD 21201

_____ (Fold Here) _____

Seal here with Tape (Do not Staple)